Management of Fractured Endodontic Instruments

Theodor Lambrianidis
Editor

Management of Fractured Endodontic Instruments

A Clinical Guide

Springer

Editor
Theodor Lambrianidis
Department of Endodontics
Aristotle University of Thessaloniki, School of Dentistry
Thessaloniki, Greece

Illustrated by Dr. Mazinis

ISBN 978-3-319-86906-3 ISBN 978-3-319-60651-4 (eBook)
DOI 10.1007/978-3-319-60651-4

Softcover reprint of the hardcover 1st edition 2017

Printed on acid-free paper

This Springer imprint is published by Springer Nature
The registered company is Springer International Publishing AG
The registered company address is: Gewerbestrasse 11, 6330 Cham, Switzerland

To Virginia
for her continuous support and understanding

Contents

Contributors

Christos Boutsioukis, D.D.S., M.Sc., Ph.D. Department of Endodontology, Academic Centre for Dentistry Amsterdam (ACTA), Amsterdam, The Netherlands

Michael Hülsmann, D.D.S., Ph.D. Department of Preventive Dentistry, Periodontology and Cardiology, University Medicine Göttingen, Göttingen, Germany

Theodor Lambrianidis, D.D.S., Ph.D. Department of Endodontology, Dental School, Aristotle University of Thessaloniki, Thessaloniki, Greece

Emmanuel Mazinis, D.D.S., Ph.D. Private practice, Veria, Greece

Peter Parashos, BDSc, LDS, MDSc, PhD, FRACDS. Melbourne Dental School, University of Melbourne, Melbourne, Australia

Spiros Zinelis, B. Eng, Ph.D. Department of Biomaterials, School of Dentistry, National and Kapodistrian University of Athens, Athens, Greece

---

In an older version of the front matter the "Illustrated by Dr. Mazinis" had been missed out and this has now been corrected.

1 Introduction: Prevalence of Fractured Instruments

Theodor Lambrianidis

1.1 Introduction

A great variety of foreign objects may be found in the root canal compromising of cleaning and shaping procedures, with a potential impact on the treatment outcome. These foreign objects may be largely attributed to iatrogenic errors. They include:

- Fragments of the whole range of instruments used in root canal instrumentation (Crump and Natkin 1970; Lambrianidis 1984; Zeigler and Serene 1984; Ingle et al. 1985; Molyvdas et al. 1992; Hülsmann 1994; Hülsmann and Schinkel 1999; Al-Fouzan 2003; Shen et al. 2004; Tzanetakis et al. 2008; Rahimi and Parashos 2009; Cunha et al. 2014). These fragments can be nickel-titanium (NiTi), stainless steel (SS), or carbon steel instruments (Fig. 1.1).
- Fragments of ultrasonic tips.
- Fragments of irrigation needles (Fig. 1.2).
- Fragments of Lentulo spiral fillers (Fig. 1.3).
- Fragments of silver points (Fig. 1.4).
- Fragments of burs (Sternberg 1977; Meidinger and Kabes 1985; Lambrianidis 2001) (Fig. 1.5).
- Fragments of carrier-based obturators.
- Fragments of prefabricated or cast dental posts (Fig. 1.6).
- Fragments of synthetic posts.

T. Lambrianidis, D.D.S., Ph.D.
Department of Endodontology, Dental School, Aristotle University of Thessaloniki, Thessaloniki, Greece
e-mail: thlampri@dent.auth.gr

T. Lambrianidis (ed.), *Management of Fractured Endodontic Instruments*,
DOI 10.1007/978-3-319-60651-4_1

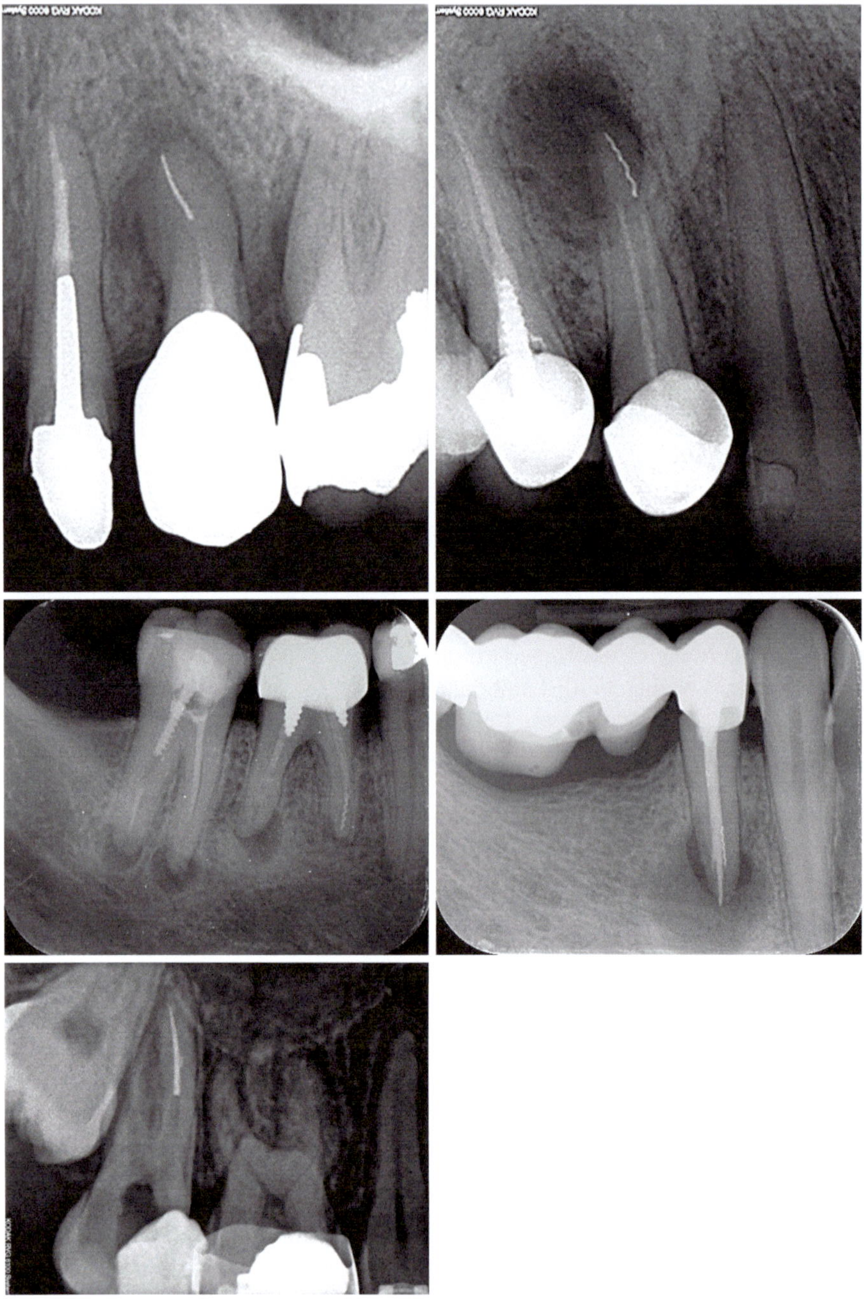

Fig. 1.1 Fragments of various endodontic instruments

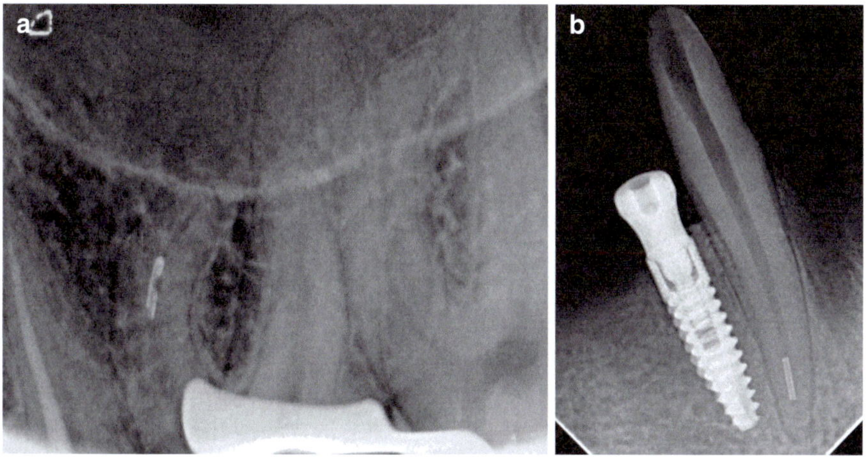

Fig. 1.2 (**a**) Fragment of an irrigation needle in the mesiobuccal root canal of a maxillary molar. (**b**) Fragment of the notched end of an irrigation needle in a mandibular canine

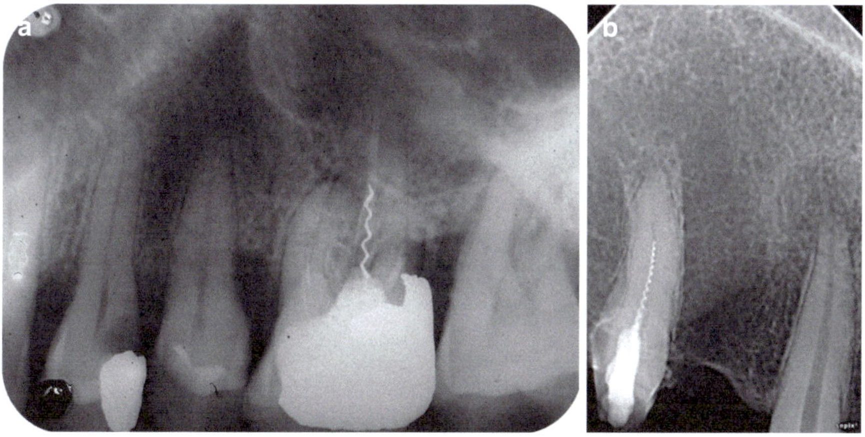

Fig. 1.3 Fragments of Lentulo spiral fillers

- Fragments of amalgam and gold fillings (Meidinger and Kabes 1985; Stamos et al. 1985) (Fig. 1.7).
- Fragments of acrylic resin.
- Fragments of temporary filling materials (Lambrianidis 1984).
- Glass beads used in chairside micro-sterilizers (Shay 1985).
- Paper points (Grossman 1974).
- Cotton wool.

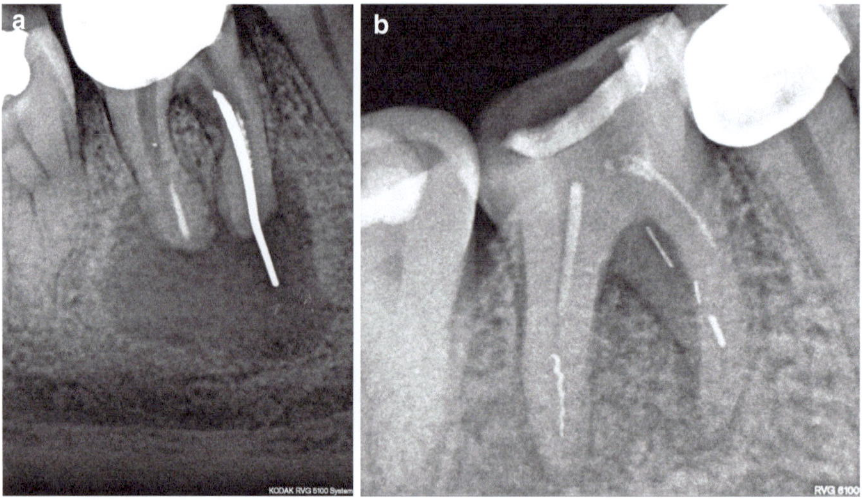

Fig. 1.4 (**a**) Root canal with an instrument fragment and a silver point fragment. (**b**) Mandibular molar with an instrument fragment in the distal canal and three metallic particles in the mesial canals, possibly fragments of silver points

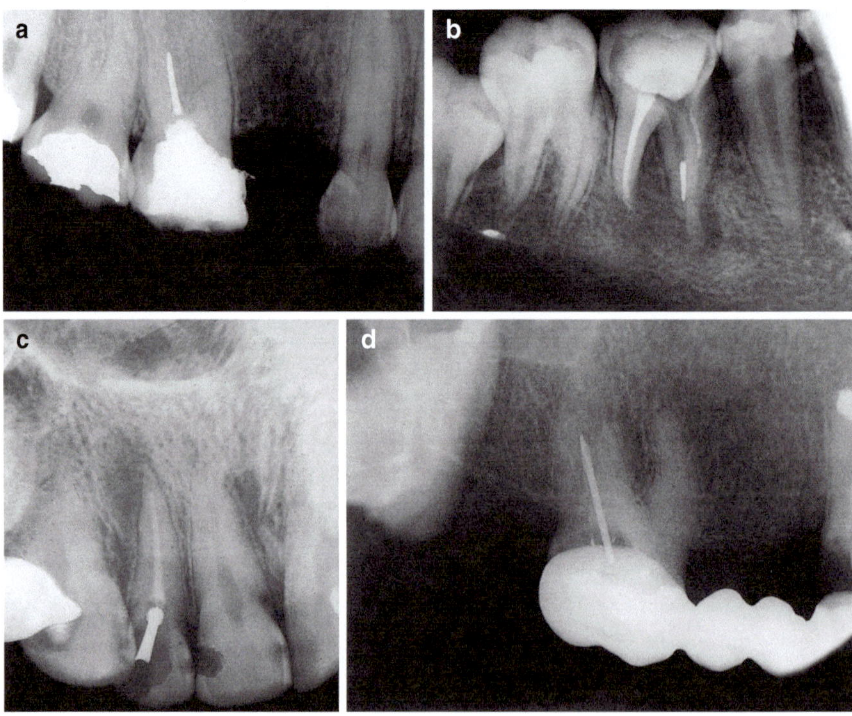

Fig. 1.5 Fragments of: (**a**) Endodontic explorer. (**b**) Spreader. (**c**) Bur. (**d**) Gates Glidden bur (with permission from Lambrianidis 2001)

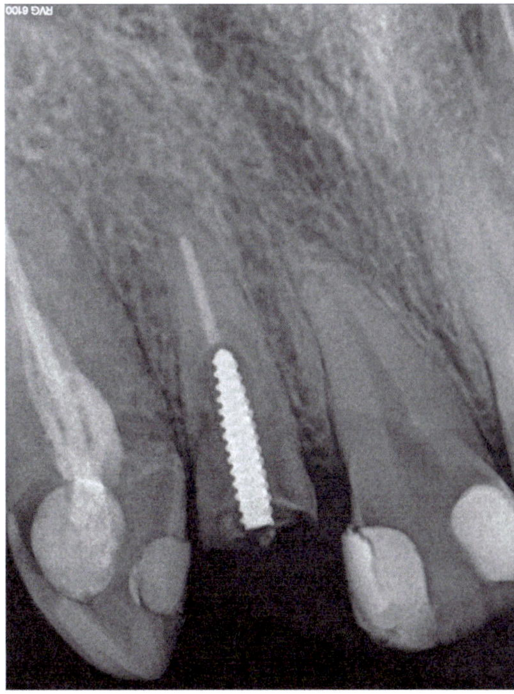

Fig. 1.6 Fragment of a prefabricated metal post

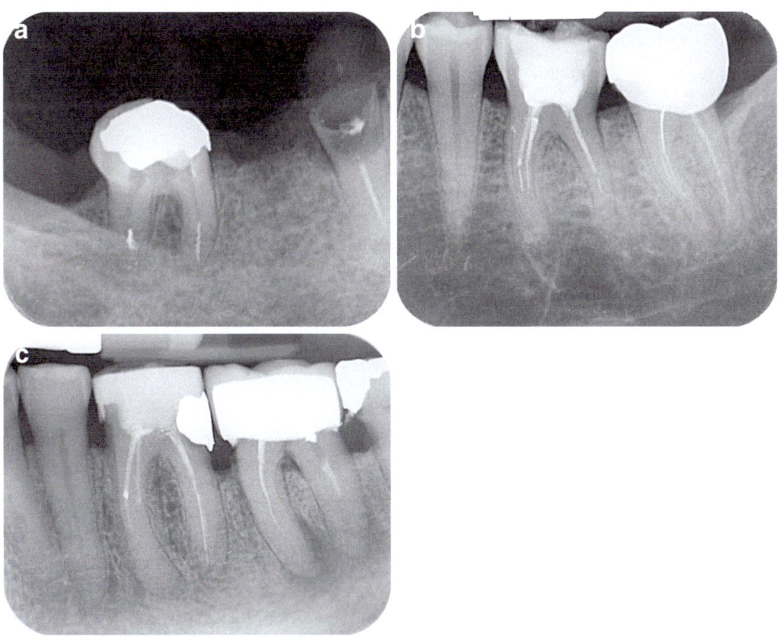

Fig. 1.7 (**a**) Amalgam particles in the distal root canal and an instrument fragment in the mesio-buccal canal of a second right mandibular molar. (**b**, **c**) Amalgam particles in the mesial root of suboptimally filled first mandibular left molars

More infrequently, the presence of foreign objects within the root canal is attributed to patient's related manipulations outside the dental surgery (Figs. 1.8 and 1.9). There are several reports related to foreign object placement into exposed pulp cavities by patients either in an effort to alleviate mid-treatment pain by exposing the chamber or as a habit. Foreign objects lodged as a habit are more commonly seen in children, as the latter often place a variety of foreign particles in their mouths. Wooden or metallic objects, such as toothpicks, sewing needles, safety pins, hat pins, dressmaker pins, stapler pins, crayons, pencil leads, toothbrush bristles, food remnants, and pieces of nails, are among the various objects of these etiologies found in the root canal of permanent teeth (Grossman 1974, Zillich and Pickens 1982, Turner 1983, Shay 1985, Chenail and Teplitsky 1987, Walvekar et al. 1995, Srivastava and Vineeta 2001, Nadkarni et al. 2002, McAuliffe et al. 2005, Aduri et al. 2009, Kalyan and Sajjan 2010, Chand et al. 2013, Patil et al. 2015). Their dimensions vary greatly. A case has been described with two objects, an 8 mm-long watch hand and a 5 mm-long pencil lead (Ozsezer et al. 2006). Moreover cases of foreign objects found in the deciduous teeth have also been described (Holla et al.

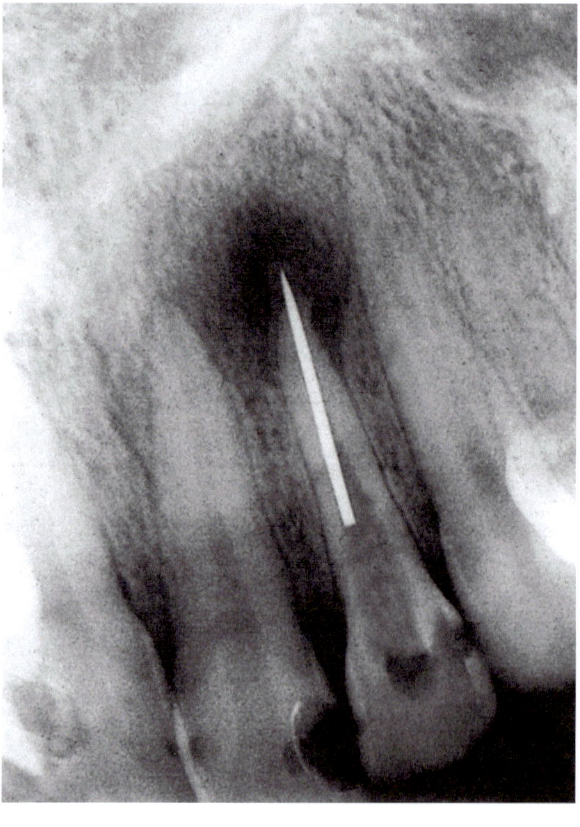

Fig. 1.8 Sewing needle in root canal (with permission from Lambrianidis 2001)

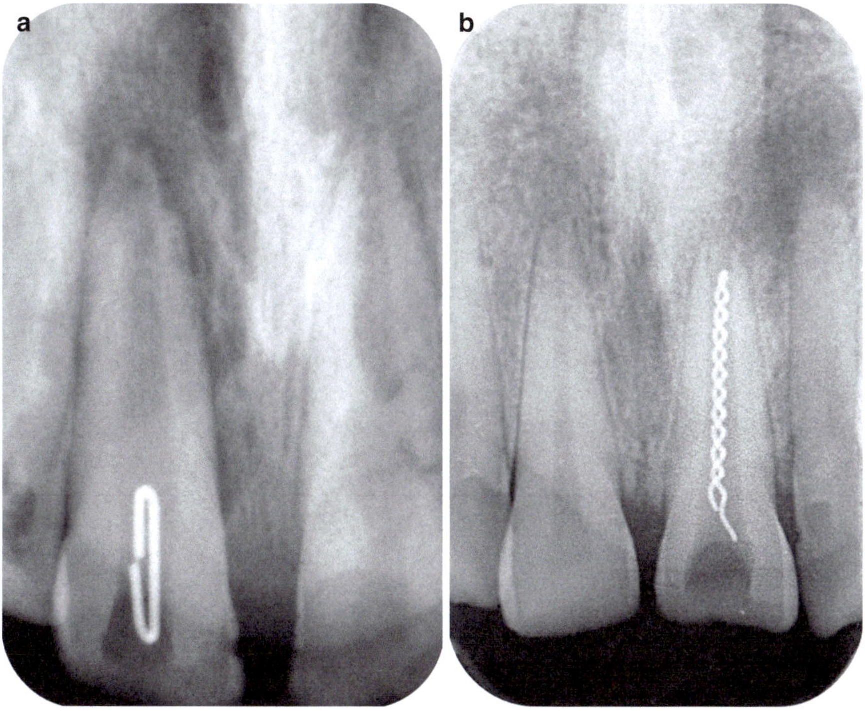

Fig. 1.9 (**a**) Stapler pin placed for fun in the root canal of a maxillary central incisor of an 8-years old boy. (**b**) Fragment of an interdental brush in an exposed maxillary central incisor of a 32-year-old man advised by his general dental practitioner to "clean" the canal with this brush after each meal

2010; Singh Dhull et al. 2013). These foreign objects, regardless of their nature, size, and location, may act as a potential source of infection. Therefore, a detailed dental history and clinical and radiographic examination are necessary to come to a conclusion about their nature, size, and location and proceed to their management accordingly.

1.2 Incidence of Fractured Instruments

In spite of the plethora of considerable metallurgical improvements in instrument design, alloy composition, and manufacturing process, file failure during instrumentation remains a primary concern. Endodontic instruments are the foreign objects most frequently found in the root canal either in retreatment cases or as a mishap in initial treatments. A literature review revealed a prevalence of retained fractured instruments of between 0.7 and 7.4% in teeth undergoing root canal treatment (RCT) (Crump and Natkin 1970; Hülsmann and Schinkel 1999; Spili et al. 2005; Iqbal et al. 2006; Parashos and Messer 2006; Cheung et al. 2007).

Instrument fracture is an undesirable and troublesome incident during RCT that frustrates both practitioners and patients. It can happen even to experienced clinicians following the most appropriate preventive measures. Instrument fracture may occur in both anterior and posterior teeth, but it is most frequently reported in molars (Iqbal et al. 2006; Wu et al. 2011; Ungerechts et al. 2014), with similar instrument fracture rates for the maxilla and the mandible (Iqbal et al. 2006; Tzanetakis et al. 2008; Ungerechts et al. 2014). Among molars, it is particularly reported as occurring in the mesial roots of mandibular molars (Molyvdas et al. 1992; Hülsmann and Schinkel 1999; Ward et al. 2003).

The vast majority of instrument fracture occurs in the apical third of the root canal (Molyvdas et al. 1992; Yared et al. 2000; Al-Fouzan 2003; Ankrum et al. 2004; Di Fiore et al. 2006; Iqbal et al. 2006; Tzanetakis et al. 2008; Ungerechts et al. 2014; Wang et al. 2014). The probability of file fracture in the apical area was estimated to be 33 times greater compared to the coronal third of the canal and almost six times greater when compared to the middle third of the root canal (Iqbal et al. 2006).

The incidence of endodontic instrument fracture is still an area of uncertainty, firstly because the numerous studies that have assessed this phenomenon offer varying and sometimes conflicting results and, secondly and most importantly, because incidence rates result from studies with several noncomparable methodologies.

The overall reported incidence rate of fractured hand instruments range between 0.25 and 6% (Crump and Natkin 1970; Hülsmann and Schinkel 1999; Spili et al. 2005; Iqbal et al. 2006). The incidence of SS hand instrument fracture among undergraduate students has been reported to be 1.8% (Kerekes and Tronstad 1979) on a tooth level and 1.3% on a root level (Sjogren et al. 1990). A lower percentage of 1% on a tooth level was reported in a retrospective investigation of the incidence of hand instrument (SS and NiTi) fracture during conservative RCT performed by undergraduate dental students over a 10-year period at the University of Bergen in Norway (Ungerechts et al. 2014). The introduction of NiTi instruments, which nowadays have become a mainstay in the vast majority of endodontic and general practices and have added a new dimension to the practice of endodontics, despite their undeniably favorable qualities, has not resulted in an elimination of the problem. The common perception is that NiTi rotary instruments have a higher failure incidence than SS hand instruments (Barbakow and Lutz 1997; Cheung et al. 2005; Iqbal et al. 2006; Wolcott et al. 2006). In contrast (Parashos and Messer 2006), based on the best available clinical evidence, they state that the frequency of fracture of rotary NiTi instruments may actually be lower than that for SS hand files. The incidence rate of fractured rotary NiTi instruments varies greatly according to the type of instrument (brand, size, taper, cross-sectional shape, and instrument design), the assessment of fracture incidence, the operator, the methodology used, and several other variables that differ among the experimental works. These differences are clearly evident in studies that have investigated the fracture incidence of rotary instruments after clinical use (Table 1.1), as well as in ex vivo studies (Table 1.2). A very low fracture incidence was found with instruments with a reciprocation motion, namely, the

Table 1.1 Summary of characteristics of the studies on reported fracture incidence of endodontic instruments after clinical use (in chronological order)

Author(s) and year of publication	Methodology						Fractured incidence (%)
	Type of instrument[a]	Type of practice	Information on operators	No of files used	No of uses	No of teeth/roots/root canals	
Bueno et al. (2017)	WaveOne primary Reciproc R25	N/A[b]	Endodontists	60 WaveOne 60 Reciproc R25	Preparation of root canals [c]in up to 3 posterior teeth	358 teeth 1130 root canals	• 2.5%(3/120) in relation to instruments used • 0.26% (3/110) in relation to r.c. treated • 0.84% (3/358) in relation to teeth
Shen et al. (2016)	WaveOne files – 137 small – 249 primary – 52 large	Four specialist clinics and one graduate program	Endodontists and postgraduate students	438 files in total	N/A	N/A	0.5% (2/438) overall instrument fracture • 0.7% (1/137) small files • 0.4% (1/249) primary files • No fractures in large files
Rodrigues et al. (2016)	Reciproc R25, R40, R50 No glide path	Private practice	Endodontists	N/A	N/A	673 r.c. in total 454 narrow (R25) 135 medium (R40) 84 large (R50)	0.44% (3/673) overall • 0.66% (3/454) narrow r.c • No fractures in medium r.c. • No fractures in large r.c.

(continued)

Table 1.1 (continued)

Author(s) and year of publication	Methodology						Fractured incidence (%)
	Type of instrument[a]	Type of practice	Information on operators	No of files used	No of uses	No of teeth/roots/root canals	
Plotino et al. (2015)	Reciproc	N/A	Three operators	1696 files	N/A	3780 r.c. (3023 initial treatments & 757 retreatments)	0.47% (8/1696) overall in relation to the number of instruments used and 0.21% (8/3780) overall in relation to the number of the r.c. treated • 0.13% (5/3023) in relation to the number of r.c. shaped in initial treatments • 0.08% (3/757) in relation to the number of r.c. shaped in retreatments
Solomonov et al. (2015)	SAF	Private practice	Endodontists and general practitioners	2517	N/A	N/A	0.6% (15/2517)
Wang et al. (2014)	Mtwo	Nanjing Stomatology Hospital	N/A	§N/A	N/A	24,108 r.c. of 11,036 teeth	• 2.2% (245/11,036) in relation to the number of teeth • 1.0% (255/24,108) in relation to the number of r.c.

Ungerechts et al. (2014)	Hand instruments (SS & NiTi)	Dent. clinic, Univ. Bergen, Norway	Undergraduate students	N/A	N/A	Retrospective review of 3854 assessment forms filled out for each RCT over a 10-year period	1.0% (38/3854) overall incidence on a tooth level
Cunha et al. (2014)	WaveOne	N/A	Four experienced and calibrated endodontists	N/A	N/A	711 posterior teeth (2215 r.c.)	0.42% (3/711) in relation to teeth treated 0.13% (3/2215) in relation to the number of r.c. shaped
Shen et al. (2012)	ProFile Vortex	Faculty Dent. Univ. British Columbia, Canada	Undergraduate students	2203 files	Singe use	N/A	0.045% (1/2203) in relation to instruments discarded
Ehrhardt et al. (2012)	Mtwo	Dept. Endod. S^{ao} Leopoldo Mandic Dent. Research Center	Six calibrated endodontists	N/A	N/A	556 mandibular and maxillary molars and bicuspids	1.98% (11/556) in relation to teeth treated
Wu et al. (2011)	ProTaper Universal rotary instruments	Dept. Endod. Stomatology School, Nanjing Medical Univ. Jiangsu, China	N/A	N/A	One file for 3 molars or 10 premolars or 30 anterior teeth or one file single use for very complex or severely curved r.c.	6154 r.c. of 2654 teeth	2.6% (70/2654) overall instrument fracture in relation to teeth treated 1.1% (70/6154) in relation to the number of r.c. shaped

(continued)

Table 1.1 (continued)

Author(s) and year of publication	Methodology						Fractured incidence (%)
	Type of instrument[a]	Type of practice	Information on operators	No of files used	No of uses	No of teeth/roots/ root canals	
Inan and Gonulol (2009)	Mtwo	Univ. Samsun, Turkey	Ten trained operators	593 files collected and examined after clinical use over 12 months	N/A Fracture determined by measuring the difference in length	N/A	16% (95/ 593)
Shen et al. (2009a)	ProTaper rotary ProTaper hand K3 files	Three Univ. endodontic clinics in China	N/A	1682 files	Instruments were discarded when they had reached the designated number of uses (different among the three clinics) or when they were worn, fractured, or with any other discernible defect	N/A	5% (79/1682) overall • 5.3% (59/1108) ProTaper rotary • 4% (11/280) ProTaper hand • 3% (9/294) K3
Shen et al. (2009b)	ProFile	Faculty Dent. Univ. British Columbia, Canada	Undergraduate students	3706 files	Each set for three uses		0.3% (12/3706) in relation to the instruments discarded

(Shen et al. (2009c)	ProFile 0.04 ProFile Series 29/0.04 ProTaper	Private practice	Endodontists	1071 ProFile 0.04 432 ProFile Series 29/0.04 1895 ProTaper	Single use	N/A	No fracture of ProFile 0.04 0.26% (5/1895) of ProTaper
Tzanetakis et al. (2008)	Ten Hero instruments Nine ProFile Six ProTaper Two GT files One Lentulo 28 in total	Dent. School, Athens, Greece	Endodontic postgraduate students	N/A	N/A	2180 teeth (4897 r.c.)	1.33% (28/2098) overall • 1.88% (18/959) in retreatment cases • 0.88% (10/1139) in initial treatments
Cheung et al. 2007)	ProTaper system	Stomatological School and Hospital, Wuhan Univ. China	Four trained dentists	726 files (401 hand and 325 engine driven)	N/A	N/A	14% (58/401) of hand-discarded instruments 14% (44/325) of engine-driven-discarded instruments
Wei et al. (2007)	ProTaper	College Stomatology, Sun Yat-sen Univ. China	Endodontic clinic	774 files	One file for 30 canals, one file single use in severely curved canals or when cutting efficiency was reduced or when any visible defect was detected	N/A	12.9% (100/774) overall incidence • 88% (88/110) flexural fatigue cases no plastic defects • 12%(12/100 torsional failure

(continued)

Table 1.1 (continued)

Author(s) and year of publication	Methodology						Fractured incidence (%)
	Type of instrument[a]	Type of practice	Information on operators	No of files used	No of uses	No of teeth/roots/ root canals	
Iqbal et al. (2006)	– 49 ProFiles series 29 – 10 ProFiles GTs – 3 LightSpeed – 5 ProTaper – 2 K3 Endo files 69 NiTi in total +12 SS	Univ. Pennsylvania, School Dent. Medicine	N/A	N/A	N/A	4865 molars and premolars	1.66% (81/4865) overall • NiTi 1.68%(69/4865) • SS 0.25% (12/4865) in relation to teeth treated
Shen et al. (2006)	ProFile ProTaper	School Stomatology, Wuhan Univ. China	Four trained dentists	166 ProFile and 325 ProTaper	N/A	N/A	7% (12/166) for ProFile • Flexural fatigue 4.8%(8/166) • Torsional fatigue 2.4% (4/166) 14%(45/325) for ProTaper • Flexural fatigue 13.2%(43/325) • Torsional fatigue 0.6% (2/325)
Wolcott et al. (2006)	ProTaper	Endodontic group practice	Five Endodontists	N/A	N/A	4652 r.c.	2.4% (113/4652) in relation to r.c. treated

Di Fiore et al. (2006)	ProFile ProTaper, GT Rotary K3Endo	N. York Univ. College Dent. Post Graduate Endodontic Clinic	11 second-year endodontic residents	6661 files in total	N/A	3181 r.c. in 1403 teeth	0.39% (26/6661) overall incidence of fracture for all instruments used • 0.82% (26/3181) in relation to the r.c. treated • 1.9% (26/1403) in relation to teeth treated
Knowles et al. (2006)	LightSpeed	Creighton Univ. Medical Center School Dent.	Graduate students	N/A	N/A	3543 canals	1.3% (46/3543) in relation to the number of r.c. shaped
Alapati et al. (2005)	ProFile ProFile GT ProTaper	The Ohio State Univ. and Univ. Texas Dental Branch at Houston	Graduate endodontic clinics	822 files	6–8 uses	N/A	8%(14/175) of discarded ProFile • 3% (16/595) of discarded ProFile GT • 23%(12/52) of discarded ProTaper
Peng et al. (2005)	ProTaper S1	Endodontic clinic, Stomatological School, China	Endodontic clinic	122 files	One file for 4 molars or 20 premolars or 50 incisors or 50 canines or 1 file for a single use in very complex, severely curved, or calcified r.c.		23% (28/122) of discarded ProTaper S1
Cheung et al. (2005)	Same material and results as (Peng et al. 2005)						

(continued)

Table 1.1 (continued)

Author(s) and year of publication	Methodology						Fractured incidence (%)
	Type of instrument[a]	Type of practice	Information on operators	No of files used	No of uses	No of teeth/roots/ root canals	
Parashos et al. (2004)	FlexMaster GT, Orifice Shapers, ProFiles, ProTaper Quantec, Quantec Flare HERO	Practices in 4 countries	14 endodontists	7159 files	N/A	N/A	5% (353/7159) overall • 1.5% (103/7159) torsional • 3.5% (250/7159) flexural) of discarded instruments
Al-Fouzan (2003)	ProFile 0.04	Private practice	Two endodontists	449 files in total	N/A	419 maxillary and mandibular first and second molars (1457 r.c.)	4.6% (21/449) in relation to instruments used **or** • 5% (21/419) in relation to molars treated • 1.4% (21/1457) in relation to r.c. treated
Arens et al. (2003)	ProFile Series 29/0.04	Private practice	Endodontists	786 files	N/A	New instruments used during a single-patient visit	0.89% (7/786) in relation to instruments used
Yared et al. (2000)	ProFile (0.06 taper)	N/A	N/A	13 sets of files (#40–15)	One set for 4 molars	52 molars	No fracture

Sattapan et al. (2000)	Quantec engine driven NiTi files	Private practice	Endodontists	378 files discarded during normal clinical use over a 6-month period	N/A	N/A	20.9%(79/378) overall • 55.7% (44/79) torsional failure with unwinding • 44.3% (35/79) flexural failure without unwinding
Ramirez-Salomon et al. (1997)	LightSpeed	Private practice	Three endodontists	N/A	N/A	162 r.c. of 52 first molars were instrumented with the recommended by the manufacturer technique	3.7% (6/162) in relation to the number of r.c. shaped

[a]Type of instrument (alphabetical order)FlexMaster (VDW GmbH, Munich, Germany)Hero instruments (Micro-Mega, Besaçon, France)K3 files (SybronEndo Orange, CA, USA)LightSpeed (LightSpeed Technology Inc., San Antonio, TX, USA)Mtwo (VDW, Munich, Germany)ProFile Vortex instrument (Dentsply Tulsa Dental Specialties, Tulsa, OK, USA)ProFile Series 29 (Dentsply Tulsa Dental Specialties, Tulsa, OK, USA)ProFile GT (Dentsply Tulsa Dental Specialties, Tulsa, OK, USA)ProTaper (Dentsply Maillefer, Ballaigues, Switzerland)Quantec Series 2000 (Tycom Corp, Irvine, CA, USA)Reciproc (VDW, Munich, Germany)SAF (ReDent-Nova, Ra'anana, Israel)Twisted files (SybronEndo, Orange, CA, USA)WaveOne (Dentsply Tulsa Dental Specialties, Tulsa, OK, USA)

[b]*N/A* not available

[c]*r.c.* root canal

Table 1.2 Summary of characteristics of the ex vivo studies on reported fracture incidence of endodontic instruments in chronological order

Author(s) year	Methodology					Fractured incidence (%)
	Type of instrument[a]	Information on operators	No of files used	No of uses	No of teeth/roots/root canals instrumented-method	
Caballero et al. (2015)	Twisted file (23 mm) size #25/0.08 and R25 Reciproc instruments (21 mm)	Single operator	Five Twisted files and five R25 Reciproc	Each instrument was used to prepare 12 r.c.[b]	After use of three r.c., the instruments were cleaned in ultrasonic bath for 5 min This procedure continued until 12 r.c. were prepared using each file None of the instruments were autoclaved before or after use	No instruments fractured during this study
De-Deus et al. (2013)	R25 Reciproc	Single operator (an endodontist)			168 mandibular molars (502 r.c.) Group A: 253 straight r.c. Group B: 249 r.c. moderate curvature	0.2% (1/502) overall in relation to the number of r.c. shaped • Group A: No fracture • Group B:0.40% (1/249)
Farmakis et al. (2013)	SAF	Endodontists with no previous experience with the SAF system	19	Repeatedly used until deformation	Every 4 min, each file was withdrawn from the r.c. and inspected for integrity. If intact, it was used in another r.c. for an additional 4 min and checked again. This was repeated until all 19 SAF files were deformed	No instruments fractured during this study

Kosti et al. (2011)	ProFile	Single operator	75	Maximum 20 r.c. or until fracture or visible plastic deformation	300 mesial r.c. of human mandibular molars Divided into three equal groups of 100 r.c. according to curvature Group A: Straight Group B: Moderately curved Group C: Severely curved	Group A: No fracture (0/22) Group B: 22% (5/23) Group C: 50% (15/30)
Patino et al. (2005)	K3 Endo files ProFile ProTaper	Single operator	N/A[c]	N/A	205 r.c. of freshly extracted human mandibular and maxillary molars K3 Endo: 56 r.c. ProFile: 55 r.c. ProTaper: 94 r.c.	12% (25/205) in relation to the number of r.c. shaped • K3 Endo 9/56 • ProFile 7/55 • ProTaper 9/94
Ankrum et al. (2004)	ProFile K3 Endo ProTaper	Single operator	N/A	N/A	45 mesial roots of extracted mandibular first and second molars and buccal roots of maxillary first and second molars	• 1.7% (1/59 files) ProFile group • 2.1% (1/48 files) K3 Endo group • 6.0% (5/84 files) ProTaper group

(continued)

Table 1.2 (continued)

Author(s) year	Methodology					Fractured incidence (%)
	Type of instrument[a]	Information on operators	No of files used	No of uses	No of teeth/roots/root canals instrumented-method	
Hülsmann et al. (2003)	LightSpeed Quantec	N/A	20 LightSpeed (including size 15 hand file) and 10 Quantec	In both groups, instruments were discarded after preparation of ten r.c.	50 mandibular molars (25 for each group)	• 25% (5/20) for LightSpeed in relation to the number of instruments used • 20% (5/25) for LightSpeed in relation to the number of molars instrumented • 30% (3/10) for Quantec in relation to the number of instruments used • 12% (3/25) for Quantec in relation to the number of molars instrumented
Martin et al. (2003)	K3 ProTaper	N/A	N/A		240 r.c. of extracted molars divided into: Group A: Curvature <30° Group B: Curvature >30° Three different rotational speeds (150,250, & 350 rpm) were evaluated. Thus 40 teeth in each subgroup	Group A: no fracture Group B: 22 (12 ProTaper & 10 K3) files fractured in total • 5 (2 K3 & 3 ProTaper) at 150 rpm • 7 (4 K3 &3 ProTaper) at 250 rpm • 10 (4 K3 & 6 ProTaper) at 350 rpm

Roland et al. (2002)	ProFile Series 29/0.04 sizes 2–6 rotary	Two operators	20 sets	Instruments were used until fracture or to a maximum of 20 uses despite visible deformation	Group A: No pre-flaring of the r.c. Group B: Pre-flaring	Group A: 38% (19/50) Group B: 6% (3/50)
Zelada et al. (2002)	ProFile	N/A	N/A	In Group A (60 teeth), files were used a maximum of 20 times In Group B (60 teeth), the files were discarded after being used 12 times	120 molars divided into: Group A: Curvature <30° Group B: Curvature >30° Evaluation of three rotational speeds (150, 250, & 350 rpm)	Group A: No fracture Group B: 12.5% of all the instrumented r.c.
Tripi et al. (2001)	GT Rotary	Single operator	– 5 GT Rotary size 35/1.2 – 5 GT Rotary size 20/1.0 – 5 GT Rotary 20/0.8 – 5 GT Rotary size 20/0.6	Each instrument was used to prepare 12 r.c. in four extracted mandibular molars		No instruments fractured during this study

[a]Type of instruments (alphabetical order)K3 files (SybronEndo Orange, CA)LightSpeed (LightSpeed Technology Inc., San Antonio, TX, USA)ProFile Series 29 (Dentsply Tulsa Dental Specialties, Tulsa, OK, USA)ProFile GT (Dentsply Tulsa Dental Specialties, Tulsa, OK, USA)ProTaper (Dentsply Maillefer, Ballaigues, Switzerland)Quantec Series 2000 (Tycom Corp, Irvine, CA, USA)Reciproc (VDW, Munich, Germany)SAF (ReDent-Nova, Ra'anana, Israel) Twisted files (SybronEndo, Orange, CA, USA)

[b]*r.c.* root canal

[c]*N/A* not available

reciprocating WaveOne files (Cunha et al. 2014) and the Reciproc instruments (Plotino et al. 2015).

This was attributed to:

- *Metallurgic composition.* They are manufactured from M-wire alloy with superior mechanical properties compared to files made from conventionally processed NiTi wires (Johnson et al. 2008; Al-Hadlaq et al. 2010; Gao et al. 2012; Pereira et al. 2012; Ye and Gao 2012).
- *Reciprocating motion.* Instruments do not complete a full 360o turn continuously. This extends cyclic fatigue instrument life compared to conventional rotation when shaping curved canals (Castello-Escriva et al. 2012; Gavini et al. 2012; De-Deus et al. 2013; Lopes et al. 2013; Pedulla et al. 2013).
- *Single use.* A prospective clinical study questioning whether these instruments could be used in more than one clinical case of multirooted teeth revealed that Reciproc and WaveOne files were used safely, by experienced endodontists, for up to three clinical cases of endodontic treatment in posterior teeth (Bueno et al. 2017). The reported fracture rate was comparable with that observed in studies on single-use reciprocating instruments (Bueno et al. 2017).

Data on the breakage of ultrasonic tips used in orthograde endodontics or in root-end preparation are consistent but very limited (Ahmad 1989; Ahmad and Roy 1994; Walmsley et al. 1996; Lin et al. 2006; Verhaagen 2012; Wan et al. 2014). In most of the manufacturers' manuals of ultrasonic devices, it is stated (Spartan 2017) *...the operator should be aware that ultrasonic tips with small diameters are subject to breakage at any time. In order to reduce the incidence of premature breakage or failure, only a very light pressure should be applied by the operator, and the suggested intensity settings should be followed....* A comparison of the breakage of three ultrasonic tips, operated with a piezoelectric ultrasonic scaler when removing dentin from extracted molars, revealed a significant difference in breakage as a function of tip type (Wan et al. 2014). SS with no coating EDS 5E tip (Essential Dental Systems, South Hackensack, NJ) was found to be more resistant to breakage than BUC 1A (Obtura Spartan, Fenton, MO, USA) and CPR 5D (Obtura Spartan), which are diamond-coated tips (Wan et al. 2014). Similarly, in an in vitro study evaluating the cutting efficiency of SS, zirconium nitride-coated, and diamond-coated ultrasonic tips used in orthograde endodontics, only the diamond-coated tips showed breakage (Lin et al. 2006). Fatigue due to continuously changing bending during oscillation and not cavitation is hypothesized to be the most likely cause of breakage of ultrasonic files (Ahmad 1989; Ahmad and Roy 1994; Verhaagen 2012). Fracture is more likely to occur when ultrasonic tips are energized in air and less likely when used in water or in the root canal with irrigant (Ahmad and Roy 1994; Verhaagen 2012). File fracture can also occur during passive ultrasonic irrigation of the root canal (Verhaagen 2012). Determination of the breakage of ten different ultrasonic tip designs used to prepare root-end cavities during endodontic surgery revealed that their breakage always occurred at a bend and was related to the degree of bending (Walmsley et al. 1996).

Also very limited data are available for the Self-Adjusting File (SAF) (ReDent-Nova, Ra'anana, Israel). A time-dependent deformation, mainly as a detachment of one of the arches or struts at connection points on the odd side of the file with no full fracture, was found when used in simulated curved root canal (Akcay et al. 2011) or in canals of extracted teeth (Farmakis et al. 2013) (Fig. 1.10). A preliminary questionnaire survey regarding prevalence and retrieval methods during clinical use responded by 15 experienced SAF users from seven countries revealed 0.6% fracture prevalence (15 files fractured out of 2517 used) with 12 fractured files (80%, 12/15) being easily retrieved (Solomonov et al. 2015).

Fracture of two, three (Figs. 1.11 and 1.12), or even more instruments in a root canal (Lambrianidis 1984, 2001; Zeigler and Serene 1984; Ingle et al. 1985) is possible during RCT or retreatment. Occasionally a variety of instrument fragments can be found in one tooth in the same or in different canals (Fig. 1.13). There are

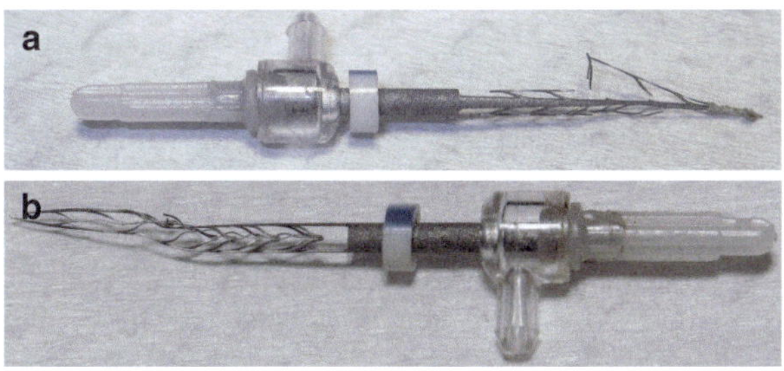

Fig. 1.10 (**a**) Self-Adjusting File that suffered on its even side (*top side*), the complete breakage of two arches and a strut, with the deformed parts still attached to the NiTi lattice and, on the odd side (*lower side*), a single-sided failure of an arch and the breakage of a strut. Pulpal tissue can be seen at the tip of the file. (**b**) Self-Adjusting File that suffered a single-sided breakage of one of the arches on the odd side and a plastic deformation of both beams (Courtesy Dr. E. Farmakis)

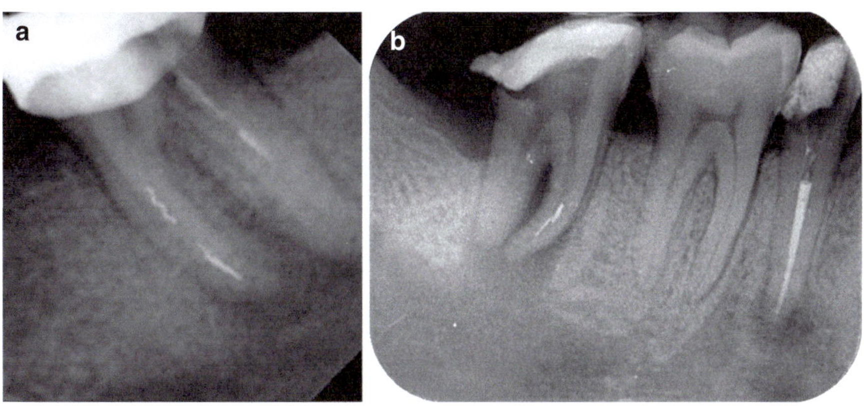

Fig. 1.11 Root canals with two fragments

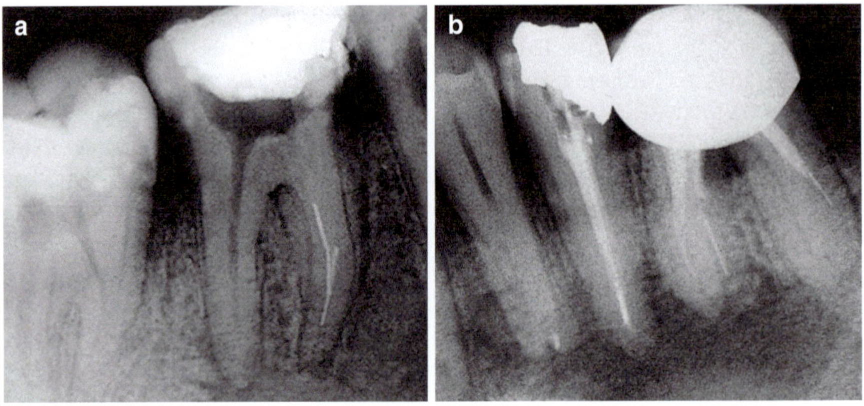

Fig. 1.12 (**a**) Root canal with three fractured instruments. (**b**) Tooth with three fragments, one in each canal (Reprinted with permission from Lambrianidis 2001)

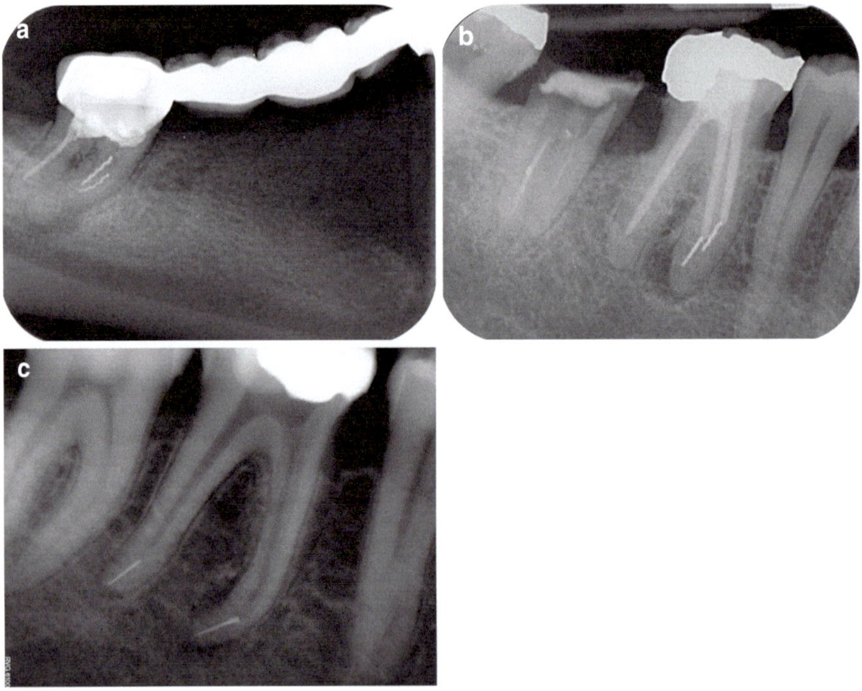

Fig. 1.13 Teeth with more than one fragment

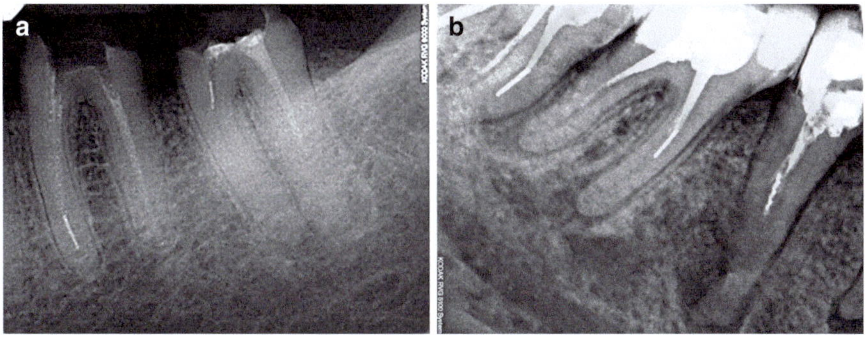

Fig. 1.14 Two and three adjacent teeth with one fragment each

also cases with fragments in adjacent teeth seen in one periapical radiograph (Fig. 1.14).

Several studies have investigated the plethora of factors implicated in endodontic instrument fracture. They will be presented in detail in Chap. 2.

References

Aduri R, Reddy RE, Kiran K. Foreign objects in teeth: retrieval and management. J Indian Soc Pedod Prev Dent. 2009;27(3):179–83.

Ahmad M. An analysis of breakage of ultrasonic files during root canal instrumentation. Endod Dent Traumatol. 1989;5(2):78–82.

Ahmad M, Roy RA. Some observations on the breakage of ultrasonic files driven piezoelectrically. Endod Dent Traumatol. 1994;10(2):71–6.

Akcay I, Yigit-Ozer S, Adiguzel O, Kaya S. Deformation of the self-adjusting file on simulated curved root canals: a time-dependent study. Oral Surg Oral Med Oral Pathol Oral Radiol Endod. 2011;112(5):e12–7.

Alapati SB, Brantley WA, Svec TA, Powers JM, Nusstein JM, Daehn GS. SEM observations of nickel-titanium rotary endodontic instruments that fractured during clinical Use. J Endod. 2005;31(1):40–3.

Al-Fouzan KS. Incidence of rotary ProFile instrument fracture and the potential for bypassing in vivo. Int Endod J. 2003;36(12):864–7.

Al-Hadlaq SM, Aljarbou FA, AlThumairy RI. Evaluation of cyclic flexural fatigue of M-wire nickel-titanium rotary instruments. J Endod. 2010;36(2):305–7.

Ankrum MT, Hartwell GR, Truitt JE. K3 Endo, ProTaper, and ProFile systems: breakage and distortion in severely curved roots of molars. J Endod. 2004;30(4):234–7.

Arens FC, Hoen MM, Steiman HR, Dietz GC Jr. Evaluation of single-use rotary nickel-titanium instruments. J Endod. 2003;29(10):664–6.

Barbakow F, Lutz F. The 'Lightspeed' preparation technique evaluated by Swiss clinicians after attending continuing education courses. Int Endod J. 1997;30(1):46–50.

Bueno CSP, Oliveira DP, Pelegrine RA, Fontana CE, Rocha DGP, Bueno CES. Fracture incidence of WaveOne and Reciproc Files during root canal preparation of up to 3 posterior teeth: a prospective clinical study. J Endod. 2017. pii: S0099-2399(17)30001-8. doi: 10.1016/j.joen.2016.12.024. Epub ahead of print.

Caballero H, Rivera F, Salas H. Scanning electron microscopy of superficial defects in Twisted files and Reciproc nickel-titanium files after use in extracted molars. Int Endod J. 2015;48(3):229–35.

Castello-Escriva R, Alegre-Domingo T, Faus-Matoses V, Roman-Richon S, Faus-Llacer VJ. In vitro comparison of cyclic fatigue resistance of ProTaper, WaveOne, and Twisted Files. J Endod. 2012;38(11):1521–4.
Chand K, Joesph S, Varughese JM, Nair MG, Prasanth S. Endodontic management of an unusual foreign body in a maxillary central incisor. J Conserv Dent. 2013;16(5):474–6.
Chenail BL, Teplitsky PE. Orthograde ultrasonic retrieval of root canal obstructions. J Endod. 1987;13(4):186–90.
Cheung GS, Peng B, Bian Z, Shen Y, Darvell BW. Defects in ProTaper S1 instruments after clinical use: fractographic examination. Int Endod J. 2005;38(11):802–9.
Cheung GS, Bian Z, Shen Y, Peng B, Darvell BW. Comparison of defects in ProTaper hand-operated and engine-driven instruments after clinical use. Int Endod J. 2007;40(3):169–78.
Crump MC, Natkin E. Relationship of broken root canal instruments to endodontic case prognosis: a clinical investigation. J Am Dent Assoc. 1970;80(6):1341–7.
Cunha RS, Junaid A, Ensinas P, Nudera W, Bueno CE. Assessment of the separation incidence of reciprocating WaveOne files: a prospective clinical study. J Endod. 2014;40(7):922–4.
De-Deus G, Arruda TE, Souza EM, Neves A, Magalhaes K, Thuanne E, et al. The ability of the Reciproc R25 instrument to reach the full root canal working length without a glide path. Int Endod J. 2013;46(10):993–8.
Di Fiore PM, Genov KA, Komaroff E, Li Y, Lin L. Nickel-titanium rotary instrument fracture: a clinical practice assessment. Int Endod J. 2006;39(9):700–8.
Ehrhardt IC, Zuolo ML, Cunha RS, De Martin AS, Kherlakian D, Carvalho MC, et al. Assessment of the separation incidence of mtwo files used with preflaring: prospective clinical study. J Endod. 2012;38(8):1078–81.
Farmakis ET, Sotiropoulos GG, Pantazis N, Kozyrakis K. The permanent deformation of the self-adjusting files when used in canals of extracted teeth. Int Endod J. 2013;46(9):863–9.
Gao Y, Gutmann JL, Wilkinson K, Maxwell R, Ammon D. Evaluation of the impact of raw materials on the fatigue and mechanical properties of ProFile Vortex rotary instruments. J Endod. 2012;38(3):398–401.
Gavini G, Caldeira CL, Akisue E, Candeiro GT, Kawakami DA. Resistance to flexural fatigue of Reciproc R25 files under continuous rotation and reciprocating movement. J Endod. 2012;38(5):684–7.
Grossman LI. Endodontic case reports. Dent Clin N Am. 1974;18(2):509–27.
Holla G, Baliga S, Yeluri R, Munshi AK. Unusual objects in the root canal of deciduous teeth: a report of two cases. Contemp Clin Dent. 2010;1(4):246–8.
Hülsmann M. Removal of fractured instruments using a combined automated/ultrasonic technique. J Endod. 1994;20(3):144–7.
Hülsmann M, Schinkel I. Influence of several factors on the success or failure of removal of fractured instruments from the root canal. Endod Dent Traumatol. 1999;15(6):252–8.
Hülsmann M, Herbst U, Schafers F. Comparative study of root-canal preparation using Lightspeed and Quantec SC rotary NiTi instruments. Int Endod J. 2003;36(11):748–56.
Inan U, Gonulol N. Deformation and fracture of Mtwo rotary nickel-titanium instruments after clinical use. J Endod. 2009;35(10):1396–9.
Ingle J, Beveridge E, Glick D, Weichman J, Abou-Rass M. Modern endodontic therapy. In: Ingle JI, Taintor FJ, editors. Endodontics. 3rd ed. Philadelphia: Lea & Febiger; 1985. p. 1–53.
Iqbal MK, Kohli MR, Kim JS. A retrospective clinical study of incidence of root canal instrument separation in an endodontics graduate program: a PennEndo database study. J Endod. 2006;32(11):1048–52.
Johnson E, Lloyd A, Kuttler S, Namerow K. Comparison between a novel nickel-titanium alloy and 508 nitinol on the cyclic fatigue life of ProFile 25/.04 rotary instruments. J Endod. 2008;34(11):1406–9.
Kalyan SR, Sajjan G. Endodontic management of a foreign body. Contemp Clin Dent. 2010;1(3):180–2.
Kerekes K, Tronstad L. Long-term results of endodontic treatment performed with a standardized technique. J Endod. 1979;5(3):83–90.

Knowles KI, Hammond NB, Biggs SG, Ibarrola JL. Incidence of instrument separation using LightSpeed rotary instruments. J Endod. 2006;32(1):14–6.
Kosti E, Zinelis S, Molyvdas I, Lambrianidis T. Effect of root canal curvature on the failure incidence of ProFile rotary Ni-Ti endodontic instruments. Int Endod J. 2011;44(10):917–25.
Lambrianidis T. Iatrogenic errors during root canal treatment. Hellenic Stomatol Rev. 1984;28:7–18. (in Greek)
Lambrianidis T. Risk management in root canal treatment. Thessaloniki: University Studio Press; 2001. p. 199–247.
Lin YH, Mickel AK, Jones JJ, Montagnese TA, Gonzalez AF. Evaluation of cutting efficiency of ultrasonic tips used in orthograde endodontic treatment. J Endod. 2006;32(4):359–61.
Lopes HP, Elias CN, Vieira MV, Siqueira JF Jr, Mangelli M, Lopes WS, Oliveira JC, Soares TG. Fatigue life of Reciproc and Mtwo instruments subjected to static and dynamic tests. J Endod. 2013;39(5):693–6.
Martin B, Zelada G, Varela P, Bahillo JG, Magan F, Ahn S, et al. Factors influencing the fracture of nickel-titanium rotary instruments. Int Endod J. 2003;36(4):262–6.
McAuliffe N, Drage NA, Hunter B. Staple diet: a foreign body in a tooth. Int J Paediatr Dent. 2005;15(6):468–71.
Meidinger DL, Kabes BJ. Foreign object removal utilizing the Cavi-Endo ultrasonic instrument. J Endod. 1985;11(7):301–4.
Molyvdas I, Lambrianidis T, Zervas P, Veis A. Clinical study on the prognosis of endodontic treatment of teeth with broken endodontic instruments. Stoma. 1992;20:63–72. (in Greek).
Nadkarni UM, Munshi A, Damle SG, Kalaskar RR. Retrieval of a foreign object from the palatal root canal of a permanent maxillary first molar: a case report. Quintessence Int. 2002;33(8):609–12.
Ozsezer E, Ozden B, Kulacaoglu N, Ozden FO. The treatment of unusual foreign objects in a root canal: a case report. Oral Surg Oral Med Oral Pathol Oral Radiol Endod. 2006;102(6):e45–7.
Parashos P, Messer HH. Rotary NiTi instrument fracture and its consequences. J Endod. 2006;32(11):1031–43.
Parashos P, Gordon I, Messer HH. Factors influencing defects of rotary nickel-titanium endodontic instruments after clinical use. J Endod. 2004;30(10):722–5.
Patil P, Pimpale S, Mandwe A, Shetty H. Sewing needle obturation of root canal: a rare case report. IJSS Case Rep Rev. 2015;1(12):31–5.
Patino PV, Biedma BM, Liebana CR, Cantatore G, Bahillo JG. The influence of a manual glide path on the separation rate of NiTi rotary instruments. J Endod. 2005;31(2):114–6.
Pedulla E, Grande NM, Plotino G, Gambarini G, Rapisarda E. Influence of continuous or reciprocating motion on cyclic fatigue resistance of 4 different nickel-titanium rotary instruments. J Endod. 2013;39(2):258–61.
Peng B, Shen Y, Cheung GS, Xia TJ. Defects in ProTaper S1 instruments after clinical use: longitudinal examination. Int Endod J. 2005;38(8):550–7.
Pereira ES, Peixoto IF, Viana AC, Oliveira II, Gonzalez BM, Buono VT, et al. Physical and mechanical properties of a thermomechanically treated NiTi wire used in the manufacture of rotary endodontic instruments. Int Endod J. 2012;45(5):469–74.
Plotino G, Grande NM, Porciani PF. Deformation and fracture incidence of Reciproc instruments: a clinical evaluation. Int Endod J. 2015;48(2):199–205.
Rahimi M, Parashos P. A novel technique for the removal of fractured instruments in the apical third of curved root canals. Int Endod J. 2009;42(3):264–70.
Ramirez-Salomon M, Soler-Bientz R, de la Garza-González R, Palacios-Garza CM. Incidence of lightspeed separation and the potential for bypassing. J Endod. 1997;23(9):586–7.
Rodrigues E, De-Deus G, Souza E, Silva EJ. Safe mechanical preparation with reciprocation movement without glide path creation: result from a pool of 673 root canals. Braz Dent J. 2016;27(1):22–7.
Roland DD, Andelin WE, Browning DF, Hsu GH, Torabinejad M. The effect of preflaring on the rates of separation for 0.04 taper nickel titanium rotary instruments. J Endod. 2002;28(7):543–5.
Sattapan B, Nervo GJ, Palamara JE, Messer HH. Defects in rotary nickel-titanium files after clinical use. J Endod. 2000;26(3):161–5.

Shay JC. Foreign body in a tooth. Oral Surg Oral Med Oral Pathol. 1985;59(4):431.
Shen Y, Peng B, Cheung GS. Factors associated with the removal of fractured NiTi instruments from root canal systems. Oral Surg Oral Med Oral Pathol Oral Radiol Endod. 2004;98(5):605–10.
Shen Y, Cheung GS, Bian Z, Peng B. Comparison of defects in ProFile and ProTaper systems after clinical use. J Endod. 2006;32(1):61–5.
Shen Y, Haapasalo M, Cheung GS, Peng B. Defects in nickel-titanium instruments after clinical use. Part 1: relationship between observed imperfections and factors leading to such defects in a cohort study. J Endod. 2009a;35(1):129–32.
Shen Y, Cheung GS, Peng B, Haapasalo M. Defects in nickel-titanium instruments after clinical use. Part 2: Fractographic analysis of fractured surface in a cohort study. J Endod. 2009b;35(1):133–6.
Shen Y, Coil JM, Haapasalo M. Defects in nickel-titanium instruments after clinical use. Part 3: a 4-year retrospective study from an undergraduate clinic. J Endod. 2009c;35(2):193–6.
Shen Y, Coil JM, Zhou HM, Tam E, Zheng YF, Haapasalo M. ProFile Vortex instruments after clinical use: a metallurgical properties study. J Endod. 2012;38(12):1613–7.
Shen Y, Coil JM, Mo AJ, Wang Z, Hieawy A, Yang Y, et al. WaveOne rotary instruments after clinical use. J Endod. 2016;42(2):186–9.
Singh Dhull K, Acharya S, Ray P, Singh DR. Foreign body in root canals of two adjacent deciduous molars: a case report. Int J Clin Pediatr Dent. 2013;6(1):38–9.
Sjogren U, Hagglund B, Sundqvist G, Wing K. Factors affecting the long-term results of endodontic treatment. J Endod. 1990;16(10):498–504.
Solomonov M, Ben-Itzhak J, Kfir A, von Stetten O, Lipatova E, Farmakis ET. Self-adjusting file (SAF) separation in clinical use: a preliminary survey among experienced SAF users regarding prevalence and retrieval methods. J Conserv Dent. 2015;18(3):200–4.
Spartan O. Instructions for use – CPR® non-surgical ultrasonic endodontic instruments. 2017 [cited 2017 1/24/2017]; Available from: https://www.obtura.com/media/msds/1012cprtips.pdf.
Spili P, Parashos P, Messer HH. The impact of instrument fracture on outcome of endodontic treatment. J Endod. 2005;31(12):845–50.
Srivastava N, Vineeta N. Foreign body in the periradicular area. J Endod. 2001;27(9):593–4.
Stamos DG, Haasch GC, Chenail B, Gerstein H. Endosonics: clinical impressions. J Endod. 1985;11(4):181–7.
Sternberg RN. Retrieval of broken instrument from root canal. Oral Surg Oral Med Oral Pathol. 1977;44(2):325.
Tripi TR, Bonaccorso A, Tripi V, Condorelli GG, Rapisarda E. Defects in GT rotary instruments after use: an SEM study. J Endod. 2001;27(12):782–5.
Turner CH. An unusual foreign body. Oral Surg Oral Med Oral Pathol. 1983;56(2):226.
Tzanetakis GN, Kontakiotis EG, Maurikou DV, Marzelou MP. Prevalence and management of instrument fracture in the postgraduate endodontic program at the Dental School of Athens: a five-year retrospective clinical study. J Endod. 2008;34(6):675–8.
Ungerechts C, Bardsen A, Fristad I. Instrument fracture in root canals – where, why, when and what? A study from a student clinic. Int Endod J. 2014;47(2):183–90.
Verhaagen B. Root canal cleaning through cavitation and micro-streaming. Enschede: University of Twente; 2012.
Walmsley AD, Lumley PJ, Johnson WT, Walton RE. Breakage of ultrasonic root-end preparation tips. J Endod. 1996;22(6):287–9.
Walvekar SV, Al-Duwairi Y, Al-Kandari AM, Al-Quoud OA. Unusual foreign objects in the root canal. J Endod. 1995;21(10):526–7.
Wan J, Deutsch AS, Musikant BL, Guzman J. Evaluation of the breakage of orthograde endodontic ultrasonic tips. J Endod. 2014;40(12):2074–6.
Wang NN, Ge JY, Xie SJ, Chen G, Zhu M. Analysis of Mtwo rotary instrument separation during endodontic therapy: a retrospective clinical study. Cell Biochem Biophys. 2014;70(2):1091–5.
Ward JR, Parashos P, Messer HH. Evaluation of an ultrasonic technique to remove fractured rotary nickel-titanium endodontic instruments from root canals: an experimental study. J Endod. 2003;29(11):756–63.

Wei X, Ling J, Jiang J, Huang X, Liu L. Modes of failure of ProTaper nickel-titanium rotary instruments after clinical use. J Endod. 2007;33(3):276–9.
Wolcott S, Wolcott J, Ishley D, Kennedy W, Johnson S, Minnich S, et al. Separation incidence of protaper rotary instruments: a large cohort clinical evaluation. J Endod. 2006;32(12):1139–41.
Wu J, Lei G, Yan M, Yu Y, Yu J, Zhang G. Instrument separation analysis of multi-used ProTaper Universal rotary system during root canal therapy. J Endod. 2011;37(6):758–63.
Yared GM, Bou Dagher FE, Machtou P. Cyclic fatigue of ProFile rotary instruments after clinical use. Int Endod J. 2000;33(3):204–7.
Ye J, Gao Y. Metallurgical characterization of M-Wire nickel-titanium shape memory alloy used for endodontic rotary instruments during low-cycle fatigue. J Endod. 2012;38(1):105–7.
Zeigler P, Serene T. Failures in Therapy. CV Mobsy: St. Louis; 1984.
Zelada G, Varela P, Martin B, Bahillo JG, Magan F, Ahn S. The effect of rotational speed and the curvature of root canals on the breakage of rotary endodontic instruments. J Endod. 2002;28(7):540–2.
Zillich RM, Pickens TN. Patient-induced blockage of the root canal. Report of a case. Oral Surg Oral Med Oral Pathol. 1982;54(6):689–90.

Factors Affecting Intracanal Instrument Fracture

2

Christos Boutsioukis and Theodor Lambrianidis

2.1 Introduction

Root canal treatment (RCT) may require the use of a variety of instruments including files and reamers, ultrasonic tips, explorers, irrigation needles, Lentulo spirals, spreaders and pluggers, heat-conducting tips, and filling material injection tips; any of these instruments may fracture inside the root canal during use, but the fracture of files and reamers is considered to be a more frequent problem. Furthermore, despite the longevity of stainless steel (SS) instruments, only a small number of studies have dealt with the factors leading to their fracture; most of the available information concerns nickel-titanium (NiTi) instruments. As a result, this chapter will discuss the parameters influencing the fracture of files and reamers with a particular focus on NiTi instruments that have dominated the interest of both clinicians and researchers for almost two decades.

Several factors have been implicated in the failure of root canal instruments, and many studies have attempted to elucidate their individual contributions. In order to facilitate the description and analysis of the relevant factors, they have been grouped together in four main categories, namely, *operator related*, *anatomy related*, *instrument related*, and *technique/use related* (Table 2.1). However, it is likely that some of these factors may actually fit in more than one category. Moreover, in accordance with the principles of evidence-based dentistry, the description and analysis of these factors have been based only on higher quality in vitro and clinical studies, while

C. Boutsioukis, D.D.S., M.Sc., Ph.D. (✉)
Department of Endodontology, Academic Centre for Dentistry Amsterdam (ACTA), Gustav Mahlerlaan 3004, 1081 LA Amsterdam, The Netherlands
e-mail: c.boutsioukis@acta.nl

T. Lambrianidis, D.D.S., Ph.D.
Department of Endodontology, Dental School, Aristotle University of Thessaloniki, Thessaloniki, Greece

T. Lambrianidis (ed.), *Management of Fractured Endodontic Instruments*,
DOI 10.1007/978-3-319-60651-4_2

Table 2.1 Outline of the factors affecting intracanal instrument fracture

Factors affecting intracanal instrument fracture	
Operator related	Skill, proficiency, judgment
Anatomy related	Access cavity
	Root canal anatomy
Instrument related	Material
	Design
	Manufacturing process and errors
Technique/use related	Motors operating parameters
	Instrumentation technique
	Reuse and sterilization
	Irrigants

unreliable in vitro models clearly deviating from in vivo conditions have been excluded (Hülsmann 2013).

2.2 Operator-Related Factors

Just like many other dental procedures, RCT involves a series of delicate and meticulous manipulations requiring adequate training and dexterity; preparation of root canals is perhaps one of the most technically demanding phases, so it doesn't come as a surprise that factors pertaining to the operator's skill and proficiency have been ranked as the most important among those contributing to instrument fracture (Parashos et al. 2004; Cheung 2009).

Practitioners need to choose from a constantly expanding variety of instruments, each one having its own design and mechanical properties and being accompanied by its own guidelines for use; this process can already create some confusion. Once the choice has been made, the clinician needs to become familiar with the instruments, their specific mode of use, and the manufacturer's recommendations. For example, switching from hand instrumentation by SS files to rotary instrumentation by NiTi files can be rather challenging; NiTi files provide less tactile feedback regarding the morphology of the canal, so a different kind of awareness is required.

Proper in vitro training is necessary in order to bridge this gap (Yared et al. 2001, 2002; McGuigan et al. 2013). Despite wide variability among clinicians, it appears that the handling of instruments is characteristic for each clinician (Regan et al. 2000) so it could be modified through training. Avoiding aggressive penetration in the root canal by applying too much apically directed force on the instrument (Saber 2008), sensing when a rotary instrument is about to bind inside a root canal so that it is withdrawn before torsional overload occurs, and recognizing the stress applied to the instruments during preparation of very curved root canals that could lead to a fatigue failure are skills that can be developed through practicing on extracted teeth and fine-tuned through the gradual accumulation of clinical experience. Even so, a clinician's performance may still vary to some extent over time depending on workload and physical fatigue (Briseno et al. 1993). Finally, the operator has to develop his/her judgment in order to discard an instrument that shows a dubious defect or that has been used in a difficult-to-prepare root canal.

2.3 Anatomy-Related Factors

2.3.1 Access Cavity

The definition of an "adequate" access cavity has undergone several changes throughout the years. A completed access cavity should still allow unobstructed visual access to all root canals and act as a funnel to guide the instruments into the canal, straight to the apex, or to the point of first curvature (Peters 2008). Interference by the cavity walls or by unremoved dentin shoulders in the coronal third of the root canal can increase the stress imposed on the instruments during preparation by increasing the number and severity of curvatures that must be negotiated (iatrogenic S curve) (Roda and Gettleman 2016); this could lead to instrument failure (Figs. 2.1, 2.2, and 2.3). Conversely, expanding the access cavity beyond the confines of the pulp chamber could also hinder the entrance of files into the root canals and lead to accidental bending of the tips.

Nowadays, the extensive use of the dental operating microscope that provides superior magnification and illumination has facilitated more conservative access cavities specifically designed for each case according to the pulp chamber morphology in an effort to conserve as much tooth structure as possible. The extensive occlusal tapering of the cavity wall circumferentially has been replaced by selective tapering of the cavity walls only where necessary, depending on the location of the root canal orifices and the direction and shape of the canals (Peters 2008). Taken to

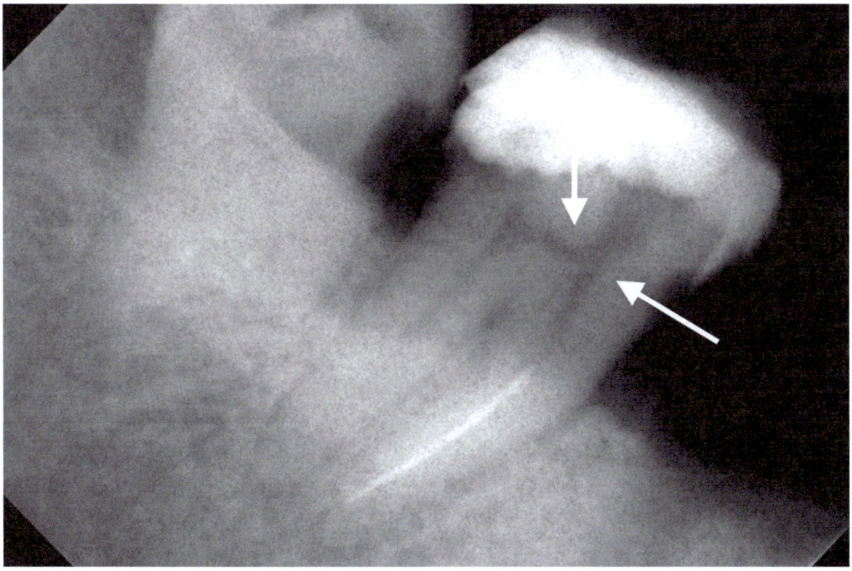

Fig. 2.1 Fractured instrument in the mesial root of a mandibular molar due to inadequate access cavity preparation. Note the presence of pulp chamber roof (*short arrow*) and insufficient shoulder removal (*long arrow*) that impeded straight-line access to the coronal third of the canal

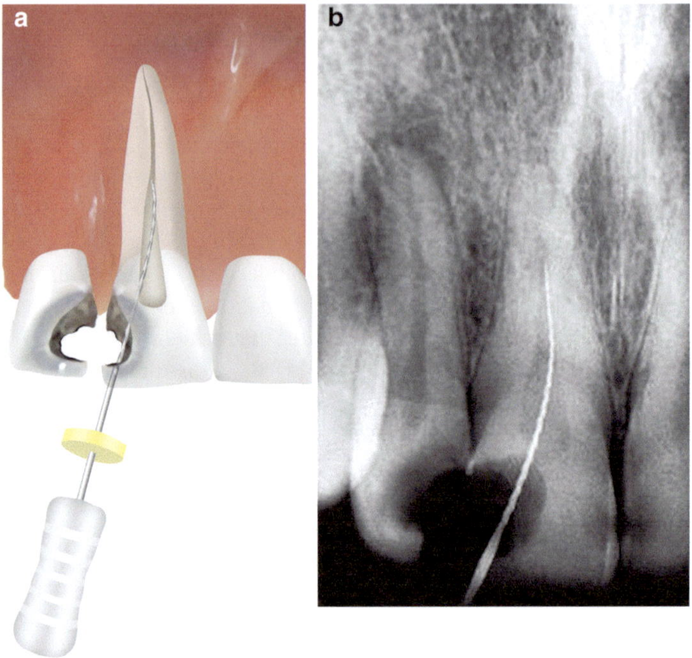

Fig. 2.2 Improper access cavity through a mesial or distal carious lesion. Instruments penetrating through such lesions cannot follow a straight-line path to the apex, which may eventually result in a variety of iatrogenic errors, including instrument fracture

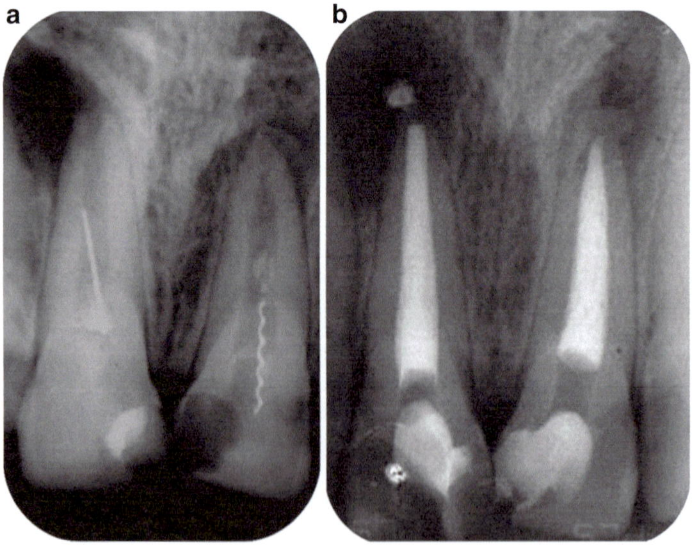

Fig. 2.3 (**a**) Two fractured instruments, one in each maxillary central incisor, were identified in the preoperative radiograph. The instruments fractured possibly due to incorrect access cavity preparation through existing carious lesions. (**b**) Following conventional access cavity preparation, the fragments were retrieved and RCT was completed. (**c**, **d**) Three- and twelve-month recall radiographs revealed uneventful healing

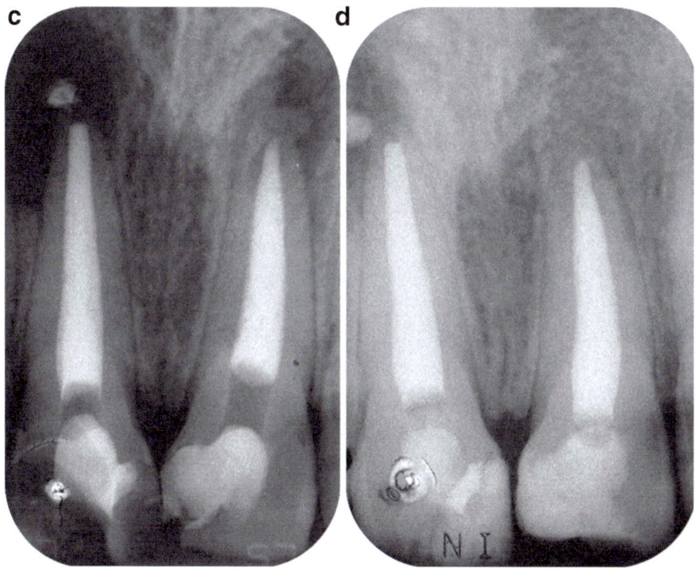

Fig. 2.3 (continued)

its extremes, this trend has led to the concept of *minimally invasive access cavities* which advocates removal of only a minimum amount of hard dental tissue (Gluskin et al. 2014; Krishan et al. 2014; Eaton et al. 2015; Moore et al. 2016), even if subsequent treatment procedures become far more challenging. Nevertheless, anecdotal evidence indicates that such miniature access cavities do not seem to increase the chance of instrument fracture, at least when treatments are performed under the microscope by experienced and skillful clinicians.

SS instruments possess several advantages regarding their placement in the root canal as compared to NiTi files that require considerably more attention to gaining straight-line access. SS files can be pre-bent enabling their introduction into difficult-to-access canals; with the exception of controlled-memory files (Coltene Endo 2014), NiTi instruments are very difficult to pre-bent accurately. In addition, stiff hand-operated SS files also provide superior tactile feedback regarding obstacles as opposed to the flexible NiTi files that are usually attached to a handpiece.

2.3.2 Root Canal Anatomy

The risk of instrument failure seems to increase in cases with complex root canal anatomy (Peters et al. 2003). Fractures appear more often in molars than premolars or anterior teeth (Iqbal et al. 2006; Wu et al. 2011; Ungerechts et al. 2014; Wang et al. 2014) and also in the mesiobuccal root canal of maxillary and mandibular molars (Iqbal et al. 2006; Wu et al. 2011) than in other root canals. These findings could be explained by the overall morphological complexity of the molar root canal system and the existence of multiple canals within each tooth, but the primary reason is most likely the curvature of these root canals.

The curvature of a root canal is described by its angle and radius (Pruett et al. 1997); the wider the angle and the smaller the radius, the more abrupt the curvature. These two parameters can vary independently of each other, so it is possible that two root canals may have the same angle but very different radii of curvature or the opposite (Fig. 2.4). In addition to the shear stress applied to the instrument during preparation of any root canal, a bending stress is concurrently applied inside a curved root canal. As the file rotates, it undergoes repeated cycles of tension and compression, with tension occurring near the outer curved surface and compression near the inner. This repeated cyclic loading may result in crack initiation and eventually in fracture (Pruett et al. 1997; Cheung 2009).

Ex vivo studies have suggested that root canal curvature may increase the failure rate of rotary NiTi instruments (Li et al. 2002, Zelada et al. 2002, Martin et al. 2003, Di Fiore et al. 2006, Kosti et al. 2011) due to both torsional overload and cyclic fatigue (Pruett et al. 1997; Zelada et al. 2002; Kosti et al. 2011), and clinical studies have corroborated these findings (Wu et al. 2011; Wang et al. 2014). The risk of fracture seems to increase as the angle increases, especially beyond 30° (Zelada et al. 2002, Martin et al. 2003, Kitchens et al. 2007), and also as the radius decreases (Haikel et al. 1999; Booth et al. 2003; Patino et al. 2005), and it appears that the radius has a more pronounced effect on this process.

Moreover, an early curvature in the coronal or middle third of the root canal is more likely to lead to failure compared to an apical curvature (Peters and Paque 2010; Lopes et al. 2013) because the diameter of the instrument at the area where

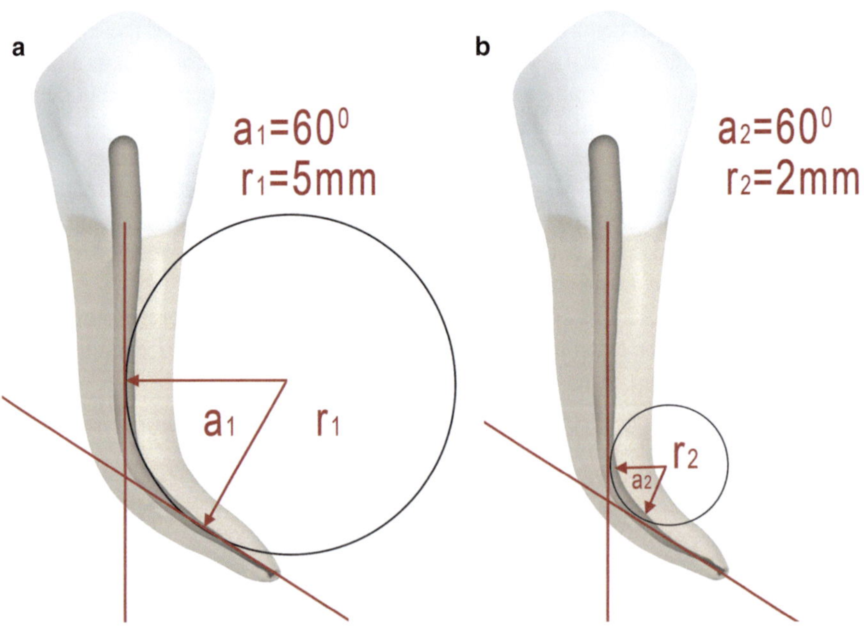

Fig. 2.4 Angle and radius of curvature measured according to Pruett et al. (1997). The two root canals have the same angle ($a_1 = a_2 = 60°$) but different radii of curvature ($r_1 = 5$ mm, $r_2 = 2$ mm)

flexural fatigue is concentrated (point of maximum flexure) is larger in the former two cases. This is consistent with the authors' anecdotal observation that NiTi instruments seem to fracture more easily when the tip binds in an acutely curved root canal compared to a straight one. Therefore, it is widely recommended that instruments should not be held at a static position inside a curved root canal but should rather be moved continuously in an axial direction in order to avoid concentrating the flexural fatigue on a specific part of the instrument (Gambarra-Soares et al. 2013). Furthermore, instruments should be discarded after a single use in very complex, calcified, or sharply curved canals.

2.4 Instrument-Related Factors

Raw materials, design, and manufacturing process can have a significant impact on instrument fracture (Alapati et al. 2005; McSpadden 2007). A noteworthy example was described several decades ago when a large number of alarmed dentists complained about fracturing of SS reamers of a certain size manufactured by a single company. These incidents were attributed to manufacturing errors (Lilley and Smith 1966) that were subsequently corrected.

Early studies have provided some support to the widespread notion that rotary NiTi instruments seem to fracture more often than hand SS instruments during clinical use (Iqbal et al. 2006). Arguably, manufacturing of NiTi instruments is much more complicated compared to that of SS instruments (Thompson 2000), and manufacturers continuously explore metallurgical modifications to the NiTi alloy, new instrument designs and additional treatments in an ongoing effort to improve the material properties, minimize inherent defects, and increase the instrument resistance to permanent distortion or fracture; still, details about proprietary manufacturing methods are rarely revealed.

Owing to the shape memory of the NiTi alloy, most such instruments are milled rather than twisted (Shen et al. 2013a), a process that allows creation of complex shapes through computer-aided design and manufacturing (CAD-CAM) technology (Thompson 2000) but that can also result in surface imperfections such as milling grooves, cracks, pits, and regions of metal rollover (Fig. 2.5) (Marsicovetere et al. 1996; Eggert et al. 1999; Kuhn et al. 2001; Tripi et al. 2001; Martins et al. 2002; Alapati et al. 2003, 2004, 2005; Valois et al. 2005; Alexandrou et al. 2006a, b; Chianello et al. 2008). It has been hypothesized that these irregularities may render the instruments more prone to fracture (Alapati et al. 2003) because they could act as stress concentration points and enable the initiation of cracks; propagation of these cracks requires less stress and could eventually lead to failure (Sawaguchi et al. 2003; McSpadden 2007). Several methods, such as implantation of argon, boron, or nitrogen ions, thermal nitridation, plasma immersion, deep dry cryogenic treatment, and electropolishing, have been applied to reduce these surface imperfections and consequently improve the resistance of instruments to failure (Anderson et al. 2007; Cheung et al. 2007a; Condorelli et al. 2010; Praisarnti et al. 2010), but the results are inconclusive in most cases [for an extensive review, see Gutmann and Gao (2012)].

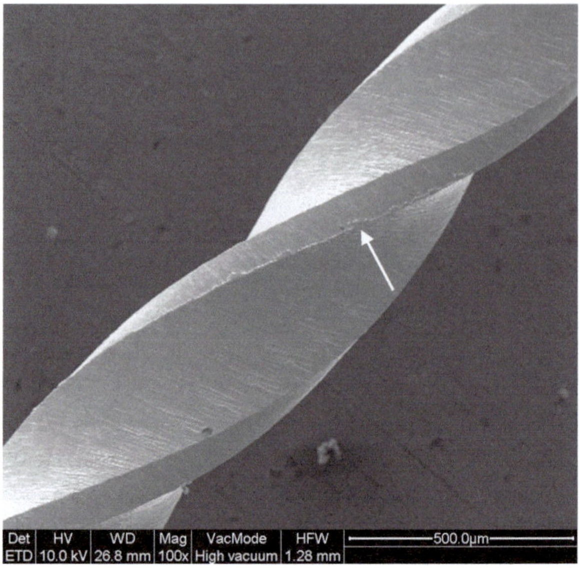

Fig. 2.5 Metal rollover at the edge of an unused Profile NiTi instrument (Dentsply Maillefer, Ballaigues, Switzerland). (Magnification ×100) (Courtesy Dr. S. Zinelis)

Rather than applying surface modifications on the milled instruments, additional thermomechanical processing of either the raw NiTi alloy or the completed instruments (Gambarini et al. 2008; Johnson et al. 2008; Larsen et al. 2009; Gao et al. 2012; Shen et al. 2013a, b; Zhao et al. 2013, 2016; Plotino et al. 2014; Capar et al. 2015) seems to be more effective and appears to increase the flexibility of the files and their fatigue resistance (Zinelis et al. 2007; Plotino et al. 2014, 2017; Kaval et al. 2016). However, it should be noted that, in general, more flexible NiTi files are also considered less resistant to torsional loading (Peters and Paque 2010; Shen et al. 2013a).

Some issues may also arise from the quality of the raw material (NiTi alloy). Oxide particles may be incorporated into the alloy during production, and later, during stress application, they could serve as nucleating sites for micro-voids that may be related to the failure process (Alapati et al. 2005). The relative concentration of these particles may indicate the metallurgical quality of the alloy (Alapati et al. 2005).

The cross-sectional area of an instrument could also affect instrument fracture (McSpadden 2007). This area is determined by a number of other parameters, including the size and taper of the instrument and its specific design (Schäfer et al. 2003; Parashos et al. 2004). Increasing the cross-sectional area by either increasing the size or the taper will increase the resistance to torsional failure (Yared et al. 2003, Guilford et al. 2005, Ullmann and Peters 2005), but it will concurrently decrease the resistance to cyclic fatigue (Haikel et al. 1999, Gambarini 2001c, Hübscher et al. 2003, Ullmann and Peters 2005, Plotino et al. 2006, Kitchens et al. 2007, Peters and Paque 2010), although indications to the contrary have also been reported (Hilfer et al. 2011). In the absence of definite evidence about the primary cause of instrument fracture in vivo (torsional overload, flexural fatigue, or a combination of both), it is noteworthy that smaller files seem to fracture more frequently during clinical use (Inan and Gonulol 2009).

The instrument design can further reduce the cross-sectional area of an instrument by increasing the number or depth of the flutes (Schäfer and Tepel 2001,

McSpadden 2007); deeper flutes seem to facilitate stress concentration (Xu et al. 2006), but the shank-to-flute ratio (Fig. 2.6) does not seem to be a contributing factor in the occurrence of fractures (Biz and Figueiredo 2004). Abrupt variations in the cross-sectional shape could also serve as stress concentration points and may promote crack initiation (Xu et al. 2006, McSpadden 2007). Finally, wide metal areas coming in contact with the dentinal wall (e.g., radial lands) (Fig. 2.7) increase

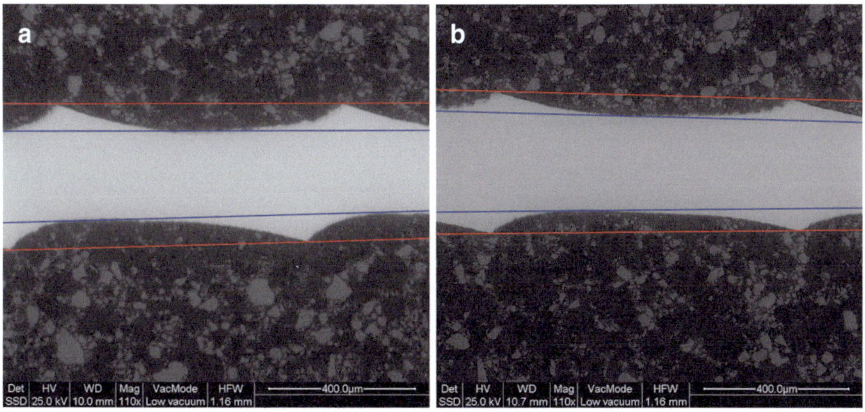

Fig. 2.6 Longitudinal sections of different files depicting the width of the shank (between the *blue lines*) in comparison with the flute depth (between the *blue* and *red line* on either side). (**a**) Smaller shank-to-flute ratio. (**b**) Larger shank-to-flute ratio (magnification ×110) (Courtesy Dr. S. Zinelis)

Fig. 2.7 Cross section of a rotary NiTi file depicting wide metal areas that come in contact with the dentinal wall during instrumentation (radial lands)

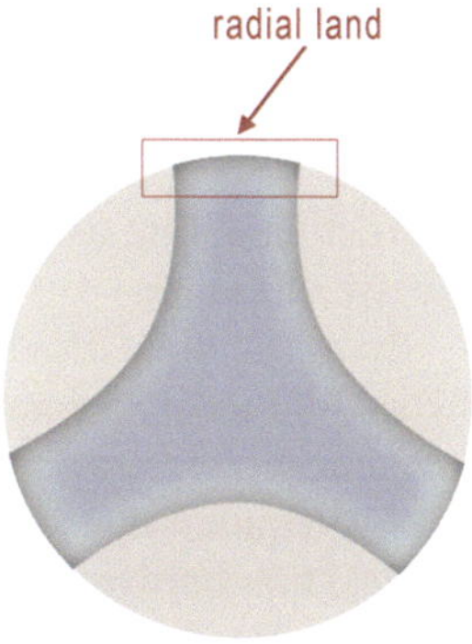

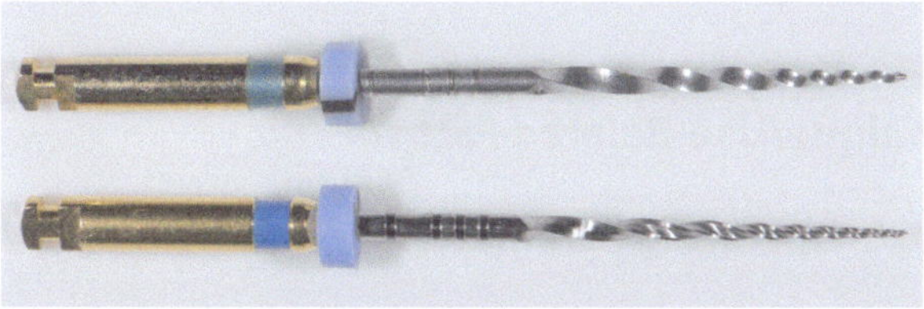

Fig. 2.8 Unused counterfeit (*top*) and original Protaper Universal F3 files (Dentsply Maillefer, Ballaigues, Switzerland) (*bottom*). Despite resemblance, differences in the design and diameter of the cutting part are noticeable (Courtesy Dr. G. Tsakiris)

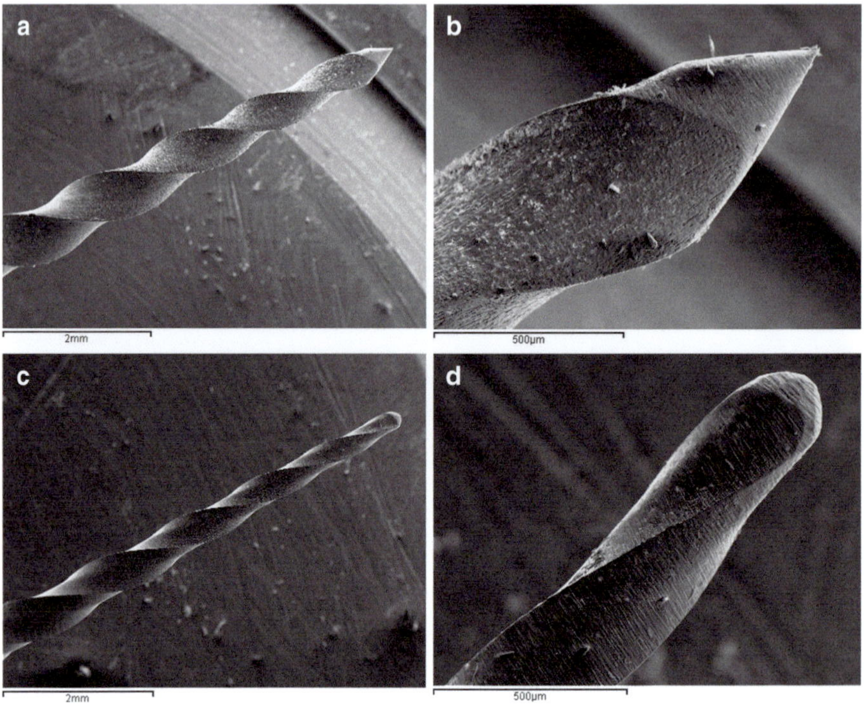

Fig. 2.9 Differences in design and surface smoothness between unused counterfeit (*top row*, **a**, **b**) and original Protaper Universal F2 files (Dentsply Maillefer, Ballaigues, Switzerland) (*bottom row*, **c**, **d**). A large amount of debris is visible on the counterfeit instrument. Its tip is larger and incorrectly manufactured as active (**b**), contrary to the original instrument's tip which is smaller and non-cutting (**d**) (magnification ×20, ×100) (Courtesy Dr. G. Tsakiris)

the friction during use (Haikel et al. 1999, Xu et al. 2006) and could also increase the risk of failure.

Even if original files are manufactured according to the highest quality standards by well-established companies, it is prudent to examine all new instruments under magnification for gross manufacturing defects prior to the first use. This precaution is also required due to the circulation of counterfeit instruments resembling the original files only in macroscopic appearance (Figs. 2.8 and 2.9). Counterfeit instruments seem to have more variations in their design and shape and also more surface imperfections than original ones (Tsakiris 2016), and their use should be avoided.

2.5 Technique/Use-Related Factors

2.5.1 Motors-Operating Parameters

Nowadays electric motors are almost unanimously recommended over air-driven motors for rotary instrumentation mainly because they can maintain a constant rotational speed and also limit the maximum torque applied to the instruments; both parameters can be easily adjusted by the operator (Fig. 2.10). Air-driven motors lack such precise controls and may be also affected by air-pressure differences. Nevertheless, the instrument fracture rate may be similar for both types of motors (Bortnick et al. 2001).

The widespread adoption of electric motors has occurred in parallel with the prevalence of the low-speed low-torque instrumentation concept (Gambarini 2001b). Manufacturers of rotary NiTi files recommend a specific rotational speed, usually in the range from 250 to 600 revolutions per minute (rpm), but its effect on instrument failure is controversial; several studies have found no influence on instrument fracture (Pruett et al. 1997, Yared et al. 2002, Zelada et al. 2002, Herold et al. 2007, Kitchens et al. 2007), while others have reported an increase in fractures with increasing speed (Li et al. 2002, Martın et al. 2003). In addition, fatigue failure seems to occur more often with motor-driven NiTi files compared with the same files used by hand, possibly because handheld files rotate at a much lower speed (Cheung et al. 2007b). Interestingly, even studies that found that cyclic fatigue is unaffected by rotational speed recognize that, since an instrument has a finite fatigue life (number of revolutions to failure), a higher rotational speed should consume this life span in a shorter time (Pruett et al. 1997), although it may also accelerate the preparation of the root canal. The rotational speed may also alter the tactile feedback provided by the instruments. Many canal irregularities can be felt through the instrument at low speed, but higher speed may result in almost total loss of any sensation, at least in vitro (Poulsen et al. 1995). In general, it is advisable to adhere to the manufacturer's recommendations regarding the rotational speed.

Torque is a less straight forward parameter than rotational speed. It is a measure of the turning force applied to the instrument in order for the instrument to overcome friction and continue rotating. Since electric motors strive to maintain a

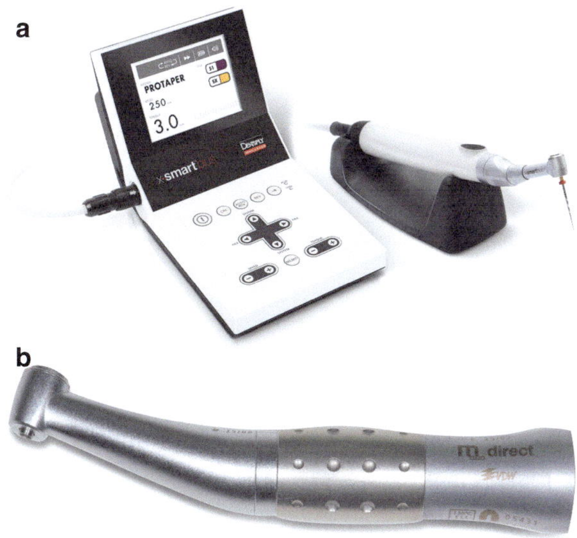

Fig. 2.10 (**a**) Electric motor featuring speed and torque control (X-Smart Plus, Courtesy Dentsply Maillefer, Ballaigues, Switzerland). (**b**) Gear-reduction contra-angle handpiece with predefined torque levels which can be attached to a conventional electric or air-driven motor (Mtwo Direct, VDW, Munich, Germany)

constant rotational speed, the torque applied to the instrument can vary continuously depending on friction, which is, in turn, determined by the contact area between the instrument blades and dentin (Fig. 2.11) and the handling of the instrument. The contact area is mainly affected by the size, taper, and cross-sectional shape of both the instrument and the root canal; a wider contact area increases friction, so higher torque is necessary in order for a larger instrument to rotate inside a narrow root canal (Kobayashi et al. 1997, Sattapan et al. 2000a). For instance, the contact area increases considerably when instruments of the same taper but of progressively larger size are used consecutively in the same root canal; every subsequent instrument after the first one is subjected to excessive friction and requires much higher driving torque to rotate (a situation called "taper lock") (Fig. 2.12) that could lead to a torsional failure. Erroneous handling of instruments such as aggressive insertion of the instrument inside the root canal also increases friction and the required torque. The maximum torque that can be applied is limited by the instrument's ability to withstand the applied stress without undergoing plastic deformation or fracture (Gambarini 2000, 2001a, b).

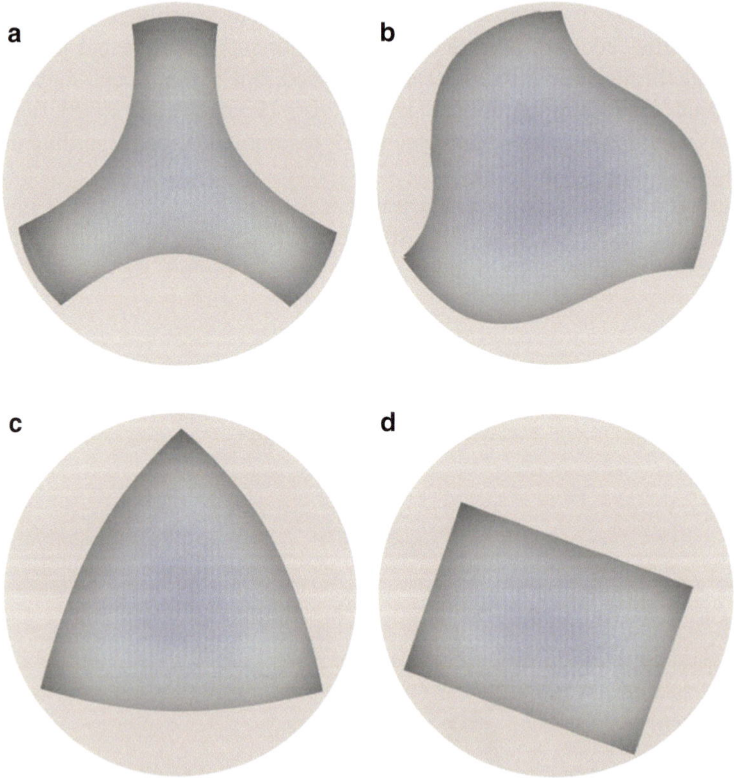

Fig. 2.11 Cross section of rotary NiTi files having a large (**a**, **b**) or small (**c**, **d**) contact area with the root canal wall, which affects friction and the torque needed to drive the instrument

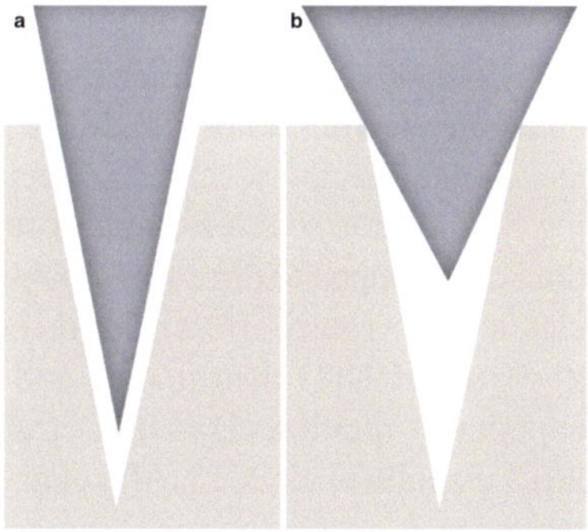

Fig. 2.12 (**a**) Using instruments of the same taper but of progressively larger size to prepare a root canal results in excessive friction due to the wider contact area with the dentinal wall ("taper lock") and requires higher driving torque that could lead to a torsional failure. (**b**) Taper lock can be prevented when sequentially used instruments have different tapers

The maximum torque at failure differs among instruments (Kobayashi et al. 1997, Gambarini 2001a, b), and it increases together with the cross-sectional area of the instrument (Yared et al. 2003; Guilford et al. 2005; Ullmann and Peters 2005); larger files can withstand higher torque without fracturing. Therefore, the applied torque should be always maintained within the narrow range that allows the instrument to rotate and cut dentin without exceeding its own plastic deformation or fracture limit (Gambarini 2000); this range is difficult to determine clinically. Manufacturers typically provide the proper maximum torque value for each instrument (Gambarini 2001a). This value is usually lower for the smaller and less tapered instruments and higher for the bigger and more tapered ones (Gambarini 2001a), which means that smaller instruments should be used taking special care not to force them aggressively inside the root canal. In addition, the recommended values refer to unused instruments and may need to be reduced for reused instruments (Gambarini 2001a).

Torque control electric motors allow the operator to determine a maximum torque value to be applied to the instrument during rotation; upon exceeding this value, the motor stops and usually reverses the rotation (auto-reverse) to disengage the instrument from dentin. Obviously, different torque limits should be used for each instrument, according to the manufacturer's recommendations (Kobayashi et al. 1997, Gambarini 2001a, b). Nevertheless, it remains unclear whether low-torque motors are able to prevent or even reduce instrument fractures. Some studies have reported benefits for both experienced (Gambarini 2001b) and inexperienced operators such as students and dentists at their initial learning phase (Yared and Kulkarni 2002), while others found no improvement compared to high-torque air-driven motors (Bortnick et al. 2001). Just like lowering the speed, low-torque instrumentation may also improve the tactile feedback, but it could also reduce the instrument's cutting efficiency to some extent and hinder its advance in the root canal; this might occasionally mislead an inexperienced operator to force the instrument which could result in locking, deformation, or even fracture (Yared et al. 2002).

Motor-driven NiTi instruments were initially used only in continuous rotation, contrary to the earlier reciprocating SS instruments that were introduced more than 60 years ago (Frank 1967, Klayman and Brilliant 1975, Hülsmann et al. 2005). The idea of reciprocation was reintroduced by Yared (2008) who proposed root canal preparation using only a very small hand instrument and a single reciprocating NiTi file. Evidently, reciprocation has evolved a lot since its reintroduction. Nowadays, elaborate electric motors allow for precise and independent setting of the clockwise and counterclockwise angles of reciprocation, and, contrary to the earlier reciprocating SS files, the rotation angle of modern NiTi files in the cutting direction is larger than in the opposite direction, enabling the so-called partial or asymmetrical reciprocation with a rotary effect (Plotino et al. 2015). This motion is believed to prolong the life span of NiTi instruments and their resistance to cyclic fatigue compared to continuous rotation (De-Deus et al. 2010, Varela-Patino et al. 2010, Gavini et al. 2012, Pedulla et al. 2013, Ahn et al. 2016), although the method used to quantify the resistance to cyclic fatigue is markedly different in continuous rotation and in reciprocation and the results may not be directly comparable. The difference between the nominal and actual rotation speed could also affect these results (Fidler 2014).

2.5.2 Instrumentation Technique

The instrumentation technique has an influence on instrument failure (Roland et al. 2002). For instance, hand-operated NiTi files used clinically in a modified balanced force movement seem to fail mainly due to torsional overload, while motor-driven files of the same type appear to fracture mostly because of cyclic fatigue (Cheung et al. 2007b). The crown-down approach has been recommended for the vast majority of rotary NiTi instruments in order to reduce friction and minimize the fracture risk (Peters 2004), even though this may not be necessary for other types of NiTi files that are advocated as "single-length" instruments and should be advanced to working length irrespective of size (Plotino et al. 2007; Ehrhardt et al. 2012). Most currently available reciprocating files are also used in a single-file single-length manner (De-Deus et al. 2013; Rodrigues et al. 2016).

Regarding the technique, light apical pressure, continuous axial movement (pecking motion), and brief use inside the root canal are almost unanimously recommended (Parashos and Messer 2006) in order to prevent torsional overload and prolong the fatigue life (Sattapan et al. 2000a; Li et al. 2002; Rodrigues et al. 2011; Gambarra-Soares et al. 2013). Moreover, the handpiece should not be tilted away from the root canal axis at the orifice in order to avoid increasing friction. In general it is advisable for inexperienced users of a particular system to adhere to the recommended instrument sequence, but files from different systems can be combined in hybrid protocols to cope with individual clinical needs; the latter requires a certain level of expertise.

Due to the non-cutting tip of most NiTi files, it is of particular importance to ensure that the root canal will allow free rotation of the tip even at its narrowest point in order to avoid locking and eventual torsional failure (Sattapan et al. 2000b; Peters 2004). This almost uniform requirement can be met by creating a continuous smooth pathway to the apical terminus of the root canal (glide path) before using the main series of rotary NiTi instruments. A glide path can be prepared by small-size hand SS instruments (Blum et al. 1999; Patino et al. 2005; Lopes et al. 2011) or by specially designed rotary NiTi instruments (Fig. 2.13) (Alves et al. 2012; Lopes

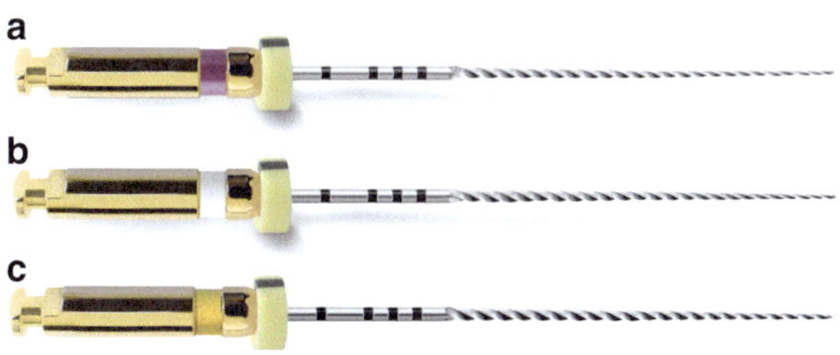

Fig. 2.13 Specially-designed rotary NiTi files for preparation of a glide path (Pathfiles, Dentsply Maillefer, Ballaigues, Switzerland) (Courtesy Dentsply Maillefer)

et al. 2012; De-Deus et al. 2016; Alovisi et al. 2017). The latter may present some advantages according to some studies (Paleker and van der Vyver 2016; Alovisi et al. 2017) but not according to others (Alves et al. 2012) and still suffer from the typical limitations of NiTi instruments. It has been claimed that reciprocating NiTi files are able to reach working length safely without a previously established glide path and without increasing the instrument failure rate during both in vitro (De-Deus et al. 2013) and clinical use (Rodrigues et al. 2016). However, operators are advised to follow the manufacturers' recommendations regarding the need for a glide path.

2.5.3 Reuse and Sterilization

Due to the increased cost of root canal instruments and especially of NiTi files, the question of whether they can be reused is always pertinent. The number of times that a file can be safely used is still a topic of ongoing debate. Manufacturers claim that the only predictable way to prevent failure is by discarding rotary instruments on a regular basis; in some cases, special features are embedded in the NiTi instrument handle to prevent their reuse after sterilization and enforce a single-use policy. However, these recommendations and policies may be influenced to some extent by the commercial interest involved.

Grossman (1981) recommended using small hand SS instruments no more than twice. More recently, single use of all rotary NiTi instruments has been suggested as a precaution (Pruett et al. 1997; Arens et al. 2003), while others advocate this strict rule only concerning the smaller files (Haapasalo and Shen 2013), possibly because any defects may be more difficult to detect. A survey found that discarding after a certain number of uses is a common practice among both general dentists and endodontists (Madarati et al. 2008), and the type of alloy, the design and size of the instrument, and the case difficulty are parameters frequently taken into account in order to decide when to discard an instrument (Cheung et al. 2005).

The evidence behind these recommendations is conflicting. Prolonged clinical use of NiTi rotary files seems to reduce their resistance to cyclic fatigue during subsequent in vitro tests (Gambarini 2001b, c; Bahia and Buono 2005; Plotino et al. 2006), so larger files should be discarded earlier than smaller ones when preparing curved root canals because their resistance to cyclic fatigue is lower (Bahia and

Buono 2005). However, instrument failure is a complex and multifactorial problem, and it seems impossible to predict when an instrument will fracture during clinical use based on simplified in vitro tests. The number of uses before failure varies widely (Parashos et al. 2004; Kosti et al. 2011), and fracture can occur even during the first use in the hands of experienced clinicians (Arens et al. 2003). In addition, instruments may fracture following clinical use for fewer times than identical instruments that present no defects or fracture. Therefore, it appears that other variables such as the operator proficiency and the root canal anatomy may be far more significant determinants of the instrument fracture rate (Parashos et al. 2004).

This apparent discrepancy could be explained by the fact that NiTi instrument failure during clinical use seems to occur because of a single overloading event (e.g., inadvertent locking in the root canal) rather than a fatigue accumulation process (Spanaki-Voreadi et al. 2006); in vitro failures during preparation of root canals seem to occur by a similar mechanism (Kosti et al. 2011). Interestingly, even authors concluding that files should not be reused because their resistance to cyclic fatigue is reduced actually managed to prepare up to ten clinical cases using the same set of instruments without any intracanal fracture (Gambarini 2001c). Furthermore, contrary to earlier views about the effect of repetitive loading on the NiTi instrument fatigue life (Sattapan et al. 2000b), more recent studies found that mild torsional preloading (not causing permanent deformation) can actually improve both the torsional strength (Oh et al. 2017) and the resistance to cyclic fatigue during subsequent loading (Cheung et al. 2013); this effect could reduce the fracture risk during clinical use, but the result may differ among various types of files (Ha et al. 2015). Therefore, taking all evidence into account, multiple uses of NiTi instruments are clinically acceptable from a mechanical point of view (Parashos et al. 2004), but it is impossible to recommend a safe number of uses. These findings are at variance to the failure of SS instruments that seems to occur mostly because of fatigue accumulation, during both in vitro (Kosti et al. 2004) and clinical use (Zinelis and Margelos 2002), and justifies frequent discarding.

All endodontic instruments should be carefully examined under magnification prior to reuse for signs of wear. Regarding SS instruments, any shiny marks, uneven spacing between the flutes, areas of unwinding, sharp bending, or any other kind of permanent distortion or corrosion (Fig. 2.14) are indications of excessive fatigue and should serve as warnings of impending fracture; any such instruments should be discarded.

Similar deformations of NiTi instruments should also be regarded as a signal to discard them (Fig. 2.15). However, their original shape can be more complex or asymmetric and may include flutes with reverse direction combined with straight areas, varying helical angles or pitch, and off-center cross section (Peters et al. 2016); these features should not be confused with indications of impending fracture. In addition, instruments made of the so-called "controlled memory" alloy may normally undergo some unwinding during use, and this should only be considered an indication to discard the instrument if rewinding in the opposite direction appears or the file does not regain its original shape upon heat treatment (Fig. 2.16) (Coltene Endo 2014). Therefore, the clinician must bear in mind the original shape of the

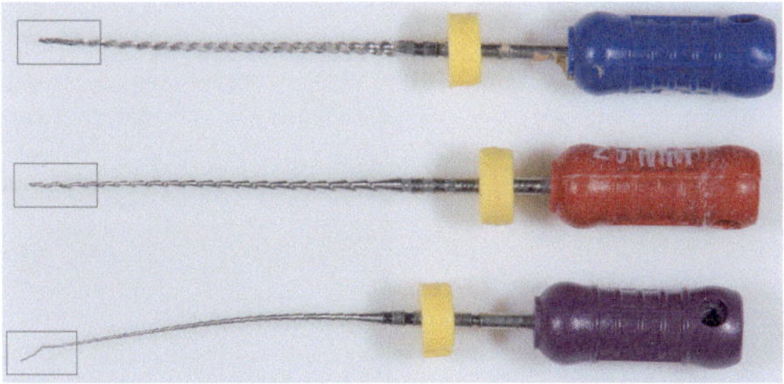

Fig. 2.14 Hand SS instruments with permanent distortion, sharp bend, or damage of the cutting part that needs to be discarded

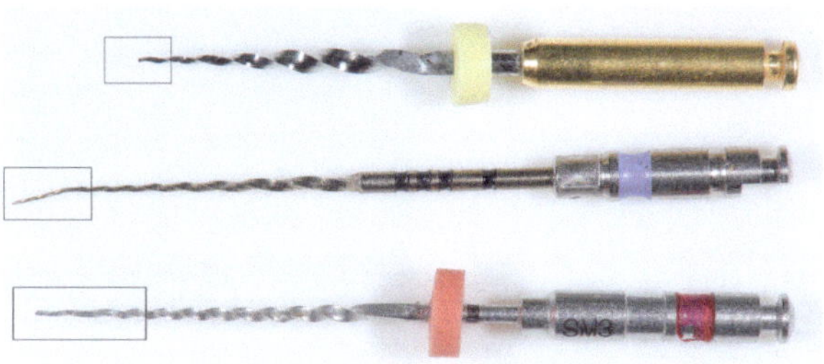

Fig. 2.15 Defects of rotary NiTi instruments signaling impending fracture; these instruments need to be discarded

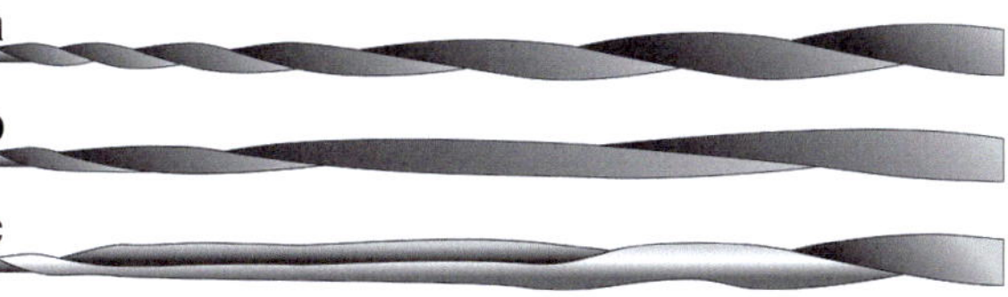

Fig. 2.16 Controlled-memory rotary NiTi files (Hyflex CM, Coltene, Altstätten, Switzerland) before (**a**) and after use (**b**, **c**). Despite unwinding (**b**), such instruments don't need to be discarded and can regain their original shape upon heat treatment. On the contrary, instruments showing rewinding in the opposite direction (**c**) should be discarded (Courtesy COLTENE Group)

instrument and any specific guidelines by the manufacturer in order to identify correctly which instruments should be discarded. Still, NiTi instruments may commonly fracture even without any visible deformation (Sattapan et al. 2000b; Martın et al. 2003; Peng et al. 2005; Shen et al. 2006, 2009).

Examination under high magnification has also revealed dentin debris embedded into machining grooves or surface cracks of used instruments (Fig. 2.17) (Zinelis and Margelos 2002; Alapati et al. 2004), and it has been hypothesized that this debris may accelerate crack propagation (Alapati et al. 2004). However, the presence of debris could also be a random observation without any involvement in the fracture process since there is no proven cause-effect relationship (Parashos and Messer 2006).

Instruments need to be cleaned and sterilized before their first use (unless they are delivered by the manufacturer in sealed presterilized packages) and also before every reuse; the effect of this process on instrument failure is still controversial.

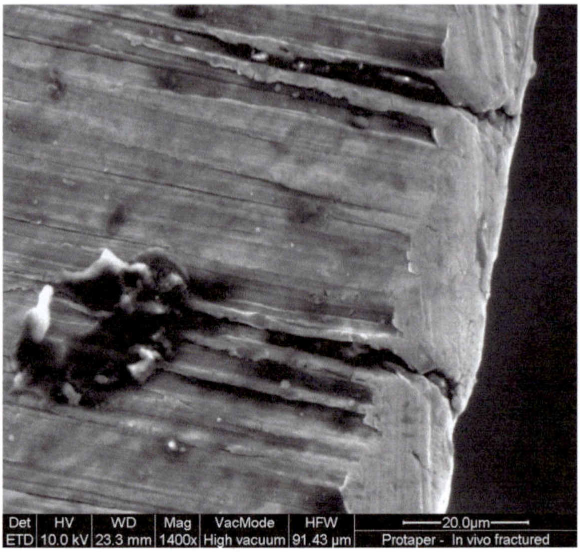

Fig. 2.17 Dentin debris embedded into surface cracks of a rotary NiTi file (magnification ×1400) (Courtesy Dr. S. Zinelis)

Regarding SS instruments, a small reduction in the torsional strength has been reported after 10 cycles of immersion in 5% sodium hypochlorite followed by autoclave sterilization, especially for larger files (Mitchell et al. 1983); a similar small effect was found after 10–40 autoclave sterilization cycles without immersion in sodium hypochlorite (Hilt et al. 2000), but in both cases the difference may not be clinically significant. Other studies did not find any such difference (Iverson et al. 1985).

Multiple sterilization cycles may induce surface alterations on NiTi files, including corrosion and defects (Valois et al. 2008; Spagnuolo et al. 2012), and may also increase their surface roughness (Alexandrou et al. 2006a, b) possibly because of changes in the passive titanium oxide layer that covers the surfaces (Rapisarda et al. 1999, Thierry et al. 2000). However, these surface alterations have not been clearly linked to instrument fracture, so they may not be clinically relevant (Eggert et al. 1999).

Both dry heat and autoclave sterilization don't seem to have a negative effect on the cyclic fatigue resistance of several types of NiTi files (Yared et al. 1999, 2000; Hilfer et al. 2011; Plotino et al. 2012; Elbatal et al. 2016; Zhao et al. 2016), but this is not true for all types (Plotino et al. 2006; Hilfer et al. 2011; Elbatal et al. 2016). Inconsistent results have been also published regarding the torsional strength, with some files showing no effect (Svec and Powers 1999; Casper et al. 2011; King et al. 2012) and others showing a decrease (Canalda-Sahli et al. 1998; King et al. 2012).

Although its clinical relevance has been questioned (Mize et al. 1998), a possible beneficial effect of sterilization on instruments has also been reported; both resistance to cyclic fatigue and torsional strength of certain types of files were found to increase following sterilization (Silvaggio and Hicks 1997; Craveiro de Melo et al. 2002; Viana et al. 2006; Plotino et al. 2012; Zhao et al. 2016), especially after repeated cycles (Casper et al. 2011), so dry heat or autoclave sterilization could act as a form of heat treatment.

One additional parameter that should be considered before deciding to reuse root canal instruments is the cleaning and sterilization efficacy of the available methods (Sonntag and Peters 2007; Walker et al. 2007; Hartwell et al. 2011), but this parameter is beyond the scope of the present chapter.

2.5.4 Irrigants

Instruments may come in contact with irrigants in two different occasions, namely, inside the root canal during use and, afterward, during reprocessing. Although the same solutions may be used for both purposes, the exposure conditions can be different. First of all, instrumentation should never be performed in a dry root canal; excessive friction could lead to instrument failure. Manufacturers still recommend the use of gel-based lubricants in conjunction with NiTi files in order to reduce the stress applied to the instrument (Anderson et al. 2006); these gels are advised to be repeatedly applied either directly on the cutting part of the instrument or in the pulp chamber, and in addition to lubrication, they could also soften root dentin to facilitate instrumentation (Zehnder 2006). It is noteworthy that several of these gel-based lubricants are also produced by the instrument manufacturers advocating their routine use.

Experimental evidence does not support the use of these gels. They fail to reduce the friction between the instrument and the root canal wall, and in some cases friction may even be increased compared to a dry root canal (Peters et al. 2005; Boessler et al. 2007). Aqueous solutions or distilled water are much more effective for this purpose (Peters et al. 2005; Boessler et al. 2007), and they may also flush away dentin debris from the cutting flutes of the instruments (Zehnder 2006), a function unlikely to be performed by gels.

In addition, most of the gel-type lubricants contain various chelators, and similarly to aqueous chelator solutions, they can interact strongly with sodium hypochlorite and consume its free available chlorine very rapidly (Grawehr et al. 2003; Zehnder et al. 2005). Since chelator solutions are only marginally better than water as lubricants (Peters et al. 2005; Boessler et al. 2007), the effect may occur primarily due to mechanical lubrication and not due to chemical softening of dentin, so any liquid should suffice (Peters et al. 2005; Boessler et al. 2007). Thus, during instrumentation root canals and the pulp chamber should be flooded with irrigant and preferably with sodium hypochlorite, which can serve multiple purposes like killing bacteria and dissolving tissue remnants in addition to providing lubrication (Zehnder 2006).

The possible corrosive effect of sodium hypochlorite and of other irrigants on root canal instruments is an additional concern (Sonntag and Peters 2007). During instrumentation only the cutting part of the file is likely to contact the irrigant. Partial immersion (only the cutting part) of either SS or NiTi files in 5% sodium hypochlorite or 17% EDTA solution in vitro even for extended periods of time

(1–24 h) did not result in any detectable corrosion (Darabara et al. 2004; de Castro Martins et al. 2006) and did not reduce the fatigue resistance of the files (Smith 2007). Similar findings were reported after partial immersion in preheated (50 °C) 5% sodium hypochlorite for 5 min (Berutti et al. 2006) or repeated 5-min immersion in a 2.5% solution at room temperature (Bulem et al. 2013). In addition no signs of surface corrosion were found on hand SS files used clinically in combination with 2.5% sodium hypochlorite irrigation (Zinelis and Margelos 2002).

Total immersion of the instruments in sodium hypochlorite, which may occur during post-use cleaning prior to sterilization, seems to have a more pronounced effect, but there is a considerable discrepancy among studies. Corrosion begins to appear after immersion of NiTi instruments in 5% NaOCl either at room temperature or preheated (50 °C) for 5 min (Berutti et al. 2006; Smith 2007) or 30 min (Busslinger et al. 1998) and may increase with immersion time (Peters et al. 2007). Corrosion seems to be accompanied by a reduction in the resistance to cyclic fatigue, at least for some types of NiTi files (Berutti et al. 2006; Peters et al. 2007; Smith 2007). A lower concentration (1%) solution doesn't seem to corrode NiTi files or reduce their torsional strength or cyclic fatigue resistance after a cumulative exposure of 2.5 h, but overnight immersion (18 h) produces clear signs of corrosion (Fig. 2.18), although there are differences between various types of files (O'Hoy et al. 2003). Finally, very brief immersion in a 5% sodium hypochlorite solution at body temperature (37 °C) during a cyclic fatigue test does not seem to affect the results (Elnaghy and Elsaka 2017).

The main difference between partial and total immersion in sodium hypochlorite is whether the instrument shank is also immersed or not (O'Hoy et al. 2003; Berutti et al. 2006; Novoa et al. 2007). The shank of some types of instruments is made of a different metal than the cutting part (Peters et al. 2007; Bonaccorso et al. 2008a), and the concurrent presence of two metals in a sodium hypochlorite solution can affect the ion release and generate galvanic reactions that may accelerate the corrosion process (Berutti et al. 2006; Novoa et al. 2007; Smith 2007). This parameter could partially explain the wide range of results reported in corrosion studies.

Parameters related to the sodium hypochlorite solution may also modify its effect on instruments. Lower-pH solutions seem to be less aggressive in terms of corrosion (Novoa et al. 2007), and preheated solutions (60 °C) seem to decrease the fatigue resistance even though only minor corrosion may be found on the instruments (Peters et al. 2007). The clinical relevance of preheated solutions used as irrigants is very limited (de Hemptinne et al. 2015), but they may still be employed for post-use

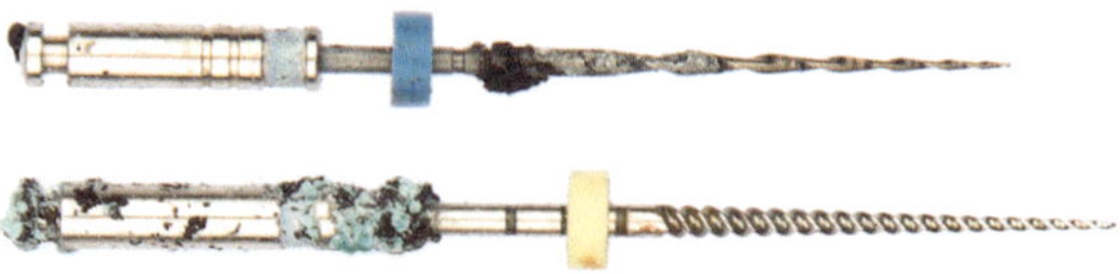

Fig. 2.18 Corrosion of rotary NiTi files immersed overnight in 3% NaOCl

disinfection of the instruments. Finally, the corrosive effect of Milton's solution (1% NaOCl, 19% NaCl) may be more pronounced than that of a normal sodium hypochlorite solution at the same concentration (O'Hoy et al. 2003).

Efforts to improve the corrosion resistance of NiTi files have been undertaken by the manufacturers, but the results are inconclusive. Surface treatment by electropolishing or physical vapor deposition may reduce corrosion during contact with normal saline (Bonaccorso et al. 2008b) but not in the presence of sodium hypochlorite (Peters et al. 2007). Nevertheless, it should be kept in mind that variations may exist in the extent of corrosion between different brands and also between individual files of the same brand (O'Hoy et al. 2003), and that, despite impressive in vitro results, there are no confirmed reports of file fracture during clinical use that can be attributed to corrosion alone.

2.6 Concluding Remarks

Contradictory findings have been reported regarding several of the parameters analyzed in this chapter. Apart from inevitable experimental errors, these discrepancies may be largely attributed to the wide variation in the testing protocols and conditions among studies; different types of instruments, evaluation of used or unused instruments, the precise conditions during use, contact with sodium hypochlorite, different cleaning and sterilization methods, varying cyclic fatigue tests, and corrosion detection methods are only a few of the parameters that differ. The possibility of interactions between different parameters cannot be excluded either. Thus, efforts should be undertaken to standardize the testing methods and conditions in order to facilitate comparisons among future studies. It has been suggested that standard testing of all types of instruments should be conducted prior to their introduction into the market by the manufacturers and should accompany the instrument as essential documentation (Hülsmann 2013).

Information about the behavior of the instruments during clinical use is limited, and it is possible that in vitro models may not mimic in vivo conditions closely. For instance, instruments are normally used inside root canals filled with an irrigant (usually sodium hypochlorite) very close to body temperature (~35 °C) (de Hemptinne et al. 2015), but several in vitro studies have ignored this fact and have conducted the tests at room temperature (20 °C). Recently it was shown that temperature is an important confounder, and an increase from 20 to 35 °C may decrease the fatigue resistance considerably (up to 85%) at least for some types of instruments (de Vasconcelos et al. 2016; Elnaghy and Elsaka 2017; Plotino et al. 2017). Thus, choosing clinically realistic conditions during in vitro testing is of paramount importance in order to obtain clinically relevant information.

Despite in vitro evidence that some of the abovementioned parameters may affect the fracture resistance of root canal instruments, it is worth noticing that results obtained with one type of instrument cannot be directly extrapolated to other types due to considerable differences in the material, the design, and the mode of use. Several instruments are currently available, and new “improved” versions are constantly being introduced, so detailed evaluation of all possible combinations is not feasible. Simple comparisons of randomly selected, popular, or new instruments to each other are manufacturer-oriented and make little scientific sense because of the large number of confounders. Instead, it would be more reasonable for future studies to isolate and study the effect of specific material-, design-, or technique-related parameters that may be significant across brands.

References

Ahn SY, Kim HC, Kim E. Kinematic effects of nickel-titanium instruments with reciprocating or continuous rotation motion: a systematic review of in vitro studies. J Endod. 2016;42(7):1009–17.

Alapati SB, Brantley WA, Svec TA, Powers JM, Mitchell JC. Scanning electron microscope observations of new and used nickel-titanium rotary files. J Endod. 2003;29(10):667–9.

Alapati SB, Brantley WA, Svec TA, Powers JM, Nusstein JM, Daehn GS. Proposed role of embedded dentin chips for the clinical failure of nickel titanium rotary instruments. J Endod. 2004;30(5):339–41.

Alapati SB, Brantley WA, Svec TA, Powers JM, Nusstein JM, Daehn GS. SEM observations of nickel-titanium rotary endodontic instruments that fractured during clinical use. J Endod. 2005;31(1):40–3.

Alexandrou G, Chrissafis K, Vasiliadis L, Pavlidou E, Polychroniadis EK. SEM observations and differential scanning calorimetric studies of new and sterilized nickel-titanium rotary endodontic instruments. J Endod. 2006a;32(7):675–9.

Alexandrou G, Chrissafis K, Vasiliadis L, Pavlidou E, Polychroniadis EK. Effect of heat sterilization on surface characteristics and microstructure of Mani NRT rotary nickel-titanium instruments. Int Endod J. 2006b;39(10):770–8.

Alovisi M, Cemenasco A, Mancini L, Paolino D, Scotti N, Bianchi CC, Pasqualini D. Micro-CT evaluation of several glide path techniques and ProTaper Next shaping outcomes in maxillary first molar curved canals. Int Endod J. 2017;50(4):387–97.

Alves O, Bueno CE, Cunha RS, Pinheiro SL, Fontana CE, de Martin AS. Comparison among manual instruments and PathFile and Mtwo rotary instruments to create a glide path in the root canal preparation of curved canals. J Endod. 2012;38(1):117–20.

Anderson DN, Joyce AP, Roberts S, Runner R. A comparative photoelastic stress analysis of internal root stresses between RC Prep and saline when applied to the Profile/GT rotary instrumentation system. J Endod. 2006;32(3):222–4.

Anderson ME, John WH, Price JWH, Parashos P. Fracture resistance of electropolished rotary nickel–titanium endodontic instruments. J Endod. 2007;33(10):1212–6..

Arens FC, Hoen MM, Steiman HR, Dietz GC Jr. Evaluation of single-use rotary nickel-titanium instruments. J Endod. 2003;29(10):664–6.

Bahia MG, Buono VT. Decrease in the fatigue resistance of nickel-titanium rotary instruments after clinical use in curved root canals. Oral Surg Oral Med Oral Path Oral Radiol Endod. 2005;100(2):249–55..

Berutti E, Angelini E, Rigolone M, Migliaretti G, Pasqualini D. Influence of sodium hypochlorite on fracture properties and corrosion of ProTaper rotary instruments. Int Endod J. 2006;39(9):693–9..

Biz MT, Figueiredo JA. Morphometric analysis of shank-to-flute ratio in rotary nickel titanium files. Int Endod J. 2004;37(6):353–8.

Blum JY, Cohen A, Machtou P, Micallef JP. Analysis of forces developed during mechanical preparation of extracted teeth using Profile NiTi rotary instruments. Int Endod J. 1999;32(1):24–31.
Boessler C, Peters OA, Zehnder M. Impact of lubricant parameters on rotary instrument torque and force. J Endod. 2007;33(3):280–3.
Bonaccorso A, Schäfer E, Condorelli GG, Cantatore G, Tripi TR. Chemical analysis of nickel-titanium rotary instruments with and without electropolishing after cleaning procedures with sodium hypochlorite. J Endod. 2008a;34(11):1391–5.
Bonaccorso A, Tripi TR, Rondelli G, Condorelli GG, Cantatore G, Schäfer E. Pitting corrosion resistance of nickel-titanium rotary instruments with different surface treatments in seventeen percent ethylenediaminetetraacetic acid and sodium chloride solutions. J Endod. 2008b;34(2):208–11.
Booth JR, Scheetz JP, Lemons JE, Eleazer PD. A comparison of torque required to fracture three different nickel-titanium rotary instruments around curves of the same angle but of different radius when bound at the tip. J Endod. 2003;29(1):55–7.
Bortnick KL, Steiman HR, Ruskin A. Comparison of nickel-titanium file distortion using electric and air-driven handpieces. J Endod. 2001;27(1):57–9.
Briseno B, Kremers L, Hamm G, Nitsch C. Comparison by means of a computer supported device of the enlarging characteristics of two different instruments. J Endod. 1993;19(6):281–7.
Bulem ÜK, Kececi AD, Guldas HE. Experimental evaluation of cyclic fatigue resistance of four different nickel-titanium instruments after immersion in sodium hypochlorite and/or sterilization. J Appl Oral Sci. 2013;21(6):505–10.
Busslinger A, Sener B, Barbakow F. Effects of sodium hypochlorite on nickel-titanium Lightspeed instruments. Int Endod J. 1998;31(4):290–4.
Canalda-Sahli C, Brau-Aguadé E, Sentis-Vilalta J. The effect of sterilization on bending and tortional properties of K-files manufactured with different metallic alloys. Int Endod J. 1998;31(1):48–52.
Capar ID, Kaval ME, Ertas H, Sen BH. Comparison of the cyclic fatigue resistance of 5 different rotary pathfinding instruments made of conventional nickel-titanium wire, M-wire, and controlled memory wire. J Endod. 2015;41(4):535–8.
Casper RB, Roberts HW, Roberts MD, Himel VT, Bergeron BE. Comparison of autoclaving effects on torsional deformation and fracture resistance of three innovative endodontic file systems. J Endod. 2011;37(11):1572–5.
Cheung GS, Peng B, Bian Z, Shen Y, Darvell BW. Defects in ProTaper S1 instruments after clinical use: fractographic examination. Int Endod J. 2005;38(11):802–9.
Cheung GS, Peng B, Bian Z, Shen Y, Darvell BW. Int Endod J. 2005;38(11):802–9.
Cheung GS, Shen Y, Darvell BW. Does electropolishing improve the low–cycle fatigue behavior of nickel- titanium rotary instrument in hypochlorite? J Endod. 2007a;33(10):1217–21.
Cheung GS, Bian Z, Shen Y, Peng B, Darvell BW. Comparison of defects in ProTaper hand-operated and engine-driven instruments after clinical use. Int Endod J. 2007b;40(3):169–78.
Cheung GS, Oh SH, Ha JH, Kim SK, Park SH, Kim HC. Effect of torsional loading of nickel-titanium instruments on cyclic fatigue resistance. J Endod. 2013;39(12):1593–7.
Chianello G, Specian VL, Hardt LCF, Raldi DP, Lage-Marques JL, Habitante SM. Surface finishing of unused rotary endodontic instruments: a SEM study. Braz Dent J. 2008;19(2):109–13.
Coltene Endo. HyFlex® CM – Controlled memory NiTi files. File sequence step by step card. 2014. Available at: http://www.hyflex.info/fileadmin/dam/DATEN/HyFlex-CM/downloads/allgemein/30001993_03-14_StepByStep_HyflexCM_DB.pdf Accessed on 27 Dec 2016.
Condorelli GG, Bonaccorso A, Smecca E, Schäfer E, Cantatore G, Tripi TR. Improvement of the fatigue resistance of NiTi endodontic files by surface and bulk modifications. Int Endod J. 2010;43(10):866–73.
Craveiro de Melo MC, Bahia MGA, Buono VTL. Fatique resistance of engine driven rotary nickel-titanium endodontic instruments. J Endod. 2002;28(11):765–9.
Darabara M, Bourithis L, Zinelis S, Papadimitriou GD. Susceptibility to localized corrosion of stainless steel and NiTi endodontic instruments in irrigating solutions. Int Endod J. 2004;37(10):705–10.

de Castro Martins R, Bahia MG, Buono VT, Horizonte B. The effect of sodium hypochlorite on the surface characteristics and fatigue resistance of ProFile nickel-titanium instruments. Oral Surg Oral Med Oral Pathol Oral Radiol Endod. 2006;102(4):e99–105.

de Hemptinne F, Slaus G, Vandendael M, Jacquet W, De Moor RJ, Bottenberg P. In vivo intracanal temperature evolution during endodontic treatment after the injection of room temperature or preheated sodium hypochlorite. J Endod. 2015;41(7):1112–5.

de Vasconcelos RA, Murphy S, Carvalho CA, Govindjee RG, Govindjee S, Peters OA. Evidence for reduced fatigue resistance of contemporary rotary instruments exposed to body temperature. J Endod. 2016;42(5):782–7.

De-Deus G, Moreira EJ, Lopes HP, Elias CN. Extended cyclic fatigue life of F2 ProTaper instruments used in reciprocating movement. Int Endod J. 2010;43(2):1063–8.

De-Deus G, Arruda TEP, Souza EM, Neves A, Magalhaes K, Thuanne E, Fidel RAS. The ability of the Reciproc R25 instrument to reach the full root canal working length without a glide path. Int Endod J. 2013;46(10):993–8.

De-Deus G, Belladonna FG, Souza EM, Alves Vde O, Silva EJ, Rodrigues E, Versiani MA, Bueno CE. Scouting ability of 4 pathfinding instruments in moderately curved molar canals. J Endod. 2016;42(10):1540–4.

Di Fiore PM, Genov KA, Komaroff E, Li Y, Lin L. Nickel-titanium rotary instrument fracture: a clinical practice assessment. Int Endod J. 2006;39(9):700–8.

Eaton JA, Clement DJ, Lloyd A, Marchesan MA. Micro-computed tomographic evaluation of the influence of root canal system landmarks on access outline forms and canal curvatures in mandibular molars. J Endod. 2015;41(11):1888–91.

Eggert C, Peters O, Barbakow F. Wear of nickel-titanium Lightspeed instruments evaluated by scanning electron microscopy. J Endod. 1999;25(7):494–7.

Ehrhardt IC, Zuolo ML, Cunha RS, De Martin AS, Kherlakian D, Carvalho MC, Bueno CE. Assessment of the separation incidence of Mtwo files used with preflaring: prospective clinical study. J Endod. 2012;38(8):1078–81.

Elbatal LM, El Batouty KM, Obeid MM. Effect of repeated autoclaving on cyclic fatigue of three nickel-titanium rotary instruments. ENDO (Lond Engl). 2016;10(1):15–22.

Elnaghy AM, Elsaka SE. Effect of sodium hypochlorite and saline on cyclic fatigue resistance of WaveOne Gold and Reciproc reciprocating instruments. Int Endod J. 2017; In press: 1–8. (doi: 10.1111/iej.12712).

Fidler A. Kinematics of 2 reciprocating endodontic motors: the difference between actual and set values. J Endod. 2014;40(7):990–4.

Frank AL. An evaluation of the Giromatic endodontic handpiece. Oral Surg Oral Med Oral Path. 1967;24(3):419–21.

Gambarini G. Rationale for the use of low-torque endodontic motors in root canal instrumentation. Endod Dent Traumatol. 2000;16(3):95–100.

Gambarini G. Advantages and disadvantages of new torque-controlled endodontic motors and low-torque NiTi rotary instrumentation. Aust Endod J. 2001a;27(3):99–104.

Gambarini G. Cyclic fatigue of nickel-titanium rotary instruments after clinical use with low- and high-torque endodontic motors. J Endod. 2001b;27(12):772–4.

Gambarini G. Cyclic fatigue of ProFile rotary instruments after prolonged clinical use. Int Endod J. 2001c;34(5):386–9.

Gambarini G, Grande NM, Plotino G, Somma F, Garala M, DeLuca M, Teslarelli L. Fatigue resistance of engine-driven rotary Nickel-Titanium instruments produced by new manufacturing methods. J Endod. 2008;34(8):1003–5.

Gambarra-Soares T, Lopes HP, Machado Oliveira JC, Chaves Souza L, Leal Vieira VT, Elias CN. Dynamic or static cyclic fatigue tests: which best determines the lifespan of endodontic files? ENDO (Lond Engl). 2013;7(2):101–4.

Gao Y, Gutmann JL, Wilkinson K, Maxwell R, Ammon D. Evaluation of the impact of raw materials on the fatigue and mechanical properties of ProFile Vortex rotary instruments. J Endod. 2012;38(3):398–401.

Gambarini G, Grande NM, Plotino G, Somma F, Garala M, De Luca M, Testarelli L. Fatigue resistance of engine-driven rotary nickel-titanium instruments produced by new manufacturing methods. J Endod. 2008;34(8):1003–5.
Gluskin AH, Peters CI, Peters OA. Minimally invasive endodontics: challenging prevailing paradigms. Br Dent J. 2014;216(6):347–53.
Grawehr M, Sener B, Waltimo T, Zehnder M. Interactions of ethylenediaminetetraacetic acid with sodium hypochlorite in aqueous solutions. Int Endod J. 2003;36(6):411–7.
Grossman LI. Endodontic practice. 10th ed. Philadelphia: Lea & Febiger; 1981. p. 200–36.
Guilford WL, Lemons JE, Eleazer PD. A comparison of torque required to fracture rotary files with tips bound in simulated curved canal. J Endod. 2005;31(6):468–70.
Gutmann JL, Gao Y. Alteration in the inherent metallic and surface properties of nickel-titanium root canal instruments to enhance performance, durability and safety: a focused review. Int Endod J. 2012;45(2):113–28.
Ha JH, Kim SK, Cheung GS, Jeong SH, Bae YC, Kim HC. Effect of alloy type on the life-time of torsion-preloaded nickel-titanium endodontic instruments. Scanning. 2015;37(3):172–8.
Haapasalo M, Shen Y. Evolution of nickel-titanium instruments: from past to future. Endod Top. 2013;29(1):3–17.
Haikel Y, Serfaty R, Bateman G, Senger B, Allemann C. Dynamic and cyclic fatigue of engine-driven rotary nickel-titanium endodontic instruments. J Endod. 1999;25(6):434–40.
Hartwell G, Bowles W, Peters O, Peikoff M, Torneck C. Joint AAE/CAE special committee on single use endodontic instruments. Final report. 2011. p. 1–5.
Herold KS, Johnson BR, Wenckus CS. A scanning electron microscopy evaluation of microfractures, deformation and separation in EndoSequence and Profile nickel-titanium rotary files using an extracted molar tooth model. J Endod. 2007;33(6):712–4.
Hilfer PB, Bergeron BE, Mayerchak MJ, Roberts HW, Jeansonne BG. Multiple autoclave cycle effects on cyclic fatigue of nickel titanium rotary files produced by new manufacturing methods. J Endod. 2011;37(1):72–4.
Hilt BR, Cunningham CJ, Shen C, Richards N. Torsional properties of stainless-steel and nickel-titanium files after multiple autoclave sterilizations. J Endod. 2000;26(2):76–80.
Hübscher W, Barbakow F, Peters OA. Root canal preparation with FlexMaster: assessment of torque and force in relation to canal anatomy. Int Endod J. 2003;36(12):883–90.
Hülsmann M. Research that matters – canal preparation, retreatment and working length studies. Int Endod J. 2013;46(4):293–5.
Hülsmann M, Peters OA, Dummer PM. Mechanical preparation of root canals: shaping goals, techniques and means. Endod Top. 2005;10(1):30–76.
Inan U, Gonulol N. Deformation and fracture of Mtwo rotary nickel-titanium instruments after clinical use. J Endod. 2009;35(10):1396–9.
Iqbal MK, Kohli MR, Kim JS. A retrospective clinical study of incidence of root canal instrument separation in an endodontics graduate program: a PennEndo database study. J Endod. 2006;32(11):1048–52.
Iverson GW, von Fraunhofer JA, Herrmann JW. The effects of various sterilization methods on the torsional strength of endodontic files. J Endod. 1985;11(6):266–8.
Johnson E, Lloyd A, Kuttler S, Namerow K. Comparison between a novel nickel titanium alloy and 508 nitinol on the cyclic fatigue life of ProFile 25/04 rotary instruments. J Endod. 2008;34(11):1406–9.
Kaval ME, Capar IC, Ertas H. Evaluation of the cyclic fatigue and torsional resistance of novel nickel-titanium rotary files with various alloy properties. J Endod. 2016;42(12):1840–3.
King JB, Roberts HW, Bergeron BE, Mayerchak MJ. The effect of autoclaving on torsional moment of two nickel-titanium endodontic files. Int Endod J. 2012;45(2):156–61.
Kitchens GG, Lieweh FR, Moon PC. The effect of operational speed on the fracture of nickel-titanium rotary instruments. J Endod. 2007;33(1):52–4.
Klayman SM, Brilliant JD. A comparison of the efficacy of serial preparation versus Giromatic preparation. J Endod. 1975;1(10):334–7.

Kobayashi C, Yoshioka T, Suda H. A new engine-driven canal preparation system with electronic canal measuring capability. J Endod. 1997;23(12):751–4.
Kosti E, Zinelis S, Lambrianidis T, Margelos J. A comparative study of crack development in stainless-steel hedstrom files used with step-back or crown-down techniques. J Endod. 2004;30(1):38–41.
Kosti E, Zinelis S, Molyvdas I, Lambrianidis T. Effect of root canal curvature on the failure incidence of ProFile rotary Ni–Ti endodontic instruments. Int Endod J. 2011;44(10):917–25.
Krishan R, Paqué F, Ossareh A, Kishen A, Dao T, Friedman S. Impacts of conservative endodontic cavity on root canal instrumentation efficacy and resistance to fracture assessed in incisors, premolars, and molars. J Endod. 2014;40(8):1160–6.
Kuhn G, Tavernier B, Jordan L. Influence of structure on nickel-titanium endodontic instruments failure. J Endod. 2001;27(8):516–20.
Larsen CM, Watanabe I, Glickman G, He J. Cyclic fatigue analysis of a new generation of nickel titanium rotary instruments. J Endod. 2009;35(3):401–3.
Li U, Lee B, Shih C, Lan W, Lin C. Cyclic fatigue of endodontic nickel-titanium rotary instruments: static and dynamic tests. J Endod. 2002;28(6):448–51.
Lilley JD, Smith DC. An investigation of the fracture of root canal reamers. Br Dent J. 1966;120(8):364–72.
Lopes HP, Elias CN, Amaral G, Vieira VT, Moreira EJL, Mangelli M, Siqueira JF. Torsional properties of pathfinding instruments. Oral Surg Oral Med Oral Pathol Oral Radiol Endod. 2011;112(5):667–70.
Lopes HP, Elias CN, Siqueira JF Jr, Soares RG, Souza LC, Oliveira JCM, Lopes WSP, Mangelli M. Mechanical behavior of pathfinding endodontic instruments. J Endod. 2012;38(10):1417–21.
Lopes HP, Vieira MVB, Elias CN, Siqueira JF Jr, Gonçalves LS, Vieira TLV. Location of the canal curvature and its influence on the resistance to fatigue fracture of two rotary nickel-titanium endodontic instruments. ENDO (Lond Engl). 2013;7(1):53–8.
Madarati AA, Watts DC, Qualtrough AJ. Opinions and attitudes of endodontists and general dental practitioners in the UK towards the intracanal fracture of endodontic instruments: part 1. Int Endod J. 2008;41(8):693–701.
Marsicovetere ES, Clement DJ, Del Rio CE. Morphometric video analysis of the engine-driven nickel-titanium Lightspeed instrument system. J Endod. 1996;22(5):231–5.
Martin B, Zelada G, Varela P, Bahillo JG, Magan F, Ahn S, Rodriguez C. Factors influencing the fracture of nickel-titanium rotary instruments. Int Endod J. 2003;36(4):262–6.
Martins RC, Bahia MGA, Buono VTL. Surface analysis of ProFile instruments by scanning electron microscopy and X-ray energy-dispersive spectroscopy: a preliminary study. Int Endod J. 2002;35(10):848–53.
McGuigan MB, Louca C, Duncan HF. Endodontic instrument fracture: causes and prevention. Br Dent J. 2013;214(7):341–8.
McSpadden J. Mastering endodontic instrumentation. Chattanooga: Cloudland Institute; 2007. p. 1–197.
Mitchell BF, James GA, Nelson RC. The effect of autoclave sterilization on endodontic files. Oral Surg Oral Med Oral Pathol. 1983;55(2):204–7.
Mize SB, Clement DJ, Pruett JP, Carnes DL. Effect of sterilization on cyclic fatigue of rotary nickel-titanium endodontic instruments. J Endod. 1998;24(12):843–7.
Moore B, Verdelis K, Kishen A, Dao T, Friedman S. Impacts of contracted endodontic cavities on instrumentation efficacy and biomechanical responses in maxillary molars. J Endod. 2016;42(12):1779–83.
Novoa XR, Martin-Biedma B, Varela-Patino P, Collazo A, Macías-Luaces A, Cantatore G, Pérez MC, Magán-Muñoz F. The corrosion of nickeltitanium rotary endodontic instruments in sodium hypochlorite. Int Endod J. 2007;40(1):36–44.
O'Hoy PY, Messer HH, Palamara JE. The effect of cleaning procedures on fracture properties and corrosion of NiTi files. Int Endod J. 2003;36(11):724–32.
Oh SH, Ha JH, Kwak SW, Ahn SW, Lee WC, Kim HC. The effects of torsional preloading on the torsional resistance of nickel-titanium instruments. J Endod. 2017;43(1):157–62.

Paleker F, van der Vyver PJ. Comparison of canal transportation and centering ability of K-files, Proglider file, and G-files: a micro-computed tomography study of curved root canals. J Endod. 2016;42(7):1105–9.

Parashos P, Gordon I, Messer HH. Factors influencing defects of rotary nickel-titanium endodontic instruments after clinical use. J Endod. 2004;30(10):722–5.

Parashos P, Gordon I, Messer HH. Factors influencing defects of rotary Nickel-Titanium endodontic instruments after clinical use. J Endod. 2004;30(10):722–5.

Patino PV, Biedma BM, Liebana CR, Cantatore G, Bahillo JG. The influence of a manual glide path on the separation rate of NiTi rotary instruments. J Endod. 2005;31(2):114–6.

Pedulla E, Grande NM, Plotino G, Gambarini G, Rapisarda E. Influence of continuous or reciprocating motion on cyclic fatigue resistance of different nickel-titanium rotary instruments. J Endod. 2013;39(2):258–61.

Peng B, Shen Y, Cheung GSP, Xia TJ. Defects in ProTaper S1 instruments after clinical use: longitudinal examination. Int Endod J. 2005;38(8):550–7.

Peters OA. Current challenges and concepts in the preparation of root canal systems: a review. J Endod. 2004;30(8):559–65.

Peters OA. Accessing root canal systems: knowledge base and clinical techniques. ENDO (Lond Engl). 2008;2(2):87–104.

Peters OA, Paque F. Current developments in rotary root canal instrument technology and clinical use: a review. Quintessence Int. 2010;41(6):479–88.

Peters OA, Peters CI, Schonenberger K, Barbakow F. ProTaper rotary root canal preparation: assessment of torque and force in relation to canal anatomy. Int Endod J. 2003;36(2):93–9.

Peters OA, Boessler C, Zehnder M. Effect of liquid and paste type lubricants on torque values during simulated rotary root canal instrumentation. Int Endod J. 2005;38(4):223–9.

Peters OA, Roehlike JO, Baumann MA. Effect of immersion in sodium hypochlorite on torque and fatigue resistance of nickel-titanium instruments. J Endod. 2007;33(5):589–93.

Peters OA, Peters CI, Basrani B. Cleaning and shaping the root canal system. In: Hargreaves K, Berman LH, editors. Cohen's pathways of the pulp. 11th ed. St. Louis: Elsevier; 2016. p. 209–79.

Plotino G, Grande NM, Sorci E, Malagnino VA, Somma F. A comparison of cyclic fatigue between used and new Mtwo Ni-Ti rotary instruments. Int Endod J. 2006;39(9):716–23.

Plotino G, Grande NM, Falanga A, Di Giuseppe IL, Lamorgese V, Somma F. Dentine removal in the coronal portion of root canals following two preparation techniques. Int Endod J. 2007;40(11):852–8.

Plotino G, Costanzo A, Grande NM, Petrovic R, Testarelli L, Gambarini G. Experimental evaluation on the influence of autoclave sterilization on the cyclic fatigue of new nickel-titanium rotary instruments. J Endod. 2012;38(2):222–5.

Plotino G, Testarelli L, Al-Sudani D, Pongione G, Grande NM, Gambarini G. Fatigue resistance of rotary instruments manufactured using different nickel-titanium alloys: a comparative study. Odontology. 2014;102(1):31–5.

Plotino G, Grande NM, Porciani PF. Deformation and fracture incidence of Reciproc instruments: a clinical evaluation. Int Endod J. 2015;48(2):199–205.

Plotino G, Grande NM, Mercadé M, Testarelli L, Gambarini G. Influence of temperature on cyclic fatigue resistance of ProTaper Gold and ProTaper Universal rotary files. J Endod. 2017;43(2):200–2.

Poulsen WB, Dove SB, del Rio CE. Effect of nickel-titanium engine-driven instrument rotational speed on root canal morphology. J Endod. 1995;21(12):609–12.

Praisarnti C, Chang JW, Cheung GS. Electropolishing enhances the resistance of nickel-titanium rotary files to corrosion-fatigue failure in hypochlorite. J Endod. 2010;36(8):1354–7.

Pruett JP, Clement DJ, Carnes DL Jr. Cyclic fatigue testing of nickel-titanium endodontic instruments. J Endod. 1997;23(2):77–85.

Rapisarda E, Bonaccorso A, Tripi TR, Condorelli GG. Effect of sterilization on the cutting efficiency of rotary nickel-titanium endodontic files. Oral Surg Oral Med Oral Path Oral Radiol Endod. 1999;88(3):343–7.

Regan JD, Sherriff M, Meredith N, Gulabivala K. A survey of interfacial forces used during filing of root canals. Endod Dent Traumatol. 2000;16(3):101–6.

Roda SR, Gettleman BH. Nonsurgical retreatment. In: Hargreaves K, Berman LH, editors. Cohen's pathways of the pulp. 11th ed. St. Louis: Elsevier; 2016. p. 324–86.

Rodrigues RC, Lopes HP, Elias CN, Amaral G, Vieira VT, De Martin AS. Influence of different manufacturing methods on the cyclic fatigue of rotary nickel-titanium endodontic instruments. J Endod. 2011;37(11):1553–7.

Rodrigues E, De-Deus G, Souza E, Silva EJ. Safe mechanical preparation with reciprocation movement without glide path creation: result from a pool of 673 root canals. Braz Dent J. 2016;27(1):22–7.

Roland DD, Andelin WE, Browning DF, Hsu GH, Torabinejad M. The effect of preflaring on the rates of separation for 0.04 taper nickel titanium rotary instruments. J Endod. 2002;28(7):543–5.

Saber SEDM. Factors influencing the fracture of rotary nickel titanium instruments. ENDO (Lond Engl). 2008;2(4):273–83.

Sattapan B, Palamara J, Messer H. Torque during canal instrumentation using rotary nickel-titanium files. J Endod. 2000a;26(3):156–60.

Sattapan B, Nervo GJ, Palamara JE, Messer HH. Defects in rotary nickel-titanium files after clinical use. J Endod. 2000b;26(3):161–5.

Sawaguchi T, Kausträter G, Yawny A, Wagner M, Eggeler G. Crack initiation and propagation in 50.9 at. pct Ni-Ti pseudoelastic shape-memory wires in bending-rotation fatigue. Metall Mater Trans A. 2003;34(12):2847–60.

Schäfer E, Tepel J. Relationship between design features of endodontic instruments and their properties. Part 3. Resistance to bending and fracture. J Endod. 2001;27(4):299–303.

Schäfer E, Dzepina A, Danesh G. Bending properties or rotary nickel-titanium instruments. Oral Surg Oral Med Oral Pathol Oral Radiol Endod. 2003;96(6):757–63.

Shen Y, Cheung GS, Bian Z, Pang B. Comparison of defects in ProFile and ProTaper systems after clinical use. J Endod. 2006;32(1):61–5.

Shen Y, Haapasalo M, Cheung GS, Peng B. Defects in nickel-titanium instruments after clinical use. Part 1: Relationship between observed imperfections and factors leading to such defects in a cohort study. J Endod. 2009;35(1):129–32.

Shen Y, Zhou HM, Zheng YF, Peng B, Haapasalo M. Current challenges and concepts of the thermomechanical treatment of nickel-titanium instruments. J Endod. 2013a;39(2):163–72.

Shen Y, Zhou HM, Wang Z, Campbell L, Zheng YF, Haapasalo M. Phase transformation behavior and mechanical properties of thermomechanically treated K3XF nickel-titanium instruments. J Endod. 2013b;39(7):919–23.

Silvaggio J, Hicks ML. Effect of heat sterilization on the torsional properties of rotary nickel-titanium endodontic files. J Endod. 1997;23(12):731–4.

Smith MS. Sodium hypochlorite's effect on nickel-titanium rotary instruments and its effect on resistance to fracture. Master Thesis. Richmond: Virginia Commonwealth University; 2007. p. 1–34.

Sonntag D, Peters OA. Effect of decontamination protocols on nickel titanium rotary surfaces. J Endod. 2007;33(4):442–6.

Spagnuolo G, Ametrano G, D'Antò V, Rengo C, Simeone M, Riccitiello F, Amato M. Effect of autoclaving on the surfaces of TiN-coated and conventional nickel-titanium rotary instruments. Int Endod J. 2012;45(12):1148–55.

Spanaki-Voreadi AP, Kerezoudis NP, Zinelis S. Failure mechanism of ProTaper Ni–Ti rotary instruments during clinical use: fractographic analysis. Int Endod J. 2006;39(3):171–8.

Svec TA, Powers JM. Effects of simulated conditions on NiTi rotary files. J Endod. 1999;25(11):759–60.

Thierry B, Tabrizian M, Savadogo O, Yahia LH. Effects of sterilization processes on NiTi alloy: surface characterization. J Biomed Mater Res. 2000;49(1):88–98.

Thompson SA. An overview of nickel-titanium alloys used in dentistry. Int Endod J. 2000;33(4):297–310.

Tripi TR, Bonaccorso A, Tripi V, Condorelli GG, Rapisarda E. Defects in GT rotary instruments after use: an SEM study. J Endod. 2001;27(12):782–5.
Tsakiris G. Surface analysis of original and counterfeit rotary instruments by scanning electron microscopy and x-ray energy dispersive spectroscopy. Postgraduate dissertation. Thessaloniki, Greece: Dental School, Aristotle University of Thessaloniki; 2016. p. 1–50 (in Greek).
Ullmann CJ, Peters OA. Effect of cyclic fatigue on static fracture loads in ProTaper nickel-titanium rotary instruments. J Endod. 2005;31(3):183–6.
Ungerechts C, Bårdsen A, Fristad I. Instrument fracture in root canals - where, why, when and what? A study from a student clinic. Int Endod J. 2014;47(2):183–90.
Valois CRA, Silva LP, Azevedo RB. Atomic force microscopy study of stainless steel and nickel-titanium files. J Endod. 2005;31(12):882–5.
Valois CR, Silva LP, Azevedo RB. Multiple autoclave cycles affect the surface of rotary nickel-titanium files: an atomic force microscopy study. J Endod. 2008;34(7):859–62.
Varela-Patino P, Ibanez-Parraga A, Rivas-Mundina B, Cantatore G, Otero XL, Martin-Biedma B. Alternating versus continuous rotation: a comparative study of the effect on instrument life. J Endod. 2010;36(1):157–9.
Viana ACD, Gonzalez BM, Buono VTL, Bahia MGA. Influence of sterilization on mechanical properties and fatigue resistance of nickel-titanium rotary endodontic instruments. Int Endod J. 2006;39(9):709–15.
Walker JT, Dickinson J, Sutton JM, Raven NDH, Marsh PD. Cleanability of dental instruments – implications of residual protein and risks from Creutzfeldt-Jakob disease. Br Dent J. 2007;203(7):395–401.
Wang NN, Ge JY, Xie SJ, Chen G, Zhu M. Analysis of Mtwo rotary instrument separation during endodontic therapy: a retrospective clinical study. Cell Biochem Biophys. 2014;70(2):1091–5.
Wu J, Lei G, Yan M, Yu Y, Yu J, Zhang G. Instrument separation analysis of multi-used ProTaper Universal rotary system during root canal therapy. J Endod. 2011;37(6):758–63.
Xu X, Eng M, Zheng Y, Eng D. Comparative study of torsional and bending properties for six models of nickel-titanium root canal instruments with different cross-sections. J Endod. 2006;32(4):372–5.
Yared G. Canal preparation using only one Ni-Ti rotary instrument: preliminary observations. Int Endod J. 2008;41(4):339–44.
Yared GM, Kulkarni GK. Failure of ProFile Ni-Ti instruments used by an inexperienced operator under access limitations. Int Endod J. 2002;35(6):536–41.
Yared G, Bou Dagher FEB, Matchou P. Cyclic fatigue of profile rotary instruments after simulated clinical use. Int Endod J. 1999;32(2):115–9.
Yared GM, Bou Dagher FE, Machtou P. Cyclic fatigue of ProFile rotary instruments after clinical use. Int Endod J. 2000;33(3):204–7.
Yared G, Bou Dagher FE, Machtou P. Influence of rotational speed, torque, and operator's proficiency on ProFile failures. Int Endod J. 2001;34(1):47–53.
Yared GM, Bou Dagher FE, Machtou P, Kulkarni GK. Influence of rotational speed, torque and operator proficiency on failure of Greater Taper files. Int Endod J. 2002;35(1):7–12.
Yared G, Kulkarni GK, Ghossayn F. An in vitro study of the torsional properties of new and used K3 instruments. Int Endod J. 2003;36(11):764–9.
Zehnder M. Root canal irrigants. J Endod. 2006;32(5):389–98.
Zehnder M, Schmidlin P, Sener B, Waltimo T. Chelation in root canal therapy reconsidered. J Endod. 2005;31(11):817–20.
Zelada G, Varela P, Martín B, Bahíllo JG, Magán F, Ahn S. The effect of rotational speed and the curvature of root canals on the breakage of rotary endodontic instruments. J Endod. 2002;28(7):540–54.
Zhao D, Shen Y, Peng B, Haapasalo M. Micro-computed tomography evaluation of the preparation of mesiobuccal root canals in maxillary first molars with Hyflex CM, Twisted Files, and K3 instruments. J Endod. 2013;39(3):385–8.
Zhao D, Shen Y, Peng B, Haapasalo M. Effect of autoclave sterilization on the cyclic fatigue resistance of thermally treated nickel-titanium instruments. Int Endod J. 2016;49(10):990–5.

Zinelis S, Margelos J. Failure mechanism of Hedstroem endodontic files in vivo. J Endod. 2002;28(6):471–3.

Zinelis S, Darabara M, Takase T, Ogane K, Papadimitriou GD. The effect of thermal treatment on the resistance of nickel-titanium rotary files in cyclic fatigue. Oral Surg Oral Med Oral Pathol Oral Radiol Endod. 2007;103(6):843–7.

3 Mechanisms of Instrument Failure

Spiros Zinelis

3.1 Introduction

The intracanal fracture of endodontic files with the possible retention of the fragment in the root canal is an unwanted complication in everyday clinical practice. The fragment removal is time consuming and technically difficult and might jeopardize the outcome of endodontic treatment. Therefore, intense research is being carried out in this field in order to reveal the causes of intracanal fracture and provide appropriate guidelines for a safer use of endodontic instruments. On the other hand, plastically deformed endodontic files are also considered failed files (as they cannot be used further) and thus should also be included in the investigation of failure mechanisms as they might provide additional information about what happens in this multivariant environment. In addition, the knowledge of failure mechanisms is of paramount importance for the development of new endodontic files. For instance, if it is known that fatigue is the fracture mechanism of an endodontic file during clinical operation, then a new alloy with higher fatigue resistance and/or fracture toughness (a property indicating the material resistance to crack propagation) might be chosen.

Numerous experimental studies have been carried out to elucidate the fracture mechanisms of endodontic files or to estimate a safe number of root canals that the files should be used for by simulating the clinical conditions (i.e. curvature of root canals in metallic blocks, use of irrigation solution, etc.). This experimental approach is used in non-dental technologies to predict the service time of components that fail as a result of wear, corrosion, fatigue or other detrimental processes. However, in the dental field, this approach often yields information with limited clinical relevance (McGuigan et al. 2013), as the controlled experimental conditions

S. Zinelis, B. Eng, Ph.D.
Department of Biomaterials, School of Dentistry, National and Kapodistrian University of Athens, Thivon 2 Goudi, 11527 Athens, Greece
e-mail: szinelis@dent.uoa.gr

T. Lambrianidis (ed.), *Management of Fractured Endodontic Instruments*,
DOI 10.1007/978-3-319-60651-4_3

do not properly mimic clinical conditions that widely vary from experimental and can yield completely different fracture mechanisms. The determination of failure mechanisms should be based on evidence collected by controlled clinical studies and the fractographic analysis of retrieved endodontic instruments. However this is a much more complicated process compared to laboratory studies, since it includes a myriad of different factors (i.e. operator skill, canal anatomy, time of uses, etc.), and it is more challenging in experimental analysis (Parashos and Messer 2006).

3.2 Failure Mechanisms of SS Files

3.2.1 Fracture Mechanisms of Hedstrom Files

The characteristic geometry of Hedstrom files (H-files) with deep flutes cannot be achieved by twisting a tapered ground wire, and thus these instruments are made by milling round wire blanks (Miserendino 1991). In order to determine the failure mechanisms, a large number of H-files of ISO sizes 08–40 discarded due to fracture or deformation were collected from different dental clinics (Zinelis and Al Jabbari 2017). Then the files were classified according to their size and macroscopic appearance, and the percentage of fractured and deformed files were determined for each file size. Figure 3.1 shows a low magnification image of a small-sized H-file (file ISO size <20). Interestingly the plastic deformation was located near the cutting tip. This finding is in accordance with previous findings on the topic indicating that in most cases the fracture is located in the apical third due to the smaller diameter and maximum curvature of the root canal (Iqbal et al. 2006). The small sizes (8–15) showed a high frequency of plastic deformation (Fig. 3.2). On the other hand, for ISO size #20 only a percentage of 20% presented plastic deformation, while the rest were discarded due to fracture. A limited percentage of less than 5% of discarded files with ISO size #25 were plastically deformed, and larger

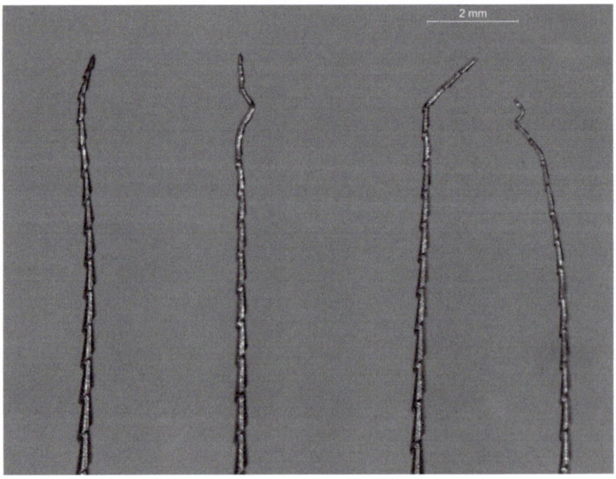

Fig. 3.1 Image showing H-files discarded after clinical use due to plastic deformation of the cutting tip

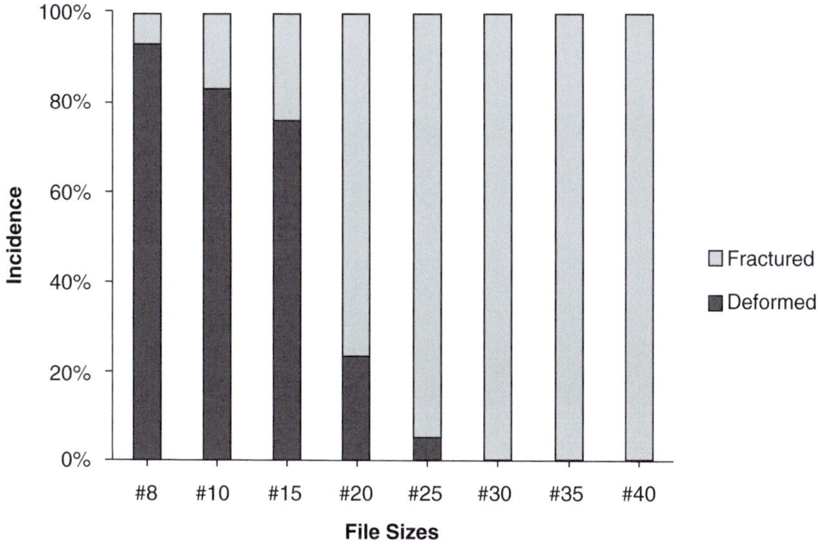

Fig. 3.2 Distribution of fractured and plastically deformed instruments within different ISO sizes of H-files after clinical use

sizes were discarded only due to fracture. Of course, these results of macroscopic classification of H-files (Fig. 3.2) should be considered indicative since the number of uses varied among the files tested. However, the results may demonstrate the most common failure type per H-file, whereas the exact quantitative estimations require a different experimental design. For small-sized H-files (ISO sizes #08 to 15), the plastic deformation observed close to the cutting tip implied that loading during clinical use exceeded the yield point of the alloy used but never reached the fracture strength.

The analysis of fractured H-files by means of optical microscopy, scanning electron microscopy (SEM) and micro-X-ray computerized tomography (micro-XCT) provided substantial information on the fracture mechanisms. SEM analysis of clinically fractured files revealed the presence of striations, which is the characteristic pattern of fatigue fracture. A crack originated from the cutting surface propagates during clinical use and causes final fracture of H-file (Fig. 3.3). The longitudinal cross-sectional analysis provided additional information on the location and orientation of these cracks in other parts of the fractured H-file. Figure 3.4 shows an optical microscope image of polished cross sections of an as-received and a multiple times used clinically fractured H-file (Fig. 3.4a, b, respectively). The as-received file is free of any internal cracks, pores or other manufacturing defects, while the in vivo fractured file presents many cracks located at the flute regions (Zinelis and Margelos 2002; Kosti et al. 2004). These cracks vary in size and are oriented perpendicular to the long axis of the file. Similarly, the analysis with the micro-XCT demonstrates no evidence of internal defects for the as-received file. However, the clinically fractured file shows

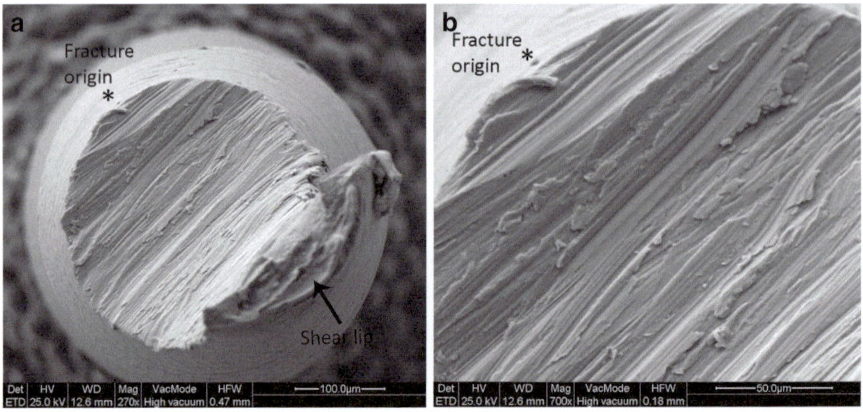

Fig. 3.3 (**a**) Secondary electron image (SEI) with the characteristic striations of fatigue fracture on the surface of clinically fractured H-file. The *asterisk* indicates the origin of fracture, while the end of the fracture is indicated on the opposite side by the shear lip. (**b**) The characteristic striations near the origin of the fracture at higher magnification

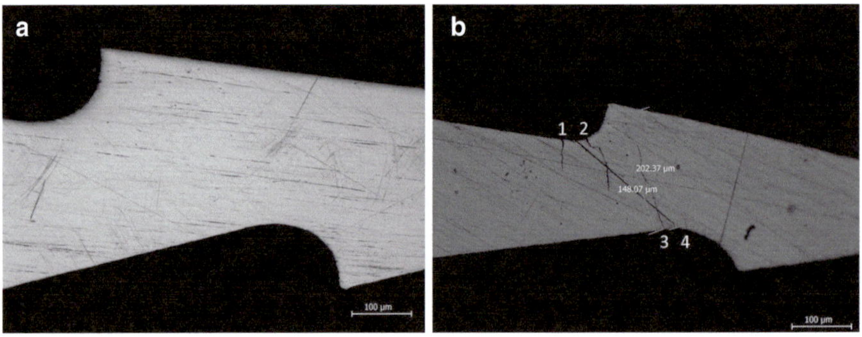

Fig. 3.4 Optical microscope photograph of the surface of an as-received (**a**) and a clinically fractured H-file (**b**). Multiple cracks (the origin is indicated by the numbers) are located on the flutes. The longest crack (#3) extends along the 73% (148.07/202.37) of the bearing cross section(4) (original magnification ×20)

extensive secondary cracking (cracks close to fracture plane) and also cracks located in the flute region (Fig. 3.5). Given that unused files are free from defects, it is clear that these cracks have originated and propagated during extensive clinical use. The origin of these cracks could be attributed to two proposed mechanisms. The first explanation suggests that the machining grooves developed during the manufacturing process with milling provide a myriad of sites for crack initiation (Luebke and Brantley 1991; Brantley et al. 1994; Luebke et al. 1995). However, the development of cracks in the flute region does not support this theory. Surface cracks from milling during the manufacturing process extend to all cutting surfaces of H-files, and thus the cracks must originate uniformly from the cutting surface and extend towards the centre of the instrument. In a second

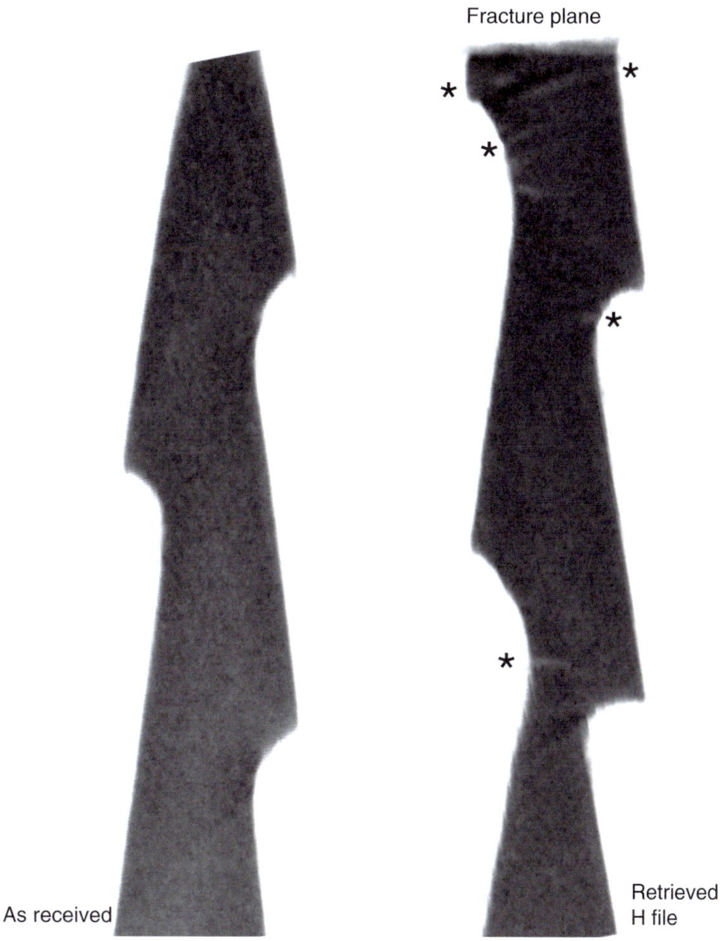

Fig. 3.5 Two-dimensional micro-XCT images of an unused and a clinically broken H-file. The as-received file is free of any internal defects, while the clinically fractured file shows many cracks close to the fracture plane and also in the flute regions (some of them are indicated by *asterisks*)

scenario, the location of cracks deep in the flutes should be attributed to the abrupt decrease in the cross-sectional diameter which has been introduced to facilitate loading of dentin debris (Zinelis and Margelos 2002). However, it seems that this acts as a stress concentration factor facilitating the initiation of surface cracks and their propagation perpendicularly to the long axis of the instrument (Zinelis and Margelos 2002; Kosti et al. 2004).

The determination of fatigue fracture as the main failure mechanism based on clinical data has important clinical and technological implications. From a clinical standpoint, it means that fracture will occur after a period of in-service use. However, cracks propagate without any macroscopic sign to warn the clinician about the deterioration of the file's mechanical properties and the upcoming fracture. Although the crown-down technique slows down the crack propagation compared to step-back technique (Kosti et al. 2004), further research is required to estimate a safe number of instrumentation procedures with H-files in such a multivariant environment as the root canal.

Experimental data based on torque testing may provide information on the resistance of H-files to plastic deformation. However, they have failed to provide any clue as to the fatigue resistance of these instruments, and thus it is proposed that the evaluation of fatigue properties should be included in future specifications. Based on the aforementioned failure mechanisms, the lifespan of H-files could be elongated by introducing different alloys in the manufacturing process. In particular the small-sized files which failed as a result of plastic deformation would benefit if they were made of an alloy with higher yield strength and increased resistance to plastic deformation, without compromising the hardness and corrosion resistance of used SS austenitic grades AISI 303 and 304 (Darabara et al. 2004). Similarly, the larger sizes which failed as a result of the fatigue mechanism might benefit from the introduction of a more fatigue-resistant alloy and the reduction of the stress concentration factor due to the abrupt decrease in the cross-sectional diameter in the flute region. However, any change in the manufacturing process should not jeopardize other desirable file properties, such as cutting efficiency, rigidity and loading of dental debris.

3.2.2 Failure Mechanisms of Stainless Steel K-Files

Although both triangular and rectangular K-files are made from the same SS alloys as H-files (Darabara et al. 2004), the ratio between fractured and deformed discarded files is completely different. K-files are discarded in huge numbers due to plastic deformation, and only a fraction of them has been fractured intraorally. Sotokawa (1988) tested 2328 discarded K-files of rectangular and triangular cross section and found a fracture rate of less than 2%. Unpublished data of our group have recorded a similar fracture rate (<3%), although in a much smaller sample size (100 approximately) of K-files discarded after clinical use. The difference from H-files could be attributed to the higher rigidity, bending and torsional resistance, because of the thicker cross section of K-files. Experimental findings showed that K-files are more resistant to torsion (higher torque resistance) and demonstrate higher angular deflection with higher twist angles before fracture (Krupp et al. 1984), although both K-files and H-files are made from the same alloys (Darabara et al. 2004).

Figure 3.6 shows representative fracture surfaces from two retrieved K-files. Both files were fractured due to overloading under torsion (Fig. 3.6a, d) although fatigue striations were also observed (Fig. 3.6b). Small flat regions were also identified in the four corners of Fig. 3.6d, although the analysis at higher magnification determined a featureless flat surface, a finding that may be attributed to the rubbing action of mutual crack surfaces. In both cases the fatigue part occupies a small

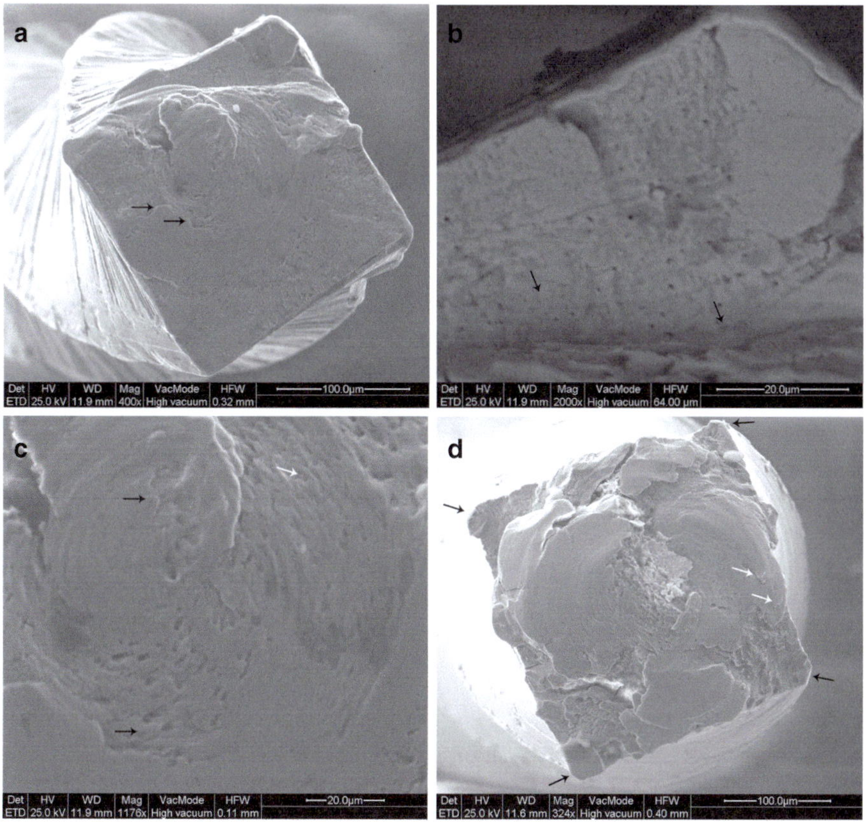

Fig. 3.6 SE images of the surface of clinically failed K-files. (**a**) A rather smooth fracture surface with shear tongues (indicated by the *arrows*). (**b**) Higher magnification of the upper right corner where a few fatigue striations (indicated by the *arrows*) have originated from the right angle of the cross section. (**c**) Higher magnification of the central area of (**a**) with the presence of shear tongues (*black arrows*) and skewed dimples (*white arrows*), a typical pattern of shear overloading. (**d**) A typical fracture surface due to shear under torsion with shear tongues (*white arrows*). The four corners (*black arrows*) show small flat regions that may be attributed to fatigue striations, although imaging at higher magnification showed featureless flat surfaces

portion of the cross-sectional area denoting low stress concentration and high overloading. Testing the K-files under simulated conditions, Sotokawa (1988) concluded that fatigue cracks originating in the corners of the cross section decrease the bearing area, leading to the catastrophic fracture of K-files. However, the limited knowledge on this topic cannot provide a conclusive fracture mechanism, and extensive further research based on clinical fractured files must be carried out in order to elucidate the fracture mechanism under clinical conditions. Given that K-files fail due to plastic deformation, the increase of yield stress in torsion would have a beneficial effect on their clinical longevity.

3.3 Failure Mechanisms of NiTi Files

Currently the "fatigue resistance" of NiTi endodontic files has attracted a lot of attention as it is considered a good criterion for comparing the in-service life of different brands (Cheung 2007). The term "fatigue resistance" stands for the number of revolutions, an instrument can sustain before fracturing and thus it is supposed that a file with a higher fatigue resistance would last longer before fatigue fracture and from this standpoint is a safer instrument. Indeed, the fatigue mechanism fits well with the intracanal conditions as the files function under bending with hundreds of revolutions per minutes (rpm) and this is a perfect environment for fatigue phenomena. However, as it was mentioned in the introductory comments, it is widely accepted that experimental findings have limited clinical relevance and therefore are incapable of foreseeing what really happens in clinical conditions.

NiTi files are also discarded from dental clinics due to plastic deformation or fracture. A number of studies have recorded the failure rate of discarded NiTi files from different dental clinics, but their results are not directly comparable due to differences in their classification protocol and other uncontrolled variables (Sattapan et al. 2000; Al-Fouzan 2003; Arens et al. 2003; Parashos et al. 2004; Alapati et al. 2005; Cheung et al. 2005, 2007; Peng et al. 2005; Spili et al. 2005; Di Fiore et al. 2006; Iqbal et al. 2006; Shen et al. 2006; Spanaki-Voreadi et al. 2006; Wolcott et al. 2006; Wei et al. 2007). Thus there is no clear picture of the incidence of plastic deformation and fracture among discarded files. However, the findings of these studies provide additional information about the nature of fracture mechanisms in vivo. The most important information is that the fracture incidence is independent of the number of uses. Testing 930 instruments of different brands, Parashos et al. (2004) found that fracture incidence is irrelevant to the number of uses (Fig. 3.7). This finding is in accordance with the outcome of a large cohort study showing that the incidence of fracture did not significantly increased if ProTaper files (Dentsply Maillefer, Ballaigues, Switzerland) were reused up to four times (Wolcott et al. 2006). The findings of both studies contradict the involvement of fatigue mechanism, as the continuous degradation of the mechanical properties of instruments should provide an increased fracture rate over successive uses.

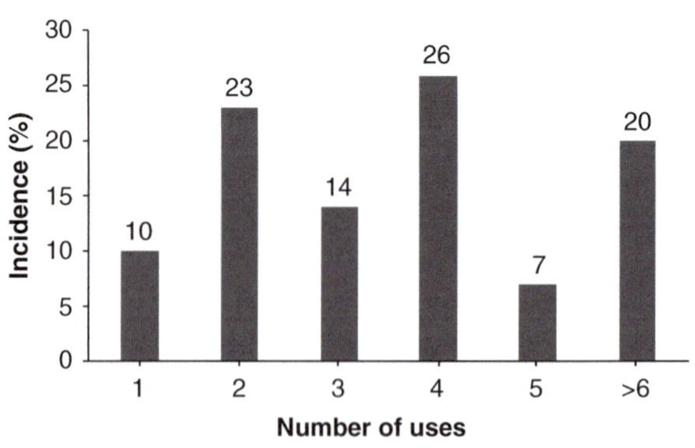

Fig. 3.7 Incidence of fracture of six brands over number of uses (Parashos et al. 2004)

The bulk of the recent literature has grouped the fracture of NiTi files into two categories commonly known as torsional fracture and flexural fatigue (Cheung 2007; McGuigan et al. 2013). Fractured instruments are classified into the aforementioned categories based on the low-power microscopic examination of their lateral surfaces. If the fractured instrument demonstrates extensive plastic deformation in the vicinity of the fracture point (mainly unscrewing or over screwing of the flutes), it is classified as a torsional fracture, while in the absence of plastic deformation, it falls into the flexural fatigue category. However, the absence or presence of plastic deformation is not a proof of fatigue fracture as other conditions such as high strain rates can eliminate the plastic deformation of ductile metals as well. Cheung et al. (2005) have argued against this criterion suggesting that only fractographic analysis can provide real information about the fracture mechanism. Nevertheless only a few studies used fractography to determine the fracture mechanism, and none of them has provided the characteristic surface pattern of the fatigue mechanism in tension, torsion, bending or other loading conditions (Alapati et al. 2005; Cheung et al. 2005, 2007; Peng et al. 2005; Spanaki-Voreadi et al. 2006; Wei et al. 2007; Shen et al. 2009b). In a few studies, the characteristic patterns of shear overloading or cleavage have been erroneously recognized as fatigue striations, while in others a tiny part of the surface covered by striations has been used to characterize the fracture mechanism.

Figure 3.8 shows characteristic fracture surface of clinically fractured NiTi files. The characteristic pattern of cleavage fracture is presented in Fig. 3.8a located mainly in the corners of the fracture surface. This type of fracture is usually associated with polycrystalline materials and is the most brittle form of fracture that can occur in metallic materials. The typical surface pattern of torsional fracture is presented in Fig. 3.8b with a smooth periphery and a fibrous central area with shallow dimples. In

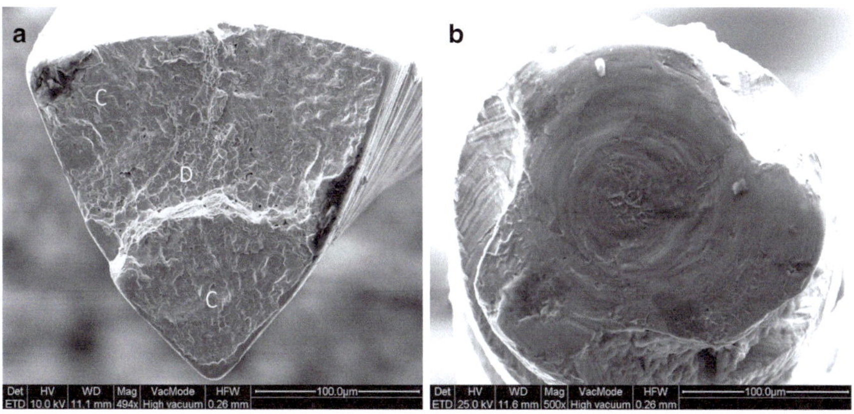

Fig. 3.8 SE images of the surfaces of clinically broken NiTi files. (**a**) The characteristic pattern of cleavage fracture is evident in areas indicated by letter C, while at the centre, there are shallow dimples (area D). (**b**) Typical fracture surface of a NiTi alloy under torsion loading with a smooth periphery and a fibrous central region

both cases the shallow dimples might be attributed to the low plastic deformation of the NiTi alloy or the high strain rate exerted during fracture which heavily constrain the extent of plastic deformation before fracture (Spanaki-Voreadi et al. 2006). However, both the aforementioned mechanisms are associated with a single overloading rather than cumulative damage over successive uses. Apart from the absence of characteristic striations, clinically fractured NiTi files also lack secondary cracking (such as in the case of SS file, Figs. 3.4 and 3.5). In general fatigue loading causes numerous cracks that propagate simultaneously, although only one leads to fracture, while the rest remain in the vicinity as secondary cracking. However, secondary cracking was never found either in the vicinity or in the full length of clinically fractured NiTi files in previous studies employing optical microscopy and micro-XCT analysis (Fig. 3.9) (Spanaki-Voreadi et al. 2006; Kosti et al. 2011).

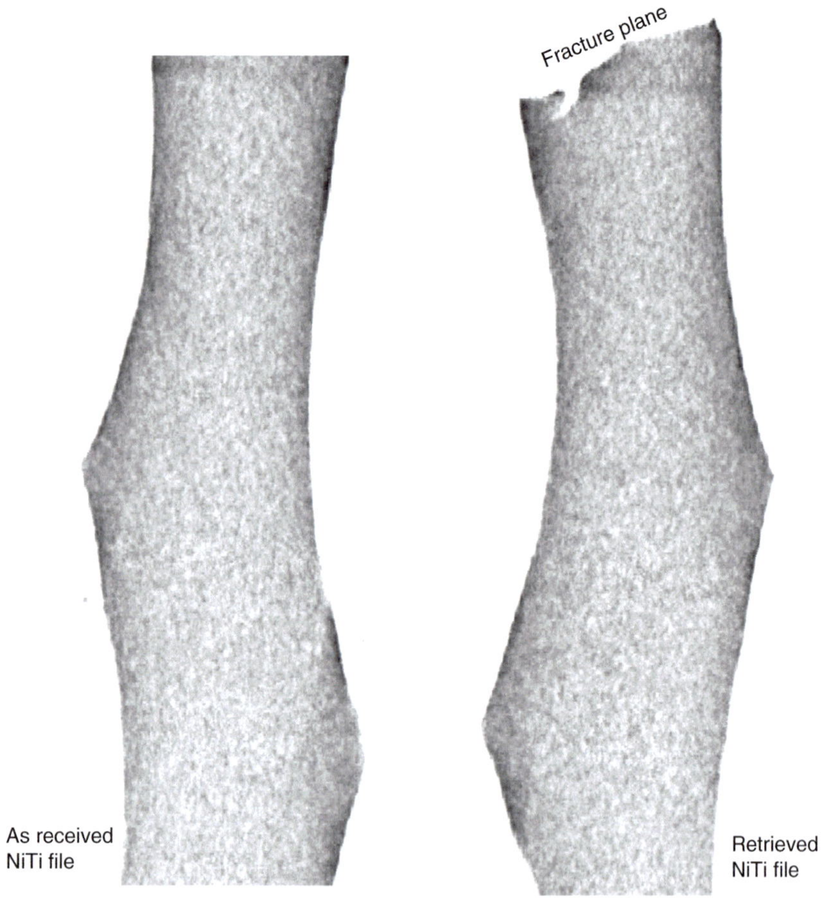

Fig. 3.9 Two-dimensional micro-XCT images of an unused and a clinically fractured NiTi file. Both files are free of internal defects or cracks originating in the cutting surface

Recently a different approach has been applied to modify the structure of NiTi alloy and consequently its mechanical properties by introducing a new generation of rotary instruments. In 2007 the M-wire was adopted for the production of NiTi files, with commercial names Profile GT series X, Profile Vortex, Profile Blue and WaveOne (Dentsply Tulsa Dental Specialties, Tulsa, OK). Contrary to the conventional files with austenite structure, M-wire instruments retain the martensite structure at room temperature. In 2008 the TF instrument (SybronEndo, Orange, CA) was introduced made out of NiTi blanks in R-phase, which originates during the austenite martensite transformation. Finally, CM wire was used in 2010 for the manufacturing of Hyflex CM (Coltene Whaledent, Cuyahoga Falls, OH) and TYPHOON (Clinician's Choice Dental Products, New Milford, CT). The CM wire underwent a proprietary thermomechanical process which eliminated the shape memory properties of the NiTi alloy (Shen et al. 2013). However limited information is available in the literature based on the retrieval analysis of clinically used new-generation rotary files. One study has examined used files of the WaveOne system and another of the Profile Vortex and Profile Vortex Blue and both concluded that intraoral fracture was due to torsional failure during service (Shen et al. 2015, 2016). Therefore, it seems that in the case of M-wire the fracture mechanism is not affected by the metallurgical and structural differences in the NiTi alloy, but the effect of CM wire and R-phase requires further investigation.

From a clinical standpoint, the fracture mechanism of single overloading fits well with the aforementioned data showing that the fracture is independent of the times of uses as this can occur at any time during the operation, while it also explains the fact that even brand new instruments have a 0.9% incidence of fracture (Arens et al. 2003). This approach also explains the general outcome of many studies showing that instrument fracture is affected more by the manner in which the instrument is used rather than by the number of uses (Parashos et al. 2004; Shen et al. 2009a). Given that the failure mechanism is not associated with cumulative damage but with a sudden overloading, probably when the tip of the instrument is locked in a constricted region of the root canal, the research aimed at determining safe number of uses for NiTi files is rather of questionable value, while the training of operators for a proper use of those instruments seems more substantial.

Conclusions

The intracanal fracture of endodontic instruments is an unpleasant complication during instrumentation with annoying consequences. H-files, K-files and NiTi files fail during operation with different failure mechanisms, implying completely different guidelines for a safer and more efficient use of these instruments in everyday clinical practice. The use of new alloys with high values in selected mechanical properties and new geometrical designs based on knowledge of the aforementioned failure mechanisms seems to be a promising area for further research and development.

References

Al-Fouzan KS. Incidence of rotary ProFile instrument fracture and the potential for bypassing in vivo. Int Endod J. 2003;36(12):864–7.

Alapati SB, Brantley WA, Svec TA, Powers JM, Nusstein JM, Daehn GS. SEM observations of nickel-titanium rotary endodontic instruments that fractured during clinical use. J Endod. 2005;31(1):40–4.

Arens FC, Hoen MM, Steiman HR, Dietz GC Jr. Evaluation of single-use rotary nickel-titanium instruments. J Endod. 2003;29(10):664–6.

Brantley WA, Luebke NH, Luebke FL, Mitchell JC. Performance of engine-driven rotary endodontic instruments with a superimposed bending deflection: V. Gates Glidden and Peeso drills. J Endod. 1994;20(5):241–5.

Cheung GS, Peng B, Bian Z, Shen Y, Darvell BW. Defects in ProTaper S1 instruments after clinical use: fractographic examination. Int Endod J. 2005;38(11):802–9.

Cheung GSP. Instrument fracture: mechanisms, removal of fragments, and clinical outcomes. Endod Top. 2007;16(1):1–26.

Cheung GS, Bian Z, Shen Y, Peng B, Darvell BW. Comparison of defects in ProTaper hand-operated and engine-driven instruments after clinical use. Int Endod J. 2007;40(3):169–78.

Darabara M, Bourithis L, Zinelis S, Papadimitriou GD. Assessment of elemental composition, microstructure, and hardness of stainless steel endodontic files and reamers. J Endod. 2004;30(7):523–6.

Di Fiore PM, Genov KA, Komaroff E, Li Y, Lin L. Nickel-titanium rotary instrument fracture: a clinical practice assessment. Int Endod J. 2006;39(9):700–8.

Iqbal MK, Kohli MR, Kim JS. A retrospective clinical study of incidence of root canal instrument separation in an endodontics graduate program: a PennEndo database study. J Endod. 2006;32(11):1048–52.

Kosti E, Zinelis S, Lambrianidis T, Margelos J. A comparative study of crack development in stainless-steel hedstrom files used with step-back or crown-down techniques. J Endod. 2004;30(1):38–41.

Kosti E, Zinelis S, Molyvdas I, Lambrianidis T. Effect of root canal curvature on the failure incidence of ProFile rotary Ni-Ti endodontic instruments. Int Endod J. 2011;44(10):917–25.

Krupp JD, Brantley WA, Gerstein H. An investigation of the torsional and bending properties of seven brands of endodontic files. J Endod. 1984;10(8):372–80.

Luebke NH, Brantley WA. Torsional and metallurgical properties of rotary endodontic instruments. 2. Stainless steel Gates Glidden drills. J Endod. 1991;17(7):319–23.

Luebke NH, Brantley WA, Sabri ZI, Luebke FL, Lausten LL. Physical dimensions, torsional performance, bending properties, and metallurgical characteristics of rotary endodontic instruments. VI Canal Master drills. J Endod. 1995;21(5):259–63.

Miserendino L. Instruments, materials and devices. In: Cohens S, Burns R, editors. Pathways of the pulp. 5th ed. St Louis: Mosby-Year Book; 1991. p. 388–432.

McGuigan MB, Louca C, Duncan HF. Endodontic instrument fracture: causes and prevention. Br Dent J. 2013;214(7):341–8.

Parashos P, Messer HH. Rotary NiTi instrument fracture and its consequences. J Endod. 2006;32(11):1031–43.

Sattapan B, Nervo GJ, Palamara JE, Messer HH. Defects in rotary nickel-titanium files after clinical use. J Endod. 2000;26(3):161–5.

Shen Y, Cheung GS, Bian Z, Peng B. Comparison of defects in ProFile and ProTaper systems after clinical use. J Endod. 2006;32(1):61–5.

Shen Y, Haapasalo M, Cheung GS, Peng B. Defects in nickel-titanium instruments after clinical use. Part 1: relationship between observed imperfections and factors leading to such defects in a cohort study. J Endod. 2009a;35(1):129–32.

Shen Y, Coil JM, McLean AG, Hemerling DL, Haapasalo M. Defects in nickel-titanium instruments after clinical use. Part 5: single use from endodontic specialty practices. J Endod. 2009b;35(10):1363–7.

Shen Y, Zhou HM, Zheng YF, Peng B, Haapasalo M. Current challenges and concepts of the thermomechanical treatment of nickel-titanium instruments. J Endod. 2013;39(2):163–72.
Shen Y, Zhou HM, Coil JM, Aljazaeri B, Buttar R, Wanh Z, Zheng YF, Haapasalo M. ProFile Vortex and Vortex Blue nickel-titanium rotary instruments after clinical use. J Endod. 2015;41(6):937–42.
Shen Y, Coil JM, Mo AJ, Wang Z, Hieawy A, Yang Y, Haapasalo M. WaveOne rotary instruments after clinical use. J Endod. 2016;42(2):186–9.
Sotokawa T. An analysis of clinical breakage of root canal instruments. J Endod. 1988;14(2):75–82.
Parashos P, Gordon I, Messer HH. Factors influencing defects of rotary nickel-titanium endodontic instruments after clinical use. J Endod. 2004;30(10):722–5.
Peng B, Shen Y, Cheung GS, Xia TJ. Defects in ProTaper S1 instruments after clinical use: longitudinal examination. Int Endod J. 2005;38(8):550–7.
Spanaki-Voreadi AP, Kerezoudis NP, Zinelis S. Failure mechanism of ProTaper Ni-Ti rotary instruments during clinical use: fractographic analysis. Int Endod J. 2006;39(3):171–8.
Spili P, Parashos P, Messer HH. The impact of instrument fracture on outcome of endodontic treatment. J Endod. 2005;31(12):845–50.
Wei X, Ling J, Jiang J, Huang X, Liu L. Modes of failure of ProTaper nickel-titanium rotary instruments after clinical use. J Endod. 2007;33(3):276–9.
Wolcott S, Wolcott J, Ishley D, Kennedy W, Johnson S, Minnich S, et al. Separation incidence of protaper rotary instruments: a large cohort clinical evaluation. J Endod. 2006;32(12):1139–41.
Zinelis S, Margelos J. Failure mechanism of Hedstroem endodontic files in vivo. J Endod. 2002;28(6):471–3.
Zinelis S, Al Jabbari Y. How Hedstroem files fail during clinical use? A retrieval study based on SEM and micro-XCT analysis. Submitted to Clinical Oral Investigation 2017.

Therapeutic Options for the Management of Fractured Instruments

4

Theodor Lambrianidis

4.1 Introduction

The endodontic management of a fractured instrument or any metallic object within the root canal is a sophisticated process that requires training, experience, and knowledge of the methods/techniques that can be used. It is a time-consuming and challenging procedure often associated with anxiety for both clinician and patient with variable success rate (see Chap. 6). Many factors must be considered before attempting to manage the instrument fragment. These include:

- The dentition: permanent or deciduous teeth?
- The location of the tooth in the dental arch and the root canal with the fragment
- The root canal anatomy, including its diameter, length, and curvature
- The thickness of the root dentin and the depth of the external concavities
- The condition of the periapical and periodontal tissues
- The stage of canal instrumentation when the fracture occurred, reflecting the extent to which microbial control was achieved
- The length of the fragment
- The location of the fragment within the canal
- The material and type of the fragment
- Fractured file's action: clockwise or counterclockwise
- Last but of course not least, the patient's wishes

T. Lambrianidis, D.D.S., Ph.D.
Department of Endodontology, Dental School,
Aristotle University of Thessaloniki, Thessaloniki, Greece
e-mail: thlampri@dent.auth.gr

T. Lambrianidis (ed.), *Management of Fractured Endodontic Instruments*,
DOI 10.1007/978-3-319-60651-4_4

4.2 Management

The optimal management of instrument fragments during RCT is retrieval in order to enable sufficient debridement and obturation of the root canal system. At present, there is no standardized procedure for safe and consistently successful instrument fragment removal in the dental literature. In each case, the chances of success should be balanced against potential complications. Fractured instruments are managed with:

- No intervention
- Non-surgical (orthograde, conservative) management
- Surgical management
- Tooth extraction

4.2.1 No Intervention

This option is applicable in two diametrically different categories of cases:

(a) *Cases in which there is no point in intervening* when the fragment is located to a nonrestorable and/or severely compromised periodontal tooth. This also applies in cases of teeth that are likely to become un-restorable subsequent to instrument management efforts. The presence of the fragment in these cases has no impact at all on the decision-making (Fig. 4.1).
(b) *Cases in which there is no need to intervene* when no clinical or radiographic signs of pathosis are present and no scheduled treatment is to be performed to include these teeth. Such characteristic examples might be the presence of a long-lasting fragment in the apical third in a symptomless tooth with no radiographic lesion or a long-lasting fragment beyond the foramen with no clinical symptoms or radiographic sign of pathosis (Fig. 4.2).

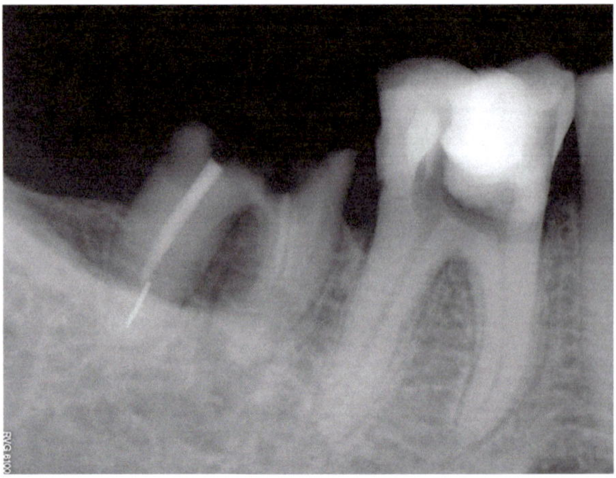

Fig. 4.1 Nonrestorable roots of a mandibular second molar with a fragment in the apical third of the distal root. Tooth extraction is the treatment of choice in this case

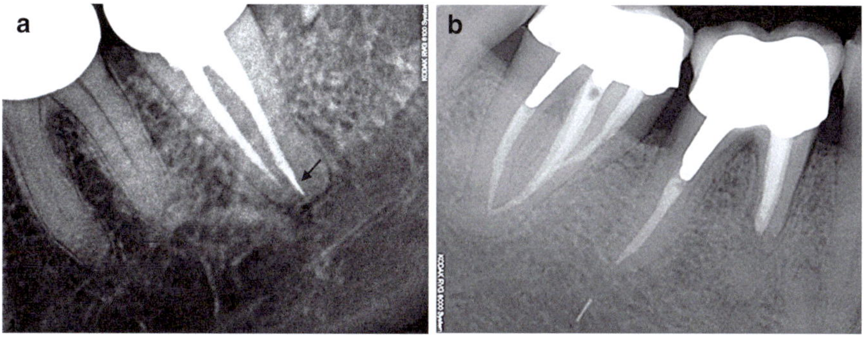

Fig. 4.2 No intervention as the treatment option for fragments revealed randomly during full-mouth periapical radiographic examination. (**a**) According to the patient's history, the instrument fracture (*arrow*) occurred during RCT 15 years earlier. Prosthetic reconstruction was performed 5 years later. (**b**) The fragment in the periapical tissues can be attributed to the RCT performed, according to the patient's history, 16 years earlier. Since then, the patient experienced no pain or discomfort in the area

4.2.2 Non-surgical Management

This approach can be divided into two phases. In the first phase as a general rule, efforts are made to retrieve the fragment and, if this is not possible, to bypass it. In cases where this is accomplished, as well as in cases where retrieval or bypassing fails and the appropriate conditions are met, the second phase follows. The second phase includes the instrumentation and obturation phase. In cases of retrieval or successful bypassing, instrumentation and obturation are performed up to the desired length; otherwise, the canal is instrumented and obturated up to the fragment, and the tooth is monitored clinically and radiographically.

4.2.3 Surgical Management

As a rule, surgical management with apicoectomy, hemisection, root amputation, or intentional reimplantation is performed when the conservative approach fails or is considered from the outset to lead to failure. It is the only reasonable alternative to extraction.

4.2.4 Tooth Extraction

This is performed when all other therapeutical options (non-surgical and surgical) have proved unsuccessful or are considered to be a failure.

4.3 Management Procedure

All procedures include the risk of creating additional errors that may eventually jeopardize the prognosis of the tooth. Therefore, the clinician should continuously reevaluate the progress of management procedures and consider alternative options when needed. The optimum management option is the retrieval of the fragment so that instrumentation and obturation can be accomplished to the desired length. There are certain steps to be followed prior to any decision and particularly initiation of efforts to retrieve the fragment. These include:

1. Steps prior to any decision:
   (a) Informing the patient
   (b) Localization of the fragment
   (c) Identification of the fragment
2. Initiation of management efforts:
   (a) In primary teeth
   (b) In permanent teeth

4.3.1 Steps Prior to Any Decision

4.3.1.1 Informing the Patient

The patient should be informed about the incident, the procedures necessary for correction, the alternative management modalities, and the impact of this iatrogenic error as well as of all alternative treatment options on prognosis. It is important to explain that the fragment itself is not a direct cause of treatment failure but rather a possible indirect one, as it prevents adequate cleaning, shaping, and filling of the apical portion of the root canal. It must also be explained to the patient that each individual case has its own unique characteristics that dictate the management approach. By explaining and discussing the procedures and their potential complications with the patient, it may be possible to alleviate many of his/her worries and reduce medicolegal consequences.

Additionally, for medicolegal reasons, a detailed history with clinical pictures and radiographic documentation is necessary. It has also been proposed that the remaining segment of the instrument should be kept in the patient's record (Cohen and Schwartz 1987). In cases of endodontic referrals related with primary or retreatment cases with fragments retained within the canal, it is of vital importance to diagnose them and consult the patient for their presence. Their presence carries a medicolegal risk, if not diagnosed preoperatively, because the iatrogenic error might be attributed to the clinician performing the new treatment. In all cases it is essential, for medicolegal reasons, to record accurately in the patient's notes all the information given to the patient.

4.3.1.2 Localization of the Fragment

Localization of the fragment provides fundamental information for decision-making regarding the potential management of the fragment. There are three different conditions under which a dentist needs to detect, identify, and localize a fragment. These are:

1. Localization of a fragment caused by the treating dentist
2. Localization of a fragment in a referral case
3. Localization of retained fragment in retreatment cases

1. Localization of a fragment caused by the treating dentist. Instrumentation must be stopped immediately after an instrument fracture. It might then be necessary for the clinician to thoughtfully interpret more than one periapical radiograph obtained with different horizontal angulations to confirm the incident, to reveal the location of the fragment in the root canal, and to appreciate the thickness of the remaining dentinal walls and, if present, the depth of an external concavity. The advantage in this case is that the exact type and size of the fragment are known as well as the exact stage of instrumentation when the error occurred.
2. Localization of a fragment in a referral case. In some cases, information obtained by the referring dentist concerning the fragment and the instrumentation stage when the fracture occurred is very illuminating, but in many cases it is not. Thorough interpretation of periapical radiograph(s) obtained before commencing any treatment is again absolutely essential.
3. Localization of retained fragment(s) in cases of root canal retreatments. In these cases, preoperative detection of retained fragments is crucial for a decision-making process regarding the treatment plan and also for medicolegal reasons. Once again periapical radiography is the principal form of radiography used. The radiographic diagnosis of fragment bypassed and retained in a root canal or retained within a canal obturated to the level of the fragment may be challenging. The material composition of the fragment, the size and length of the fragment, as well as the technical characteristics of the obturation and the type of the obturation material used (gutta-percha and sealer) are among the factors that influence the radiographic ability to detect the presence of a fragment. An ex vivo study that compared the diagnostic ability to radiographically detect, with conventional and digital radiography, fractured SS and NiTi instruments located at the apical third of root canals, filled with either AH 26 (Dentsply DeTrey GmbH, Konstanz, Germany) or Roth (Roth International Ltd., Chicago, IL, USA) sealers in extracted human teeth, showed that the type of sealer did not affect the ability to detect the retained instruments (Rosen et al. 2014). The sensitivity in detecting fractured segments of SS instruments was significantly higher than NiTi in the vicinity of both AH26 and Roth sealers. In the same study (Rosen et al. 2014), it was also found that there was no difference between the diagnostic ability of conventional and digital radiography in the detection of both NiTi and SS fragments, in the two different sealers (AH26 and Roth). Another study that compared the diagnostic efficacy of CBCT imaging and periapical radiography for the detection of retained fragments, located at the apical third of filled canal up to the fractured instrument with laterally condensed gutta-percha and AH 26 sealer or Roth sealer, revealed that CBCT imaging is inferior to periapical radiography (Rosen et al. 2016). This was attributed to the production of artifacts by the gutta-percha and the metallic nature of the fragment. The researchers concluded that the ongoing efforts in developing techniques for artifact reduction will probably result in the need to reassess these results as newer technological developments in CBCT artifact reduction algorithms become available. They also emphasize the need for further studies to assess the effect of factors, such as

various sealer types, obturation techniques, and CBCT voxel sizes, on the diagnostic efficacy for the detection of retained separated instruments in filled root canals (Rosen et al. 2016). Similarly Ramos Brito et al. (2017) compared the detection of fractured instruments in root canals with and without filling by periapical radiographs from three digital systems and CBCT images with different resolutions. They concluded that in unfilled canals, a single periapical radiograph may properly diagnose the location of a fractured instrument inside a root canal. This accuracy of periapical radiographs was lower in filled canals, while CBCT imaging showed the worst performance for the detection of fractured instruments in filled canals (Ramos Brito et al. 2017).

The updated joint position statement of the American Association of Endodontists and the American Academy of Oral and Maxillofacial Radiology on the Use of Cone Beam Computed Tomography in Endodontics 2015 Update recommends among other the following:

> *Recommendation 1: Intraoral radiographs should be considered the imaging modality of choice in the evaluation of the endodontic patient. Recommendation 8: Limited Field Of View Cone beam computed Tomography (FOV CBCT) should be the imaging modality of choice for nonsurgical retreatment to assess endodontic treatment complications, such as overextended root canal obturation material, separated endodontic instruments, and localization of perforations.* (Nair et al. 2016)

Recommendation 8 seems to be challenged, in part, by a recent work (Rosen et al. 2016) which has found CBCT to be inferior to periapical radiography for the detection of fractured endodontic instruments surrounded by endodontic sealer. It appears that artifacts originated from the gutta-percha and the endodontic instruments might have played a part. It is certain that the identification of a fractured instrument is not an easy task; factors such as the size and type of the fragment, the type of sealer, and the possible gaps around the fragment may be of significance in its identification. As research advances, a clearer view of this challenging task may evolve.

In line with Recommendation 1, it is strongly believed that periapical radiography as the principal radiographic modality for detection, identification, and localization of intracanal instrument fragments is justified. The use of CBCT to assess the canal shape and the available space around the fragment, in unfilled portions of canals, especially when the dental operating microscope does not allow direct visualization, could be justified when it is perceived to be of valuable assistance in selecting optimal management strategies.

Under all these three different conditions in which the operator is asked to detect, identify, and localize the presence of a fragment, the clamp of the isolation (metallic or plastic) might interfere with the radiographic portrayal of the fragment. Additionally, the clamp might prevent the clinician from following the course of manipulations required during management efforts and inhibit his/her ability to estimate the amount of root canal wall dentin removed. Therefore, in all cases, it is advisable, once the RCT or retreatment has started, to retain the rubber dam by placing the clamp, whenever possible, on an adjacent tooth (Fig. 4.3) or by using dental floss or rubber strips.

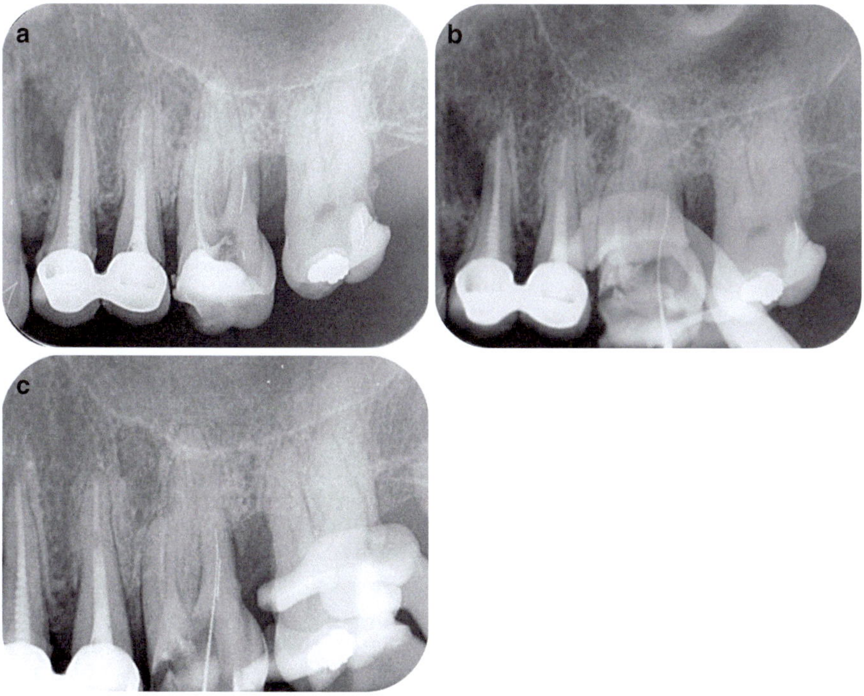

Fig. 4.3 (**a**) Preoperative radiograph of maxillary first molar with an instrument fragment in the distobuccal canal. (**b**) Placement of the plastic clamp on the tooth with the fragment during efforts to negotiate the fragment with a small file hinders management efforts. (**c**) Placement of the clamp on the adjacent second molar results in a clearer view

The potential locations of the fragment, irrespective of the type of the instrument, are the following:

- One end of the fragment protruding into the pulp chamber and the other within the root canal (Fig. 4.4).
- Both ends of the fragment within the root canal (Fig. 4.5).
- One end of the fragment within the root canal and its tip extending into the periapical area (Fig. 4.6).
- The fragment extending from the coronal third to the periapical area (Fig. 4.7).
- The fragment is lodged outside the canal in the periapical region (Fig. 4.8). Rarely, it can also be extruded in adjacent anatomical structures.

4.3.1.3 Identification of the Fragment

The type of instrument fractured and the size of the fragment must be recorded on the patient's chart. In retreatment cases with retained instrument fragment(s) or referrals with no relevant details on the patient's chart, their radiographic appearance will assist in their identification. Thus, familiarity with the radiographic appearance of instruments used within root canal and particularly NiTi and stainless steel (SS) instruments is essential.

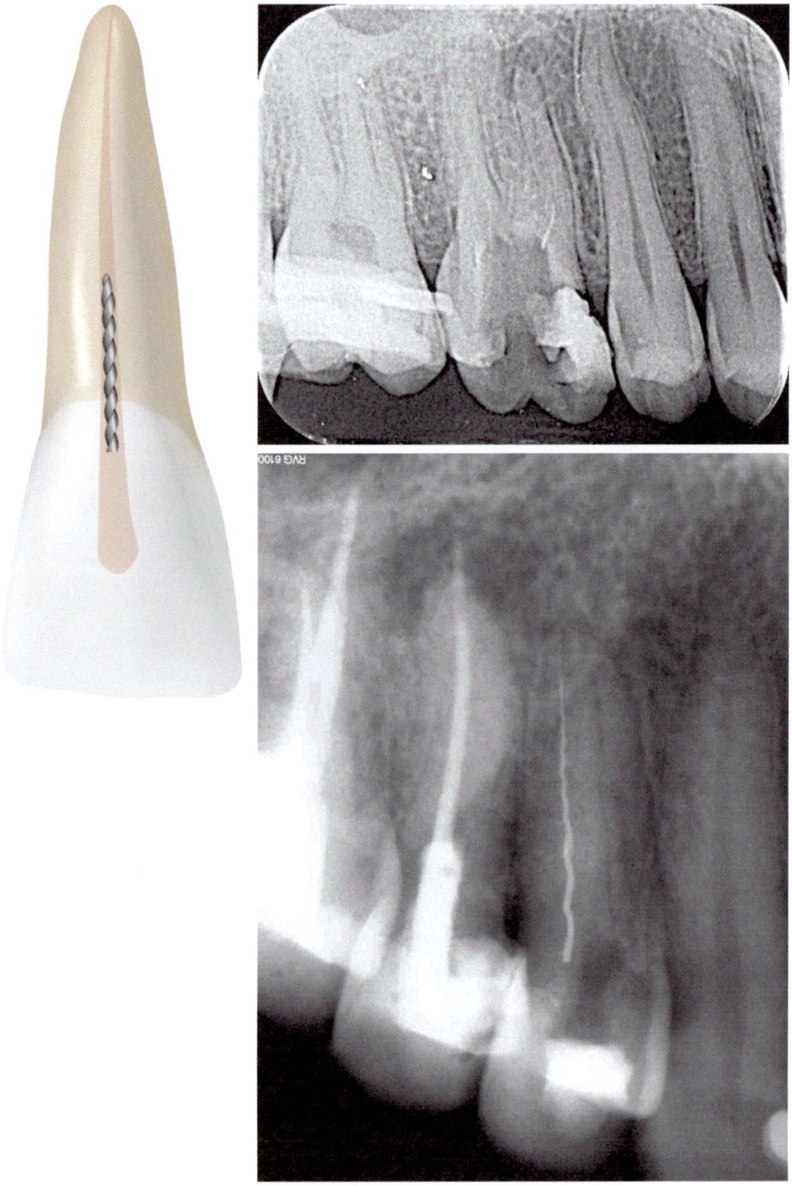

Fig. 4.4 Fragment protruding into the coronal chamber

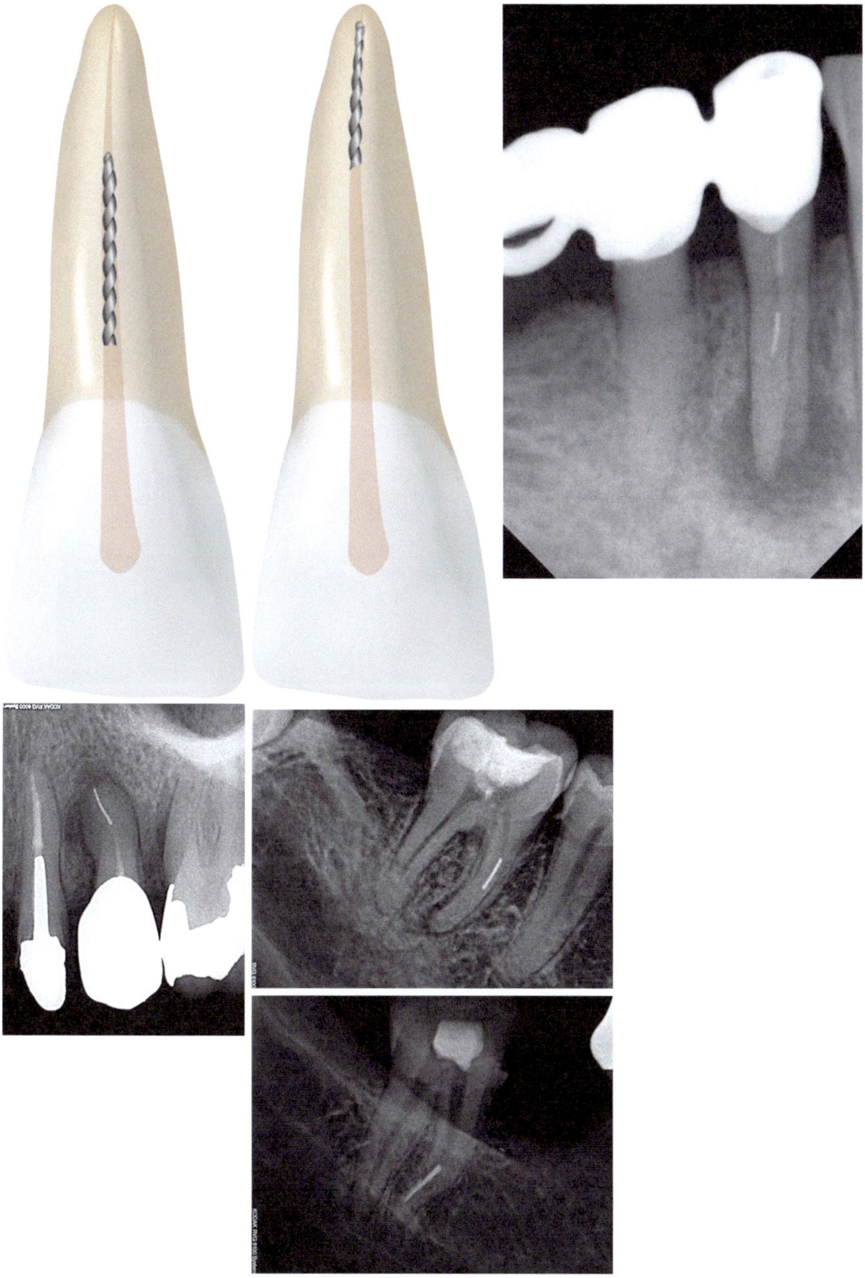

Fig. 4.5 Fragment with both ends within the root canal

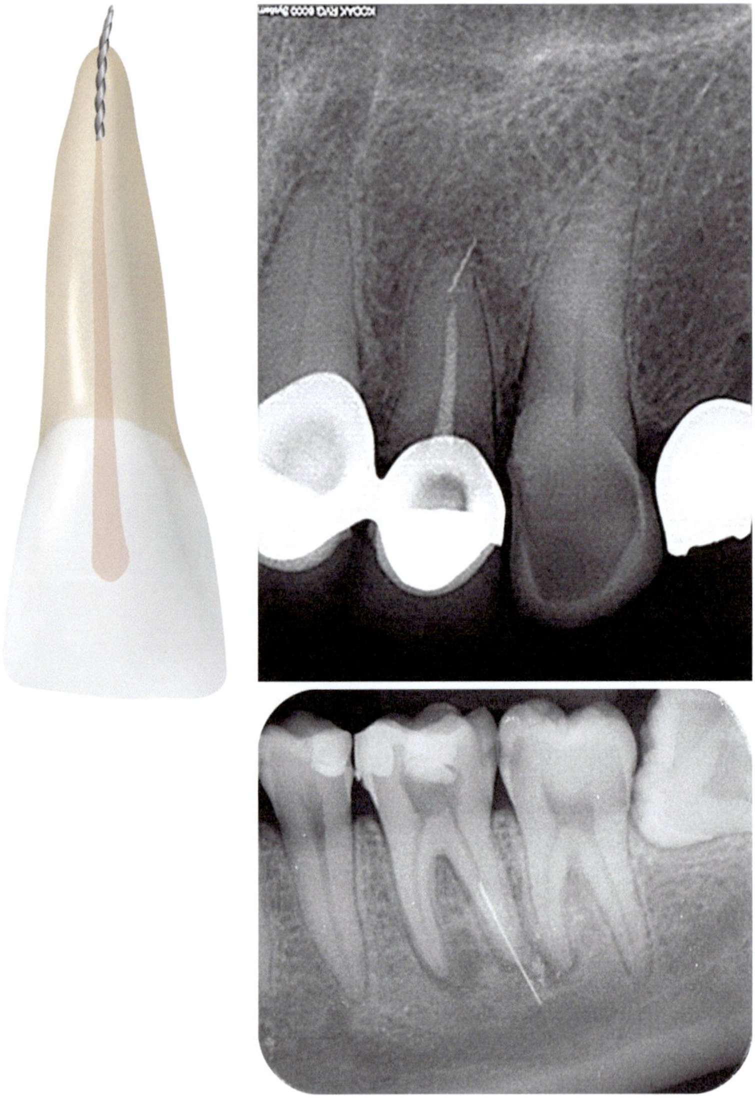

Fig. 4.6 Fragment with one end within the root canal and its tip extending into the periapical area

4.3.2 Initiation of Management Efforts

Upon completion of the patient briefing and the localization and identification of the fragment, management efforts start. It is absolutely essential before any attempt is made to ensure that there is plenty of available time for both the patient and the clinician in order to avoid additional stress on both sides. The management efforts differ in primary and permanent teeth:

1. Initiation of management efforts in primary teeth
2. Initiation of management efforts in permanent teeth

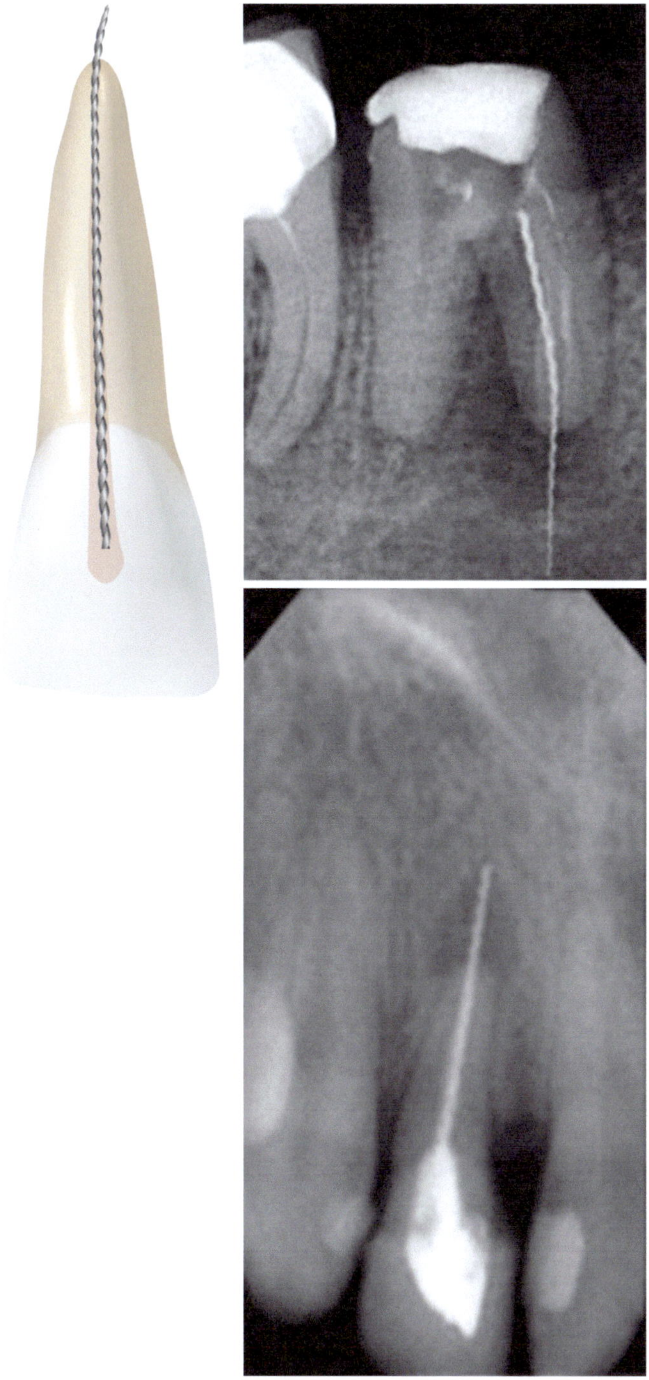

Fig. 4.7 Fragment extending from the coronal third into the periapical region

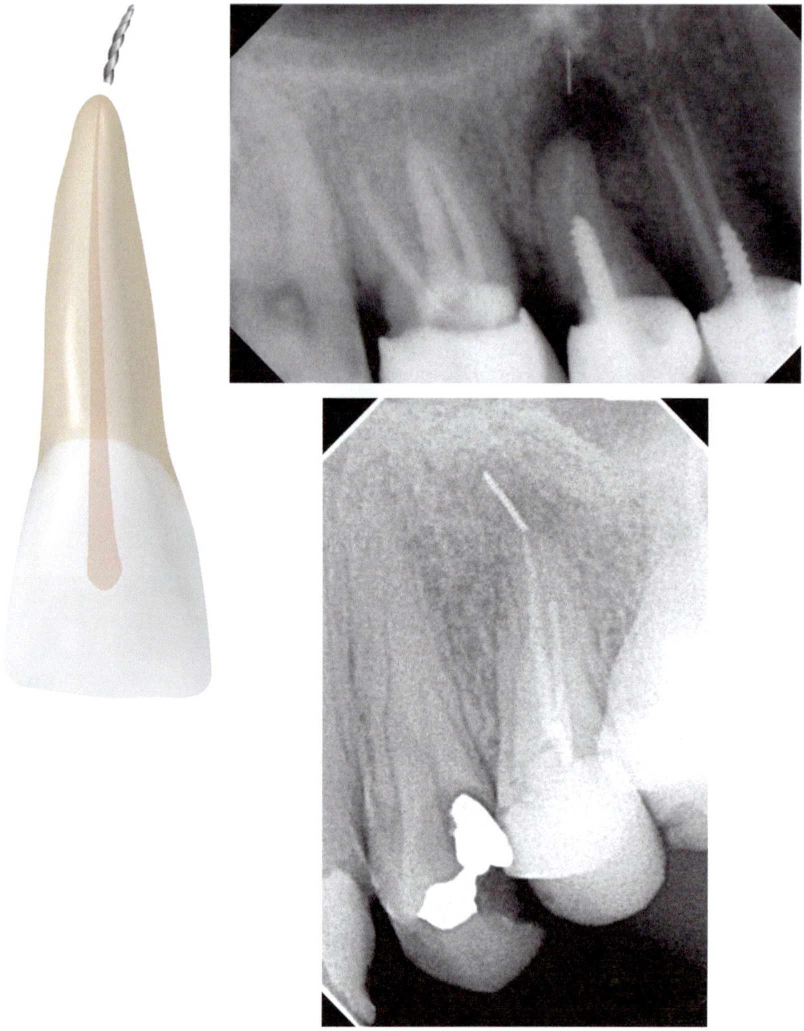

Fig. 4.8 Fragments extruded beyond the confines of the tooth

4.3.2.1 Initiation of Management Efforts in Primary Teeth

The recommended management is retrieval of the fragment or tooth extraction, depending on the fragment's location and the stage of the primary tooth's root resorption (Table 4.1). *In all cases, the clinician must very carefully consider whether removal attempts are necessary at all.* The much thinner radicular dentin, compared to that in permanent dentition, requires caution and the selection of a noninvasive or the least invasive technique for removal of the fractured instrument. In cases where retrieval is not possible but the fragment can be bypassed, instrumentation and obturation with the fragment retained within the sealing material

Table 4.1 Recommended management of fractured instruments in the primary dentition based on the location of the fragment

Location of the fragment	Management phase I	Management phase II
Fragment with one end protruding into the pulp chamber and the other in the r. c.[a] 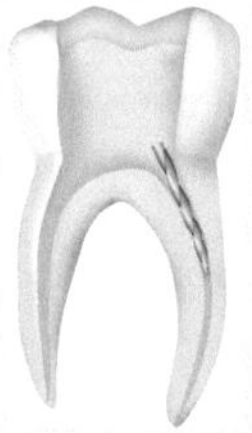	In all cases, retrieval of the fragment	RCT
Fragment with both ends within the r.c. 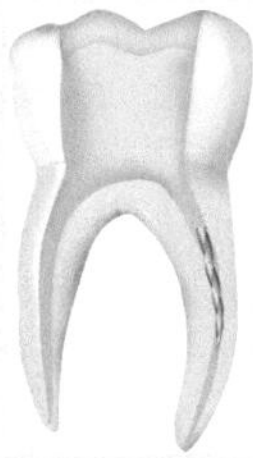	Retrieval of the fragment	RCT
	Failure to retrieve the fragment	Tooth extraction[b]
Fragment with its tip extending into the periapical area 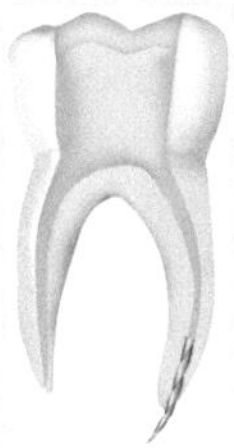	Tooth extraction[b]	
Fragment extending from the pulp chamber into the periapical area 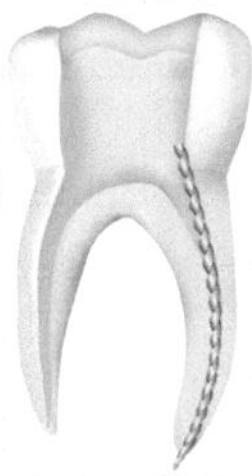	Retrieval of the fragment	RCT
	Failure to retrieve the fragment	Tooth extraction[b]
Fragment lodged outside the r.c. 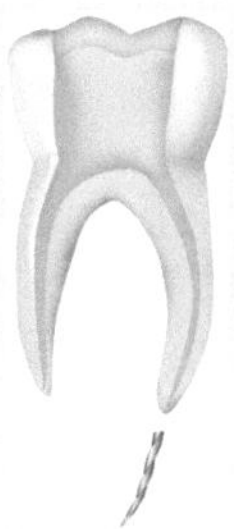	Tooth extraction[b] and removal of the fragment	

[a]*r.c.* root canal
[b]In all cases of tooth extraction, space maintenance in collaboration with the orthodontist must be thoroughly considered

and recall examinations are not recommended. Additionally, if bypassing is not possible, obturation up to the fragment and follow-up of the case are also not recommended. Patients do not always conform to recall appointments. In cases of appointment failure, there is the risk that the metallic fragment will remain in the jaw after the resorption of the root of the primary tooth. This may affect the permanent successor, and theoretically, it might even be found in the oral cavity after the exfoliation of the primary tooth and inadvertently swallowed or inhaled. Extraction followed by space maintenance is often considered the treatment of choice. Obviously the latter is decided in close collaboration with pedodontist and orthodontist.

To our knowledge, there are only three case reports with successful retrieval of fractured instruments in primary teeth with ultrasonics under the dental operating microscope (Patel et al. 2015; Pk et al. 2016). To minimize unnecessary removal of tooth structure, low intensity ultrasonic vibrations of the fragment through a DG 16 endodontic explorer was used to loosen and retrieve the fragment in two of them (Pk et al. 2016). In the third case (Patel et al. 2015), the tip of the ultrasonic instrument activated at a low power setting was placed in intimate contact with the 3 mm fragment located in the middle third of the root of a maxillary central incisor in a 5-year-old boy. A case is also presented in a book (Lambrianidis 2001) where the primary tooth with a fragment with its one end extending into the periapical tissues was extracted (Fig. 4.9). To our knowledge, there is no case in the literature with follow-up of a fragment retained in the root canal of primary tooth after the completion of RCT.

4.3.2.2 Initiation of Management Efforts in Permanent Teeth

Initially an attempt is made to retrieve the fragment (Figs. 4.10, 4.11, and 4.12), if this attempt fails to bypass it (Figs. 4.13 and 4.14) and if this attempt also fails to instrument and obturate the canal up to the fragment (Figs. 4.15, 4.16, and 4.17). In all cases, the tooth in question is scheduled for follow-up. The recommended management varies according to the fragment's location, the pulpal and periapical status at the initiation of the treatment, and the instrumentation stage when the fracture occurred (Table 4.2).

4.3.3 Retrieval of the Fragment

The retrieval of a fractured instrument or any metallic object from the root canal has been a problem for dentists for decades. Various techniques and instruments, which quite often have to be used in combination, have been advocated for retrieving fragments. Technological advances in vision and particularly the dental operating microscope seem to be a key factor in a successful outcome as it can increase visibility through the use of magnification and light, enabling clinicians to visualize the coronal portion of most fractured instruments. The combination of microscope, ultrasonics, and advances in mechanical techniques used to retrieve foreign objects from the root canal ensures safety and increased efficacy. The techniques proposed for the retrieval of fractured instruments from the root canal employ either chemical

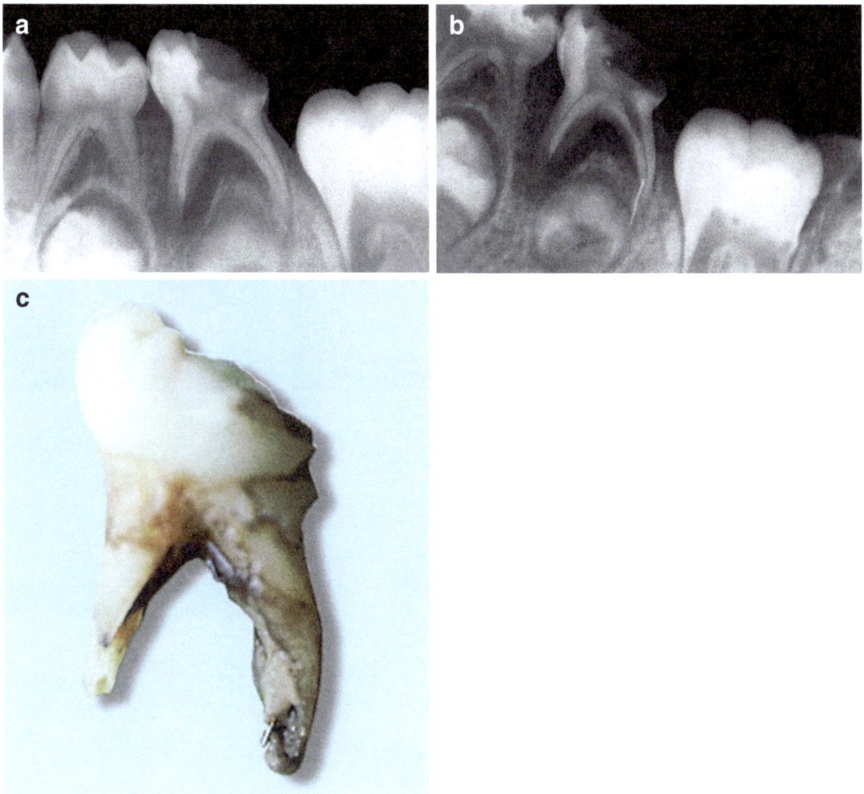

Fig. 4.9 (**a**) Preoperative radiograph. (**b**) Radiographic confirmation of the fragment's presence and identification of its location. (**c**) Extraction of tooth. The tip of the fragment protruding into periapical tissues is discernible (with permission from Lambrianidis 2001)

or mechanical means. Other methods include the electrolyte method, the softened gutta-percha technique, the use of the Multisonic Ultracleaning System, and the laser irradiation (Table 4.3).

4.3.4 Chemical Means

The use of chemical means is aimed at:

- Decalcification of root canal wall dentin around the fractured instrument with a weak acid (usually EDTA) in order to facilitate subsequent removal or bypass of the fragment with mechanical means
- Corrosion of the metallic fragment and its "dissolution" or reduction of its cross section (with iodine compounds) in order to facilitate its retrieval or bypass with mechanical means

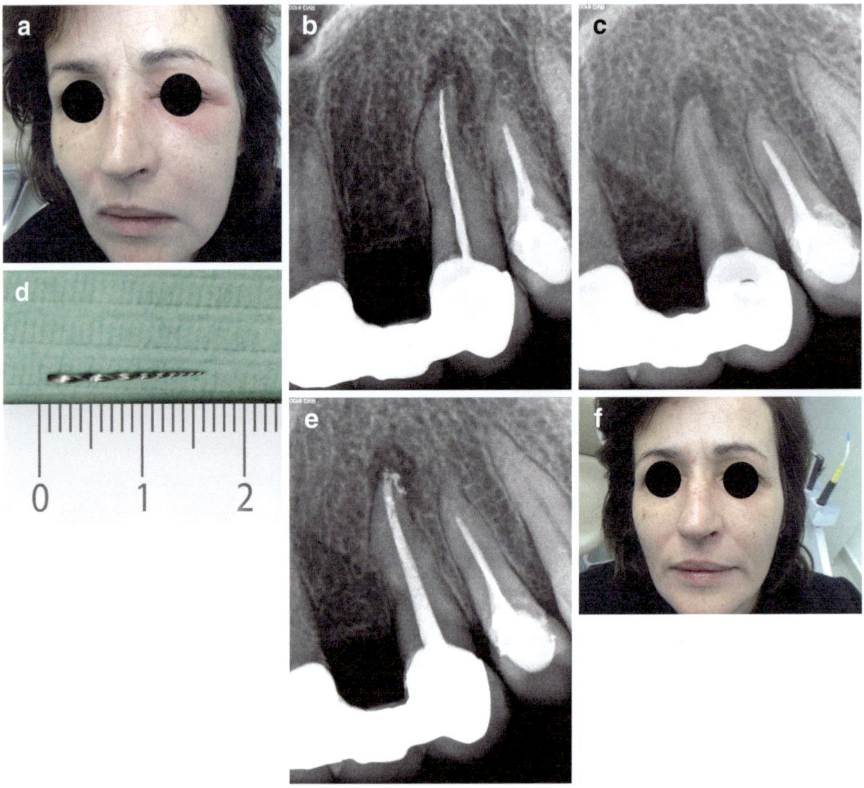

Fig. 4.10 (**a**) Clinical appearance of a healthy 45-year-old woman presented with swelling and fever lasting 3 days, despite self-administered antibiotics (amoxicillin 625 mg ×3 for 3 days). According to her dental history, she had a continuous discomfort since the RCT and bridge work performed 18 months earlier. (**b**) Preoperative radiograph revealed the presence of an endodontic instrument fragment with both ends within the root canal "covering" approximately the whole length of the canal. (**c**, **d**) Retrieval of the fragment, instrumentation, and dressing of the root canal with $Ca(OH)_2$ for 14 days. (**e**) Immediate post-obturation radiograph. (**f**) Clinical picture of the day of completion of RCT (Courtesy of Dr. K. Mastoras)

It is thus clear that the use of chemical means is not actually a technique for managing fragments within the root canal but a preparatory stage that may facilitate their management with mechanical means. Historically, potassium iodine (Lugol), crystallic iodine, iodine trichloride, crystals of iodine, iron chloride solution, and nitrohydrochloric acid have been some of the chemical proposed and most frequently used to intentionally corrode metallic objects in the root canal (Stasinopoulos 1978; Hülsmann 1993). There is a significant reduction in their use nowadays due to:

- Their ineffectiveness
- The fact that any chemical used in the root canal may be harmful to the periapical tissues if inadvertently extruded through the foramen or to the gingivae if it leaks
- The allergic reaction to iodine compounds (Schafer 2007)
- The well-known staining potential of iodine compounds

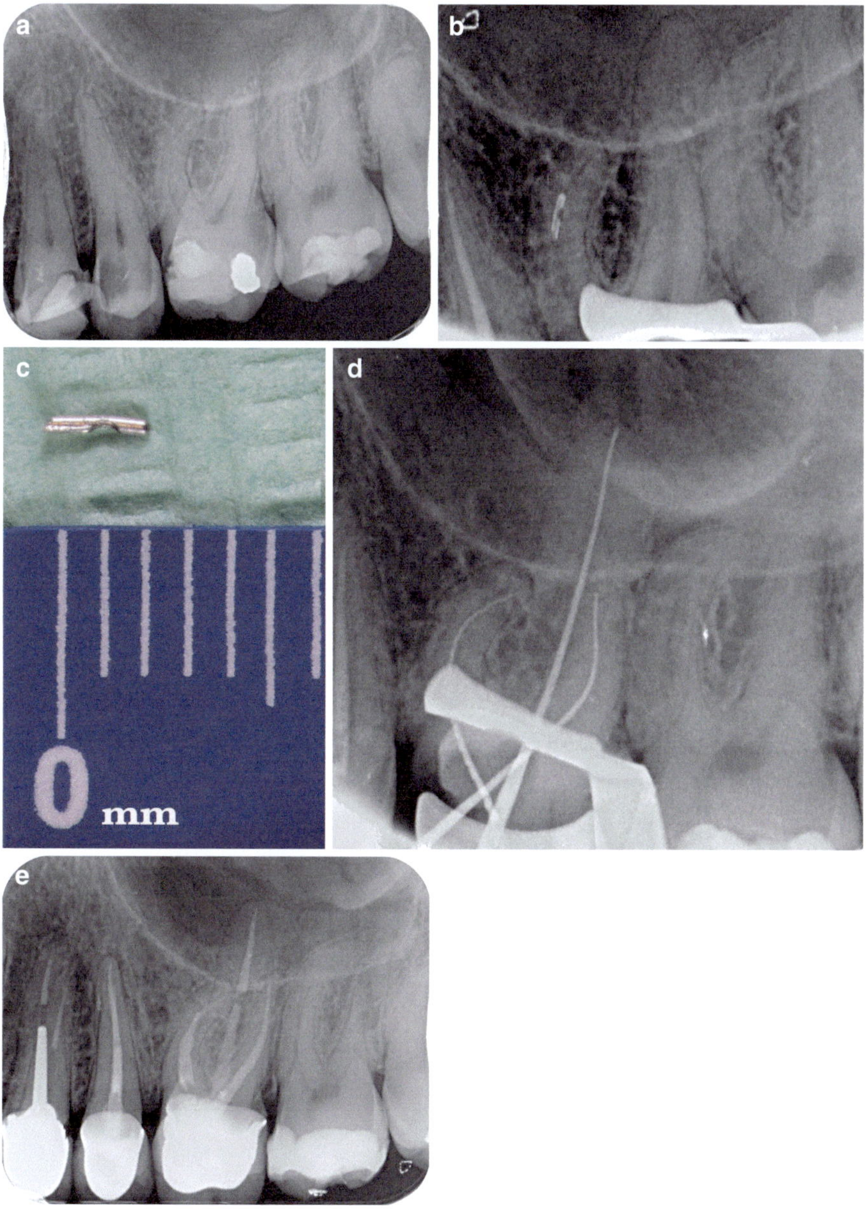

Fig. 4.11 (**a**) Preoperative radiograph of a left maxillary first molar. (**b**) Fragment of an irrigation needle in the mesiobuccal canal. (**c**) Removal of the fragment. (**d**) Working length determination radiograph. (**e**) Radiograph appearance after the completion of the RCT and the rehabilitation of the tooth (Courtesy of Dr. P. Mourouzis)

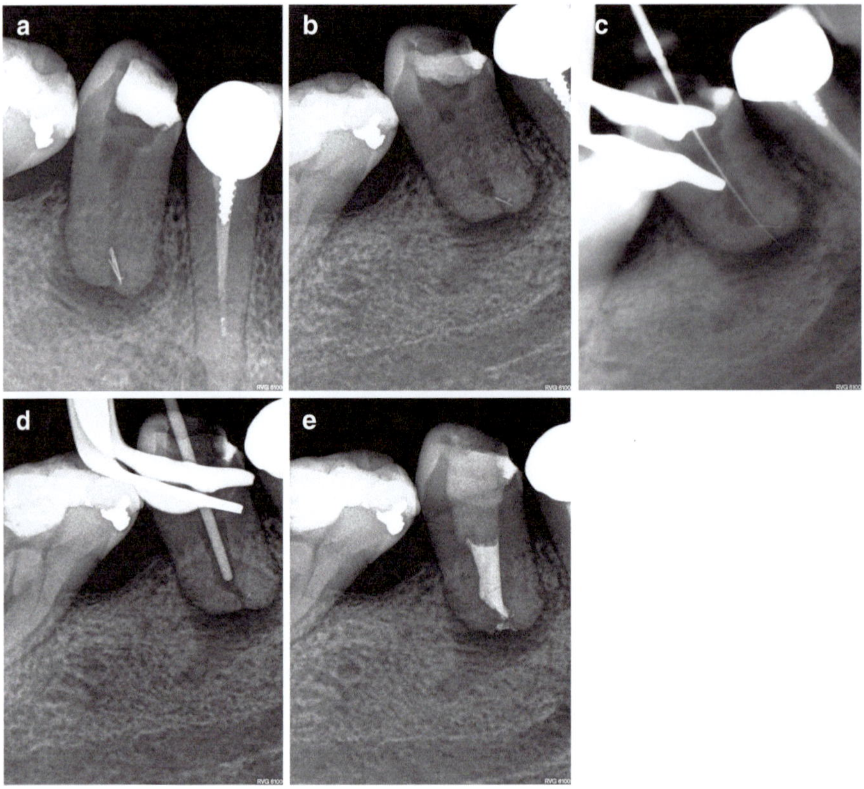

Fig. 4.12 (**a**) Preoperative radiograph showing three fractured instruments at the apical third of the root canal of a lower mandibular right second premolar tooth with a diagnosis of chronic apical periodontitis. (**b**) A staging platform was created around the most coronal aspects of the fragments by using modified Gates Glidden drills (sizes #2–4). Thereafter, an RT3 (EMS) ultrasonic tip was activated at low power settings, which trephined dentin in a counterclockwise motion around the fragments. With this action and the vibration being transmitted to the fragments, two of them began to loosen, and they were removed from the canal. (**c**) Working length determination radiograph showing one fragment inside the canal. (**d**) The third fragment, as it can be clearly seen in the master cone radiograph, was removed during copious irrigation in the course of root canal instrumentation. (**e**) Immediate post-obturation radiograph showing complete obturation of the root canal and temporary restoration with glass ionomer cement (Fuji II GC Corporation, Tokyo, Japan) and Cavit (Courtesy of Dr. T. Zarra)

4.3.5 Mechanical Means

Several mechanical approaches have been proposed for the retrieval of instrument fragments from the root canal (Table 4.3). They sometimes employ simple mechanical means such as the use of a magnet (Grossman 1974) in the expectation that it might "attract" the fragment or a barbed broach wrapped in cotton wool and introduced into the root canal in the hope that the broken piece will become enmeshed in the cotton and will thus be pulled out as the broach is withdrawn (Feldman et al.

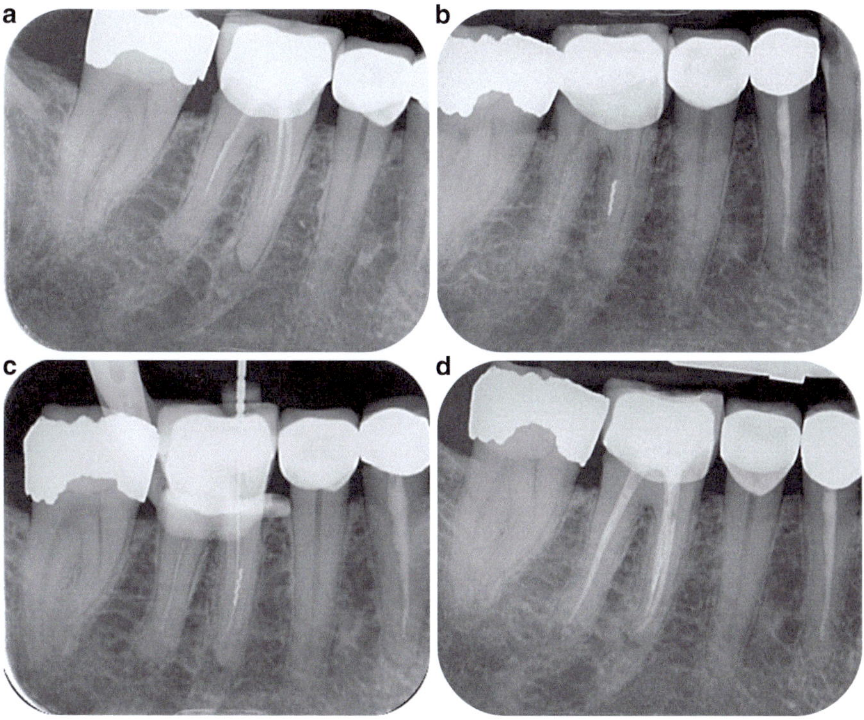

Fig. 4.13 (**a**) Preoperative radiograph. (**b**) Fragment at the middle third of the mesiolingual canal of a first mandibular molar. (**c**) Bypassing of the fragment. (**d**) Immediate post-obturation radiograph. The fragment can hardly be seen within the obturation material

1974; Stasinopoulos 1978). These two techniques and particularly the magnet have had very limited success in retrieving fragments. Furthermore, wrapped cotton wool on a barbed broach might be effective only when the fragment is loose in the straight portion of a canal.

The proposed mechanical means, regardless of how sophisticated they may be, all operate on the same basic principle, which is to *flare the canal coronal to the fragment, create space around it in order to free the fragment or at least its coronal segment, and at a second stage to retrieve it.*

Regardless of the mechanical removal means and technique or combination of techniques to be employed in all cases, there are certain common steps to be followed:

- A radiograph and in some cases more than one radiograph with different angulations are obtained to confirm the presence of the fragment, to reveal its location in relation to the root canal curvature, if present, and to estimate its size and length if unknown.
- The access cavity is redefined to allow better visualization and unobstructed manipulations.

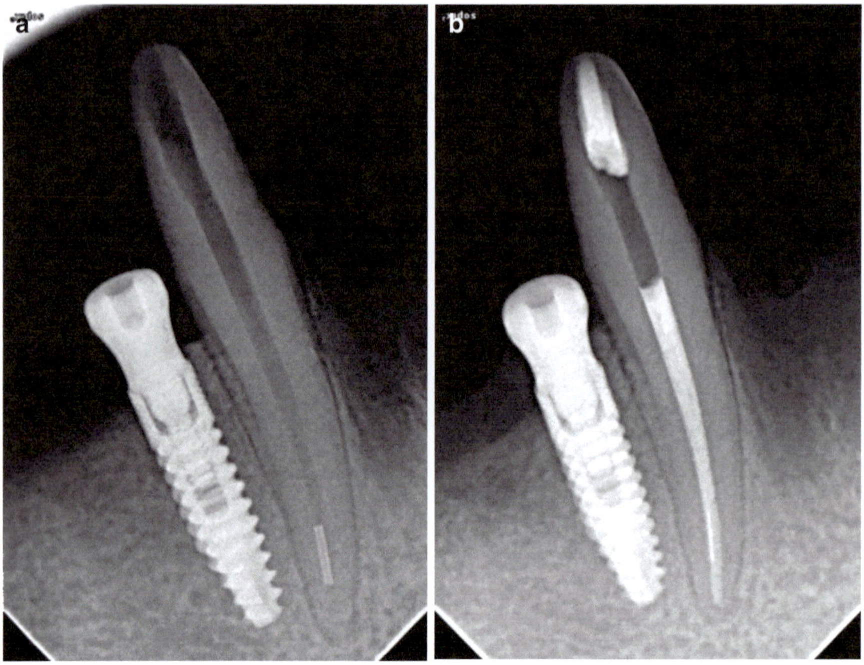

Fig. 4.14 (**a**) Fragment of the tip of a notched irrigation needle. (**b**) Bypassing the fragment and obturation of the root canal with the fragment in place (Courtesy of Dr. K. Kodonas)

- Cotton pellets are placed over other exposed orifices in multi-canal teeth to prevent dislodgment of the fragment into another root canal (see Chap. 7).
- Maintenance of constant vision during management efforts. The Stropko Irrigator (Fig. 4.18) (DCI Intl, Portland, OR) placed into a three-way syringe (DCI, Adec, Midmark, Vista, etc.) is particularly useful, but it is important to regulate the air pressure going into the three-way syringe. An SPR pressure regulator (www.stropko.com) can be utilized to reduce the airflow to between 2 and 7 psi (14–50 kPa) for a controlled precise delivery. This removes dentinal dust as it is created to maintain constant vision and ensure, even in depths of the root canal, a good drying action more effectively than paper points. Its proximal end is positioned into the three-way syringe, and its distal end has Luer Lock threads for securely attaching different length and gauged canuli. Its small tips do not impede visibility during use under the microscope. In addition to the good drying action achieved with the Stropko Irrigator, paper points are avoided and thus the risk of contamination if inadequately manipulated by the operator (Pessoa de Andrade et al. 2014) and of cellulose fiber shedding (Brown 2016) associated with their use. This shedding is of outmost importance as it is substantially documented that these cellulose fibers if inadvertently extruded beyond the foramen are associated with intense persistent periapical inflammation and treatment failure (Koppang et al. 1989; Nair et al. 1990; Sedgley and Messer 1993; Nair 2006) as they cannot be degraded by human body cells (Nair 2006).

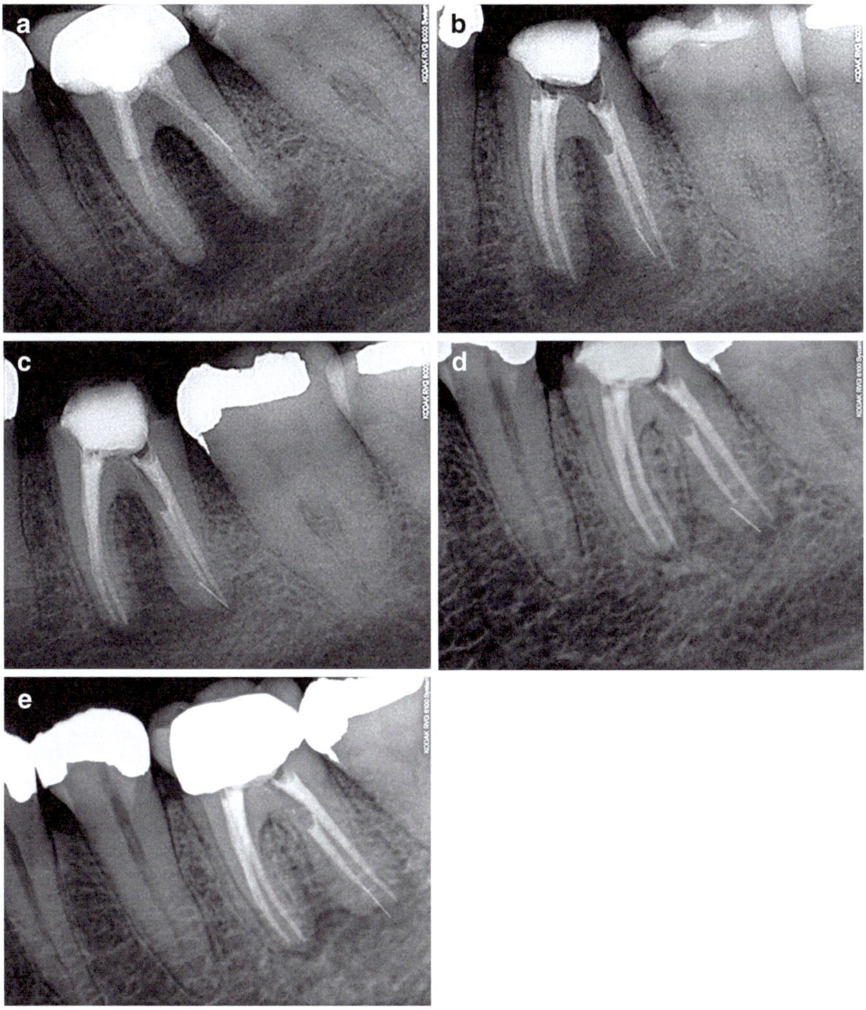

Fig. 4.15 (**a**) Preoperative radiograph of a crowned mandibular first molar with incomplete RCT and apical periodontitis. (**b**) Removal of the crown, fracture at the apical third of the distobuccal canal, of a 2 mm K-file which could not be bypassed and retrieved. This was followed eventually by instrumentation and obturation of this canal up to the fragment. (**c–e**) The scheduled recall clinical and radiographic follow-up at 3, 9, and 30 months, respectively, revealed uneventful healing

- Frequent working radiographs are mandatory to check the level of retrieval and amount of dentin loss. It must, however, always be kept in mind that radiographic evaluation of the residual dentin thickness during management efforts can be misleading because of the inherent inaccuracy of radiographic interpretation.
- Upon removal of the fragment, the canal is renegotiated with #6- to #10K-files to the apical foramen, and canal instrumentation and obturation follow. Instrumentation manipulations must be performed with caution, as the likelihood of another iatrogenic error in this clinical situation is very high.

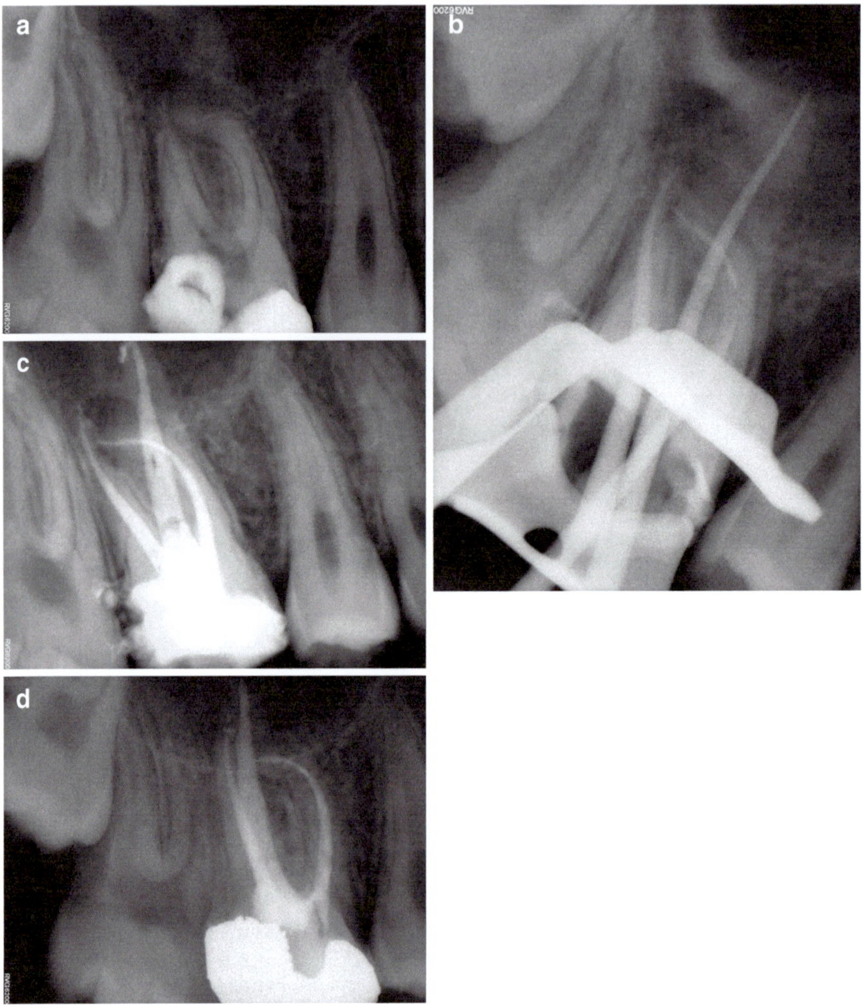

Fig. 4.16 (**a**) Preoperative radiograph. (**b**) Master cone radiograph. The fragment of the NiTi instrument can be seen at the apical third of the mesiobuccal canal. (**c**) Instrumentation and obturation up to the fragment. The fragment can hardly be identified at the immediate post-obturation radiograph. (**d**) Six-month recall radiograph (Courtesy of Dr. Ch. Beltes)

Prior to the detailed presentation of the proposed techniques, it should be noted that instrument fragments extending above the root canal orifice (Fig. 4.19) can usually be easily removed with a hemostatic forceps, Steiglitz forceps at 45° or 90° angles (Hu-Friedy), Peet silver point forceps (Silvermans, New York, NY), Endo Forceps (Roydent Dental Products, USA), Advanced Micro Endo Forceps 45° (Roydent Dental Products, USA), a Castroviejo needle holder, a Perry plier, ultrasonics, or even a spoon excavator. The micro alligator forceps commonly used by otolaryngologist can also be used.

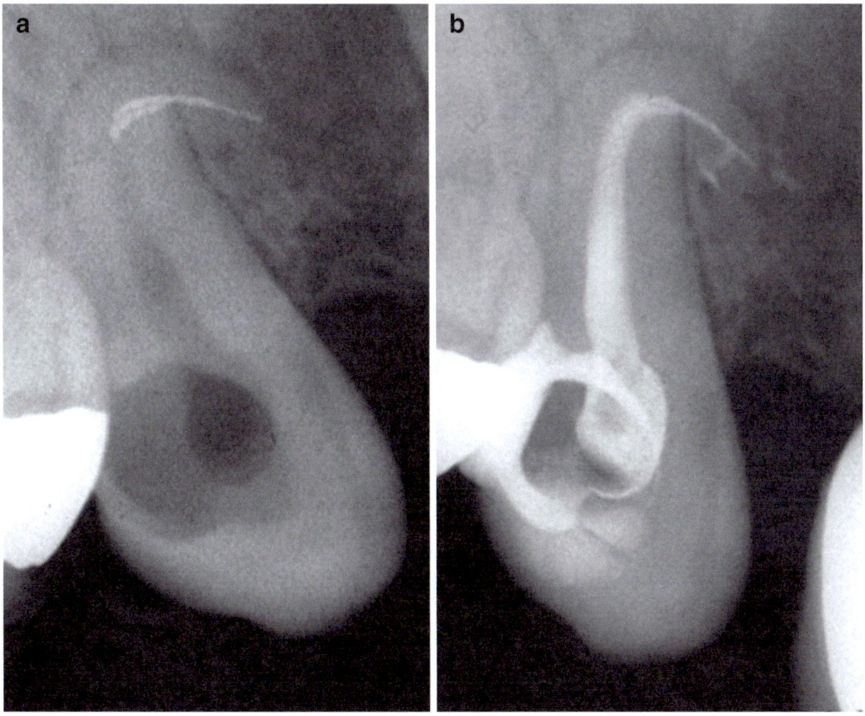

Fig. 4.17 (**a**) Two fragments of NiTi instruments at the apical third in a severely curved canal. (**b**) Instrumentation and obturation up to the fragments. Note that some sealer extruded through the apical and lateral foramina (Courtesy of Prof. P. Beltes)

4.3.6 Ultrasonics

Ultrasound is a sound energy with a frequency above the range of human hearing, which is 20 kHz. Ultrasonic vibration is currently the most widely used method for retrieving foreign objects from the root canal. The vast majority (98.5%) of endodontists practicing in the UK that responded to a questionnaire concerning their opinions and attitudes toward the intracanal fracture of endodontic instruments use ultrasonics (Madarati et al. 2008). Fragments of instruments, silver cones, or intraradicular posts (Krell and Neo 1985; Meidinger and Kabes 1985; Souyave et al. 1985; Stamos et al. 1985; Nagai et al. 1986; Jeng and ElDeeb 1987; Berbert et al. 1995; Nehme 1999; Tzanetakis et al. 2008; Cuje et al. 2010; Fu et al. 2011; Nevares et al. 2012) can be loosened by ultrasonics and then removed. It is obviously implied that the technique requires intimate contact of the vibrator tip with the metallic object to be retrieved. Initially hand files or spreaders were activated by ultrasonic devices to manage fractured instruments (Krell et al. 1984; Souyave et al. 1985; Nehme 1999). D'Arcangelo et al. (2000) reported two cases with successful removal of fragments using hand instrumentation with SS K-files and K-files mounted on the

Table 4.2 Recommended management of fractured instruments in permanent dentition based on the location of the fragment, the pulpal status, and the instrumentation stage when the fracture occurred

Location of the fragment		Management phase I	Pulpal status: Vital	Pulpal status: Non-vital	Instrumentation stage when fracture occurred: Early stage	Instrumentation stage when fracture occurred: Late stage	Management phase II
Fragment with one end protruding into the pulp chamber and the other into the r.c.[a]	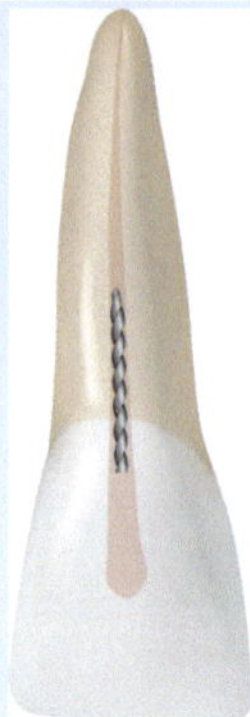	In all cases, retrieval of the fragment	(N/A)[b]	N/A	N/A	N/A	RCT
Fragment with both ends within the r.c.	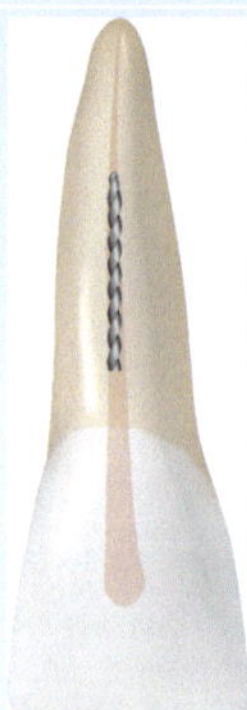 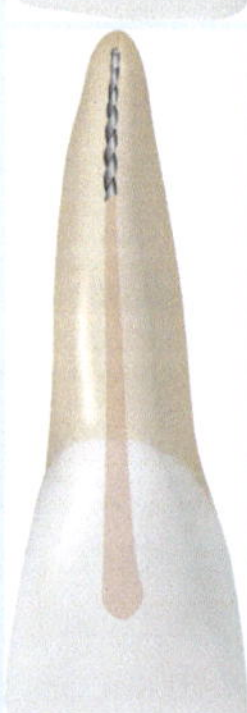	Retrieval	N/A	N/A	N/A	N/A	RCT
		Bypass	N/A	N/A	N/A	N/A	RCT. The fragment is incorporated in the filling material Follow-up[c]
		Failure to retrieve, bypass	+	–	+		Instrumentation and obturation up to the fragment Follow-up[c]
			+	–	–	+	
				+	+		
				+		+	

Table 4.2 (continued)

Fragment with its tip extending into the periapical area	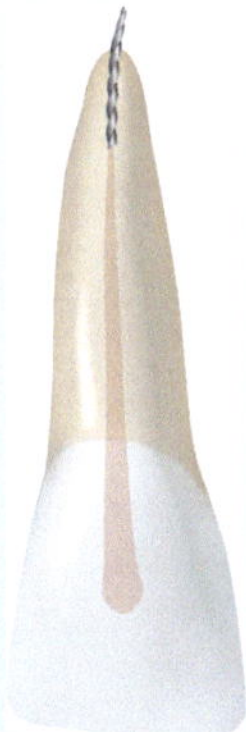	Retrieval	N/A	N/A	N/A	N/A	RCT
		Bypass	+		+		RCT. The intracanal segment of the fragment is incorporated in the filling material Follow-up[c]
			+			+	
				+	+		
				+		+	
		Failure to retrieve, bypass	+		+		Instrumentation and obturation up to the fragment Follow-up
			+			+	
				+	+		
				+		+	
Fragment extending from the pulp chamber to the periapex	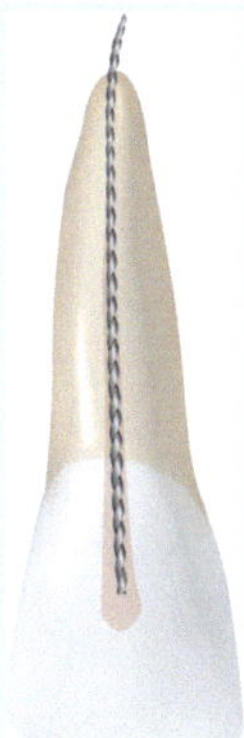	Retrieval	N/A	N/A	N/A	N/A	RCT
		Bypass	N/A	N/A	N/A	N/A	RCT. The intracanal segment of the fragment is incorporated in the filling material Follow-up[c]
		Failure to retrieve, bypass	N/A	N/A	N/A	N/A	Surgical endodontics
Fragment lodged outside the r.c.	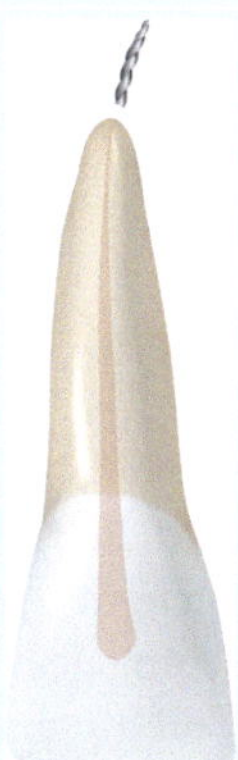	In all cases	N/A	N/A	N/A	NA	RCT Follow-up[c]

[a]*r.c.* root canal

[b]Not applicable

[c]Evidently, in all cases where the fragment remains in the root canal, follow-up is essential. This is particularly important in cases of RCT of teeth with necrotic pulp where the likelihood of surgical treatment is increased and is directly related to the instrumentation stage and technique used when instrument fracture occurred. To a large extent, this reflects the sterility of the root canal apical to the fragment. The timing and type of surgical procedure are determined by a multiplicity of factors (see "Surgical Endodontics" in this chapter)

Table 4.3 Means and techniques proposed for retrieval of instrument fragments from the root canal

Means	Techniques		
Chemical			
Mechanical means	Technique using ultrasounds		
	Endosonic filing		
	The file bypass technique		
	Holding techniques	The Masserann technique	
		The Feldman and coauthors technique	
		The Meitrac Endo Safety System	
		The Instrument Removal System (IRS)	
		The Endo Rescue	
		The Endo Extractor System	
	Tube techniques	The Endo Extractor	
		The Cancellier Extractor Kit	
		Hypodermic surgical needle	With cyanoacrylate
			With Hedstroem file
		The separated instrument removal system	
		The Micro-Retrieve & Repair System	
	Mounce extractors		
	Canal Finder System technique		
	Micro-forceps grasping technique		
	Wire loop technique		
Gutta-percha	Softened gutta-percha technique		
Multisonic Ultracleaning	Multisonic Ultracleaning System		
Electrolysis	Electrolytic technique		
Laser	Laser-assisted removal of fractured instruments		

handpiece of an ultrasonic device. In one of them, four fragments were removed. Currently most ultrasonic companies have tips specifically designed to remove fractured instruments (Fig. 4.20). Therefore, a selection of specially designed ultrasonic tips is available. They have a contra-angled design with alloy tips manufactured from a range of metal alloys, such as SS and titanium alloys, and can be coated with an abrasive such as diamond or zirconium nitride in order to increase the cutting efficiency of the tip. Tips are available in different angles, lengths, and sizes to enable use in various parts of the root canals. As a general rule, the deeper the fragment is located in the canal, the longer and thinner the ultrasonic tip that should be used. These long, thin tips must be used at very low power settings to prevent tip breakage.

Tips should be carefully chosen. Clinicians choose tips in accordance with the ultrasonic scaler they use. This is because the resonance frequency of the tips must match the working frequency of the devices. Obviously, this applies with respect to

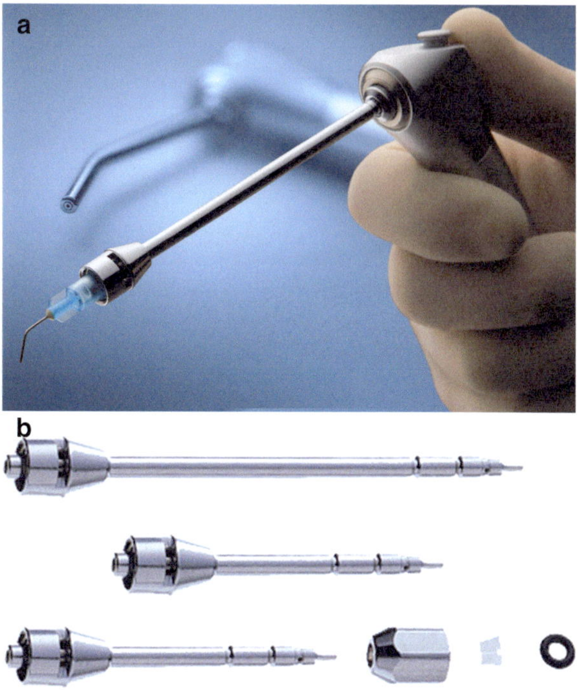

Fig. 4.18 (**a**) The Stropko Irrigator. (**b**) Stropko Irrigator (XL length, 3.5 in), Stropko Irrigator (original size, 2 in), and Stropko Irrigator Adapter (for older syringes)

devices of the same brand. Lack of compatibility will lead to tip fracture. To our knowledge, there is only one study on resonance compatibility between endodontic ultrasonic (endosonic) tips for fractured instrument removal and ultrasonic devices of different brands (Shiyakov and Vasileva 2014). The authors of this study concluded that combinations of different brands of instruments and ultrasonic devices are possible but information regarding resonance compatibility should be carefully checked.

In cases where the specific tips are not available, ultrasonic energy may be transmitted through the largest hand file reaching the fragment, an endodontic explorer or spreader, as proposed in earlier periods (Krell et al. 1984; Souyave et al. 1985; Nehme 1999).

The ultrasonic units currently available in dentistry are of two basic types with different action mechanisms. These are (Fig. 4.21):

- Magnetostrictive. Magnetostriction converts electromagnetic energy into mechanical energy.
- Piezoelectric. These are based on the piezoelectric principle, in which a crystal is used that changes dimension when an electrical charge is applied (Plotino et al. 2007). Deformation of this crystal is converted into mechanical oscillation without producing heat (Stock 1991).

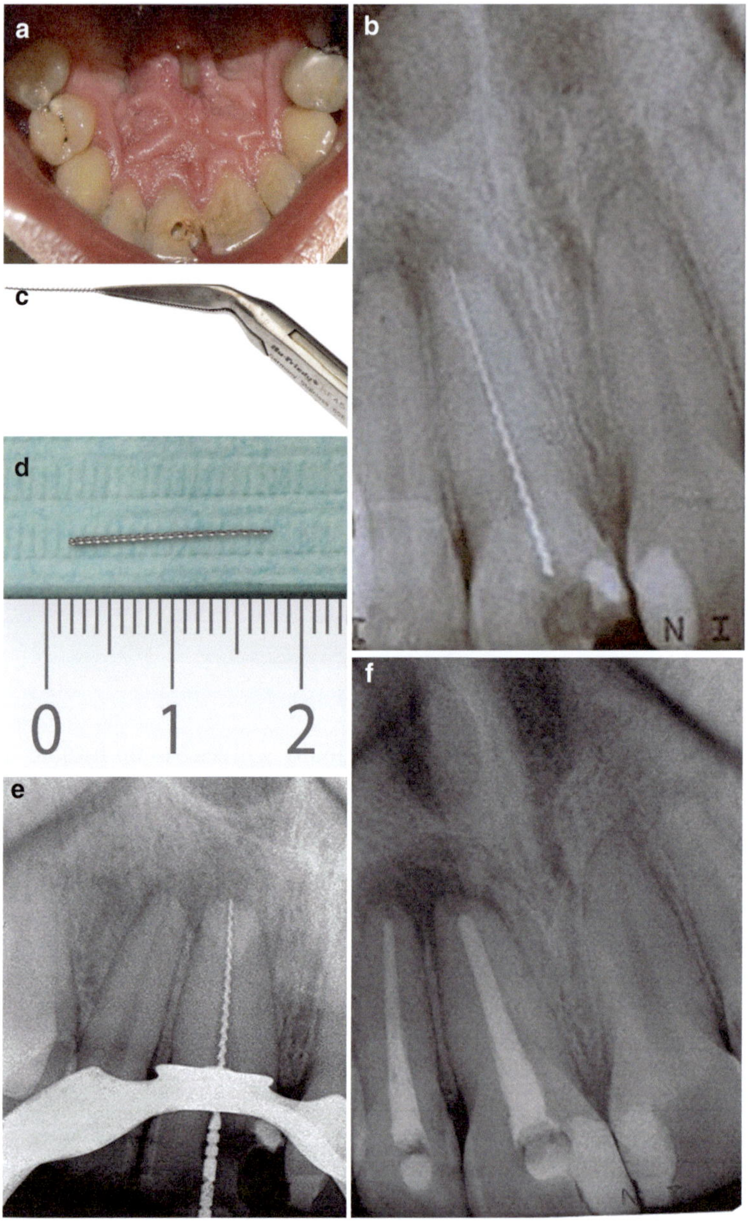

Fig. 4.19 (**a**, **b**) Clinical and radiographic examination revealed access cavity with no temporary filling in the right maxillary central incisor and a fragment of an endodontic instrument extending from the coronal orifice to the apex “covering” approximately the whole length of the root canal. The treating dentist left the access cavity unsealed and invited his patient to “clean” the canal with an instrument he had given her nearly a year before when she began treatment with him. She had fractured the instrument within the canal 3 months earlier, and since then, she had started taking antibiotics repeatedly (amoxicillin 625 mg ×3) for 4 days each time. (**c**, **d**) The fragment was retrieved with forceps. (**e**, **f**) Instrumentation, calcium hydroxide dressing for 10 days, and obturation of the root canal with the cold lateral compaction technique of gutta-percha and 811 sealer (Roth International Ltd., Chicago, IL, USA) followed (Courtesy of Dr. M. Kasambali)

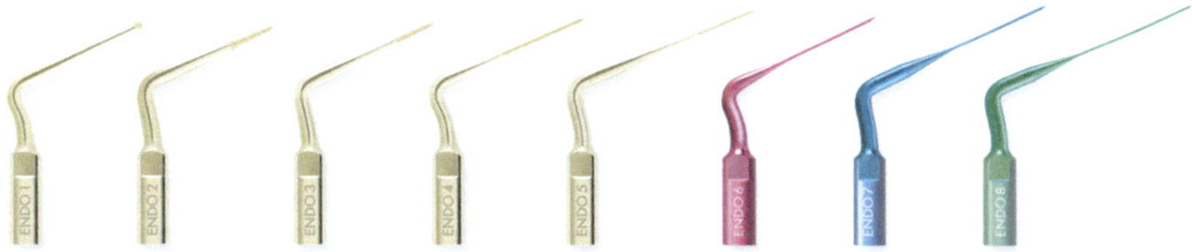

Fig. 4.20 ProUltra ENDO Tips (Dentsply Tulsa Dental, Tulsa, OK). The 1–5 Ultrasonic Endo Tips are zirconium nitride coated to harden them and improve clinical performance. These tips are designed for the removal of dentin and restorative materials along the lateral sides of the instruments. The ProUltra ENDO 6–8 have increased strength due to their titanium alloy construction and can be used to the full length of the root canal due to their longer lengths and smaller diameter

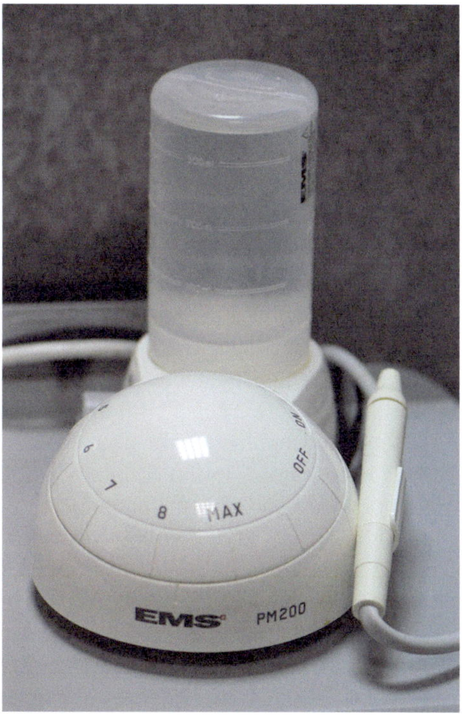

Fig. 4.21 Ultrasonic unit

Both types are clinically well accepted in dentistry. The piezoelectric type of ultrasonics is better suited to endodontic applications (Plotino et al. 2007). They offer more cycles per second, 40 versus 24 kHz, while the tips of these units work in a linear back-and-forth, "pistonlike" motion (Plotino et al. 2007). This movement is ideal for endodontics. This is particularly evident when removing posts and fractured instruments.

The stages that should be followed are (Fig.4.22):

- Instrumentation of the root canal up to the fragment. Under direct microscopic vision, circumferential staging platform around the most coronal aspect of the fragment is prepared with modified (blunted) pre-selected #2–#4 Gates Glidden bur (Fig. 4.23) used in a crown-down fashion as described by Ruddle (2004). The maximum cross-sectional diameter of the pre-selected Gates Glidden bur must be slightly larger than the diameter of the fragment at its coronal aspect. Therefore, familiarization with the sizes of Gates Glidden burs is essential (Table 4.4). The modified Gates Glidden bur is carried into the pre-enlarged canal, rotated at a reduced speed of approximately 300 rpm, and directed apically until it makes light contact with the most coronal aspect of the fractured instrument. The platform is kept centered to allow better visualization of the fragment and the surrounding dentin root canal walls; therefore, equal amounts of dentin around the fragment are preserved, minimizing the risk of root perforation. Similarly modified LightSpeed NiTi rotary instrument (Lightspeed Technology Inc., San Antonio, TX) can be used. In a comparative study, it was found that the staging platform created with the latter was more centered in curved canals than the one created by Gates Glidden burs (Iqbal et al. 2006).
- Copious irrigation to remove all debris and dentin chips. This is followed by thorough drying of the canal to facilitate excellent vision with the microscope prior to beginning ultrasonic procedures.
- The pre-selected ultrasonic tip with the appropriate length to reach the fragment and a diameter that allows it to passively fit into the previously shaped canal is placed between the exposed coronal end of the fragment and the canal wall, in intimate contact with the fragment. It is then activated at lower power settings, to trephine dentin around the fragment in a counterclockwise motion. This is continued until a couple of millimeters of the coronal end of the fragment is freed and/or some movement of the fragment is noted (Fig. 4.24). Care must be exercised at this point to touch the fragment as little as possible and avoid removing a lot of dentin from the inner, less thick canal wall. Diamond-coated tips should be avoided for this troughing phase as they are very aggressive and may remove too much of the dentin wall. Occasionally the unscrewing force thus created might dislodge the fragment, which "jumps out" of the canal (Figs. 4.25 and 4.26). In cases of fragments in long roots with limited access and slender root morphology, titanium ultrasonic tips may be used. These are longer with smaller diameters, compared to the abrasively coated instruments. Also they are flexible, can cut only at their tip, and provide a smooth, less aggressive, cutting action that promotes safety when trephining deeper within a root canal. Blind trephining of dentin even with them must be avoided as it may cause iatrogenic errors.

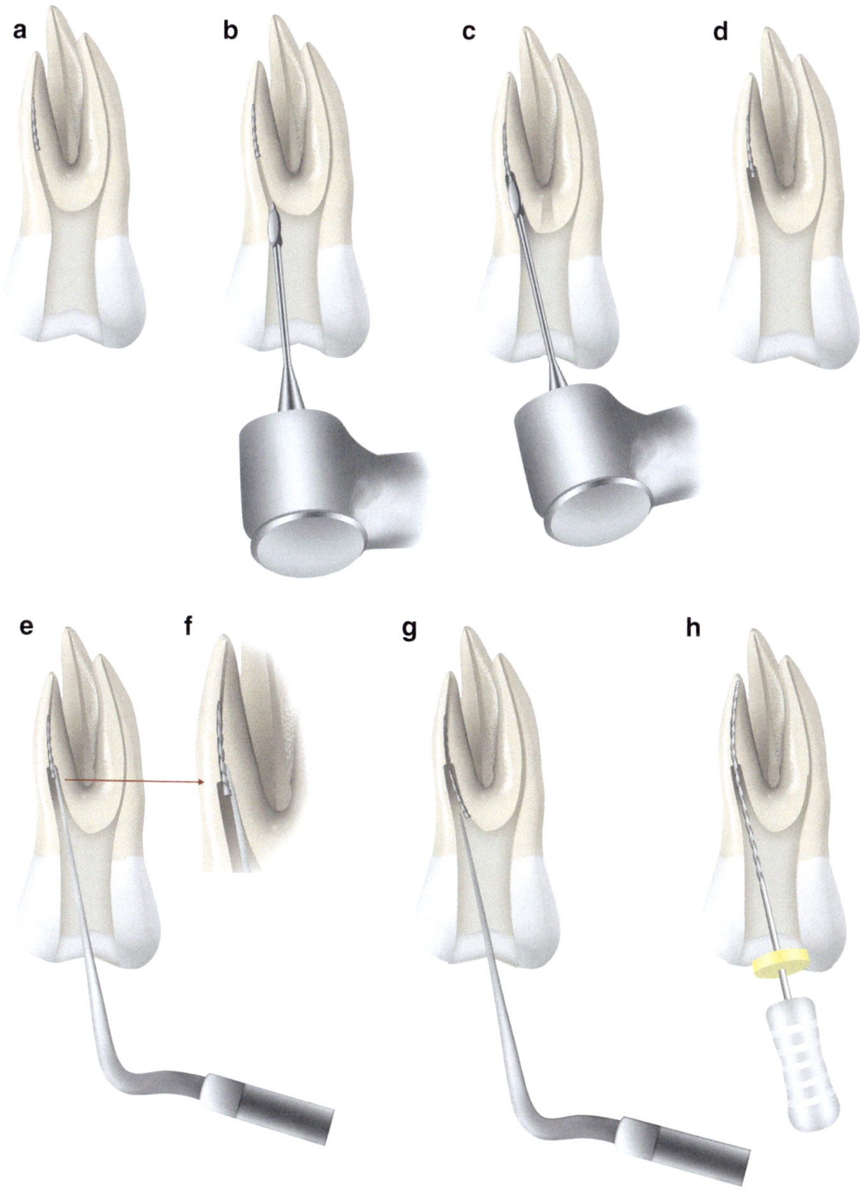

Fig. 4.22 (**a–h**) Schematic illustration of fragment retrieval with ultrasonics. (**a**) Radiographic confirmation of the presence of a fragment and recognition of its location, size, and length. (**b–d**) Instrumentation of the root canal up to the fragment and creation of a staging platform with modified Gates Glidden bur. (**e**, **f**) Exposure of the coronal segment of the fragment with dry ultrasonic troughing around the fragment with the ultrasonic tip activated at lower power settings. (**g**) Ultrasonic vibration and removal of the fragment. (**h**) Once the fragment is removed, the canal is renegotiated with an ISO size #10K-file to the apical foramen, and canal instrumentation follows

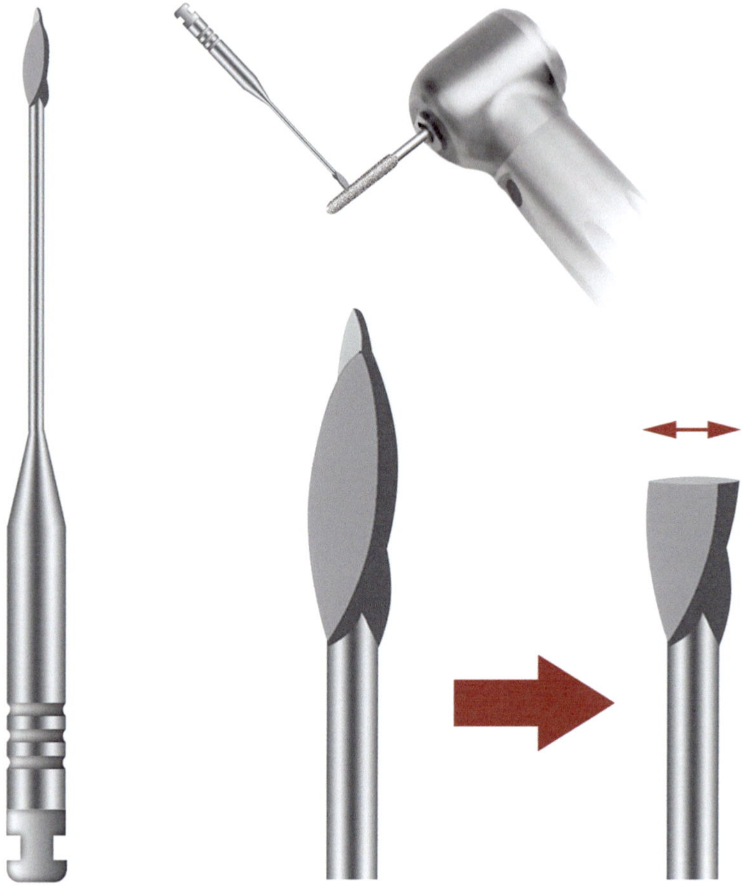

Fig. 4.23 Modified Gates Glidden bur**.** Grinding or sectioning of the non-cutting tip perpendicular to their long axis at their maximum cross-sectional diameter transforms this end into a very efficient cutting tip. Therefore, modified Gates Glidden bur must be used with great care and preferably under direct microscopic vision

Table 4.4 Sizes of Gates Glidden burs

Gates Glidden bur	Size (mm)
#1	0.50
#2	0.70
#3	0.90
#4	1.10
#5	1.30
#6	1.50

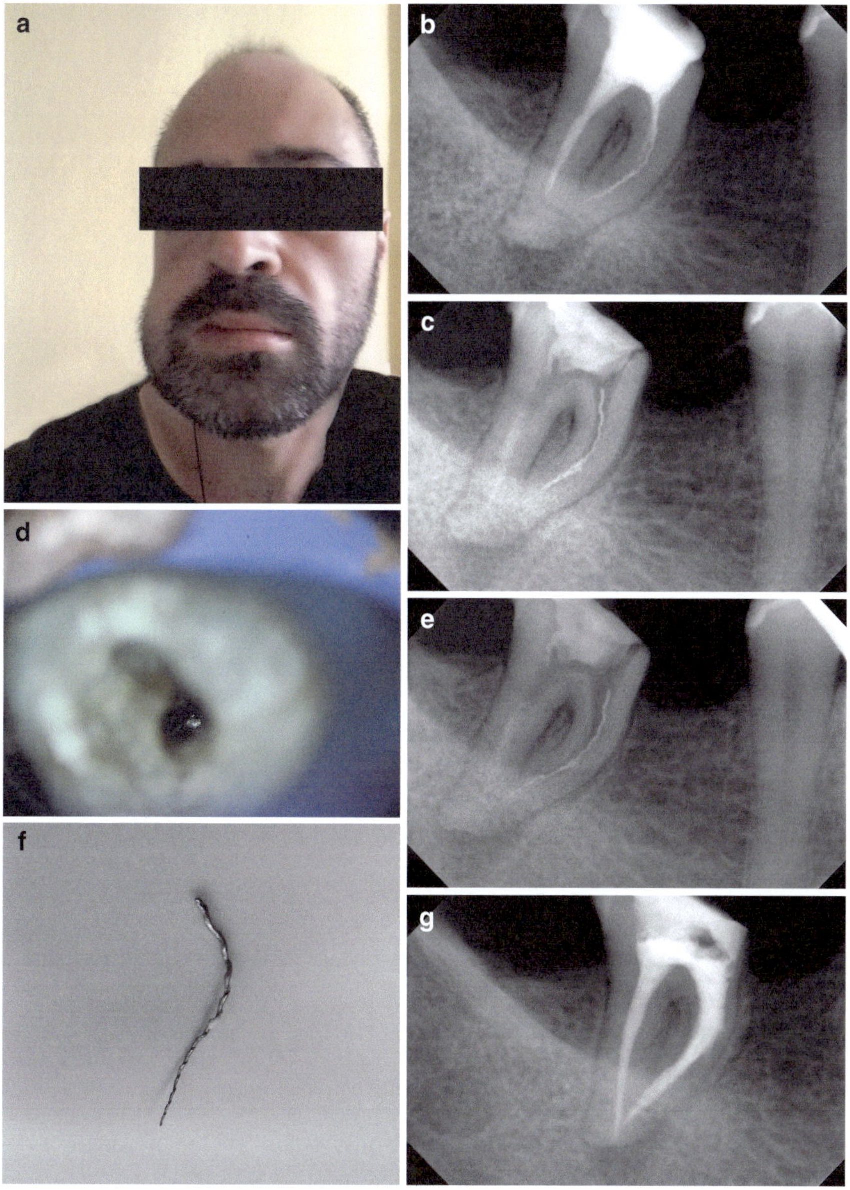

Fig. 4.24 (**a**) Clinical picture of a hospitalized patient with extensive swelling, mild to severe pain, high fever, lymphadenopathy, and nausea. (**b**) Preoperative radiograph of a lower second mandibular molar with an incomplete RCT, an apical periodontitis, and a long SS fragment in the mesial root. (**c**) Preparation of staging platform and exposure of more than 3 mm of the coronal segment of the fragment with modified Gates Glidden burs (#2–#4) and ultrasonic tips (RT3, EMS). Despite this exposure, the fragment could not be retrieved, so it was bypassed, and more preexisting obturating material was removed. (**d**) Fragment as seen through the dental operating microscope. (**e**, **f**) The fragment was eventually retrieved with an RT3 tip (EMS) activated at lower power settings. (**g**) Canals were instrumented and obturated with gutta-percha and Roth 811 sealer (Roth International Ltd., Chicago, IL, USA) with the lateral compaction technique. (**h**) Clinical picture of the patient on the day of the root canal obturation

Fig. 4.24 (continued)

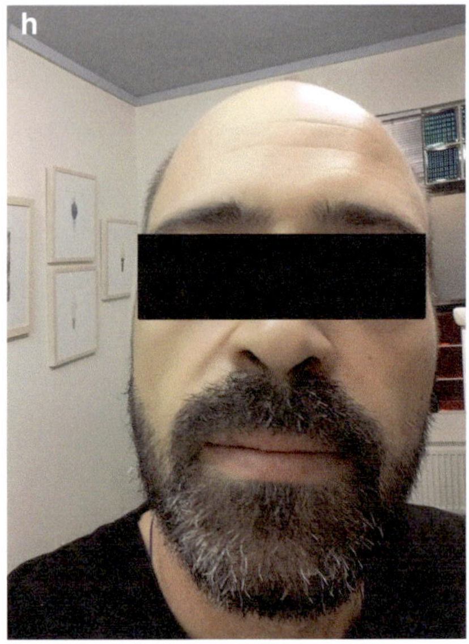

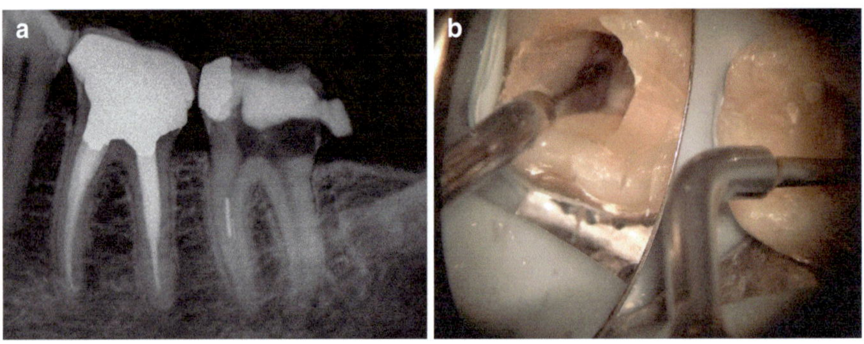

Fig. 4.25 (**a**) Preoperative radiograph of a mandibular second left molar with a fragment at the middle third of the mesiobuccal canal. (**b**) Preparation of a staging platform around the most coronal segment of the fragment with modified Gates Glidden burs (#2–#4) and ultrasonic tips (RT3, EMS) until the fragment was visible with the aid of the dental operating microscope. (**c**, **d**) The platform was kept centered, and the ultrasonic tip trephined dentin in a counterclockwise motion around the fragment until the latter began to loosen and eventually "jumped" out of the canal. (**e**) The canals were then routinely prepared and obturated with warm vertical compaction of gutta-percha and AH26 (Dentsply DeTrey GmbH, Konstanz, Germany) sealer (Courtesy of Dr. G. Dehouniotis)

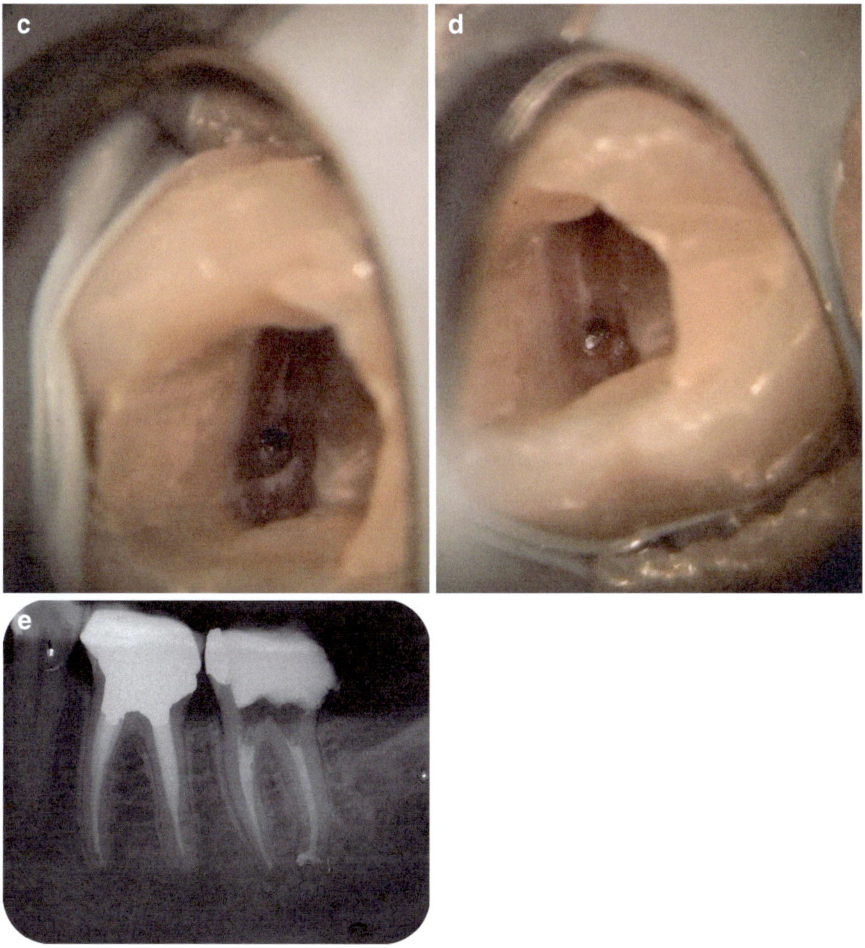

Fig. 4.25 (continued)

When trying to remove a file that has a left-handed thread, the direction would be clockwise. It is crucial to avoid unnecessary stress on the ultrasonic tip in order to prevent its fracture (Fig. 4.27). All ultrasonic work inside the root canal is conducted in a dry environment, so the clinician has continuous visualization with the microscope of the energized tip and the fragment. Blind trephining of dentin may lead to undesirable complications. The Stropko Irrigator utilized by the dental assistant is particularly useful during ultrasonic use to collimate and direct a continuous stream of air and blow out dentinal dust.

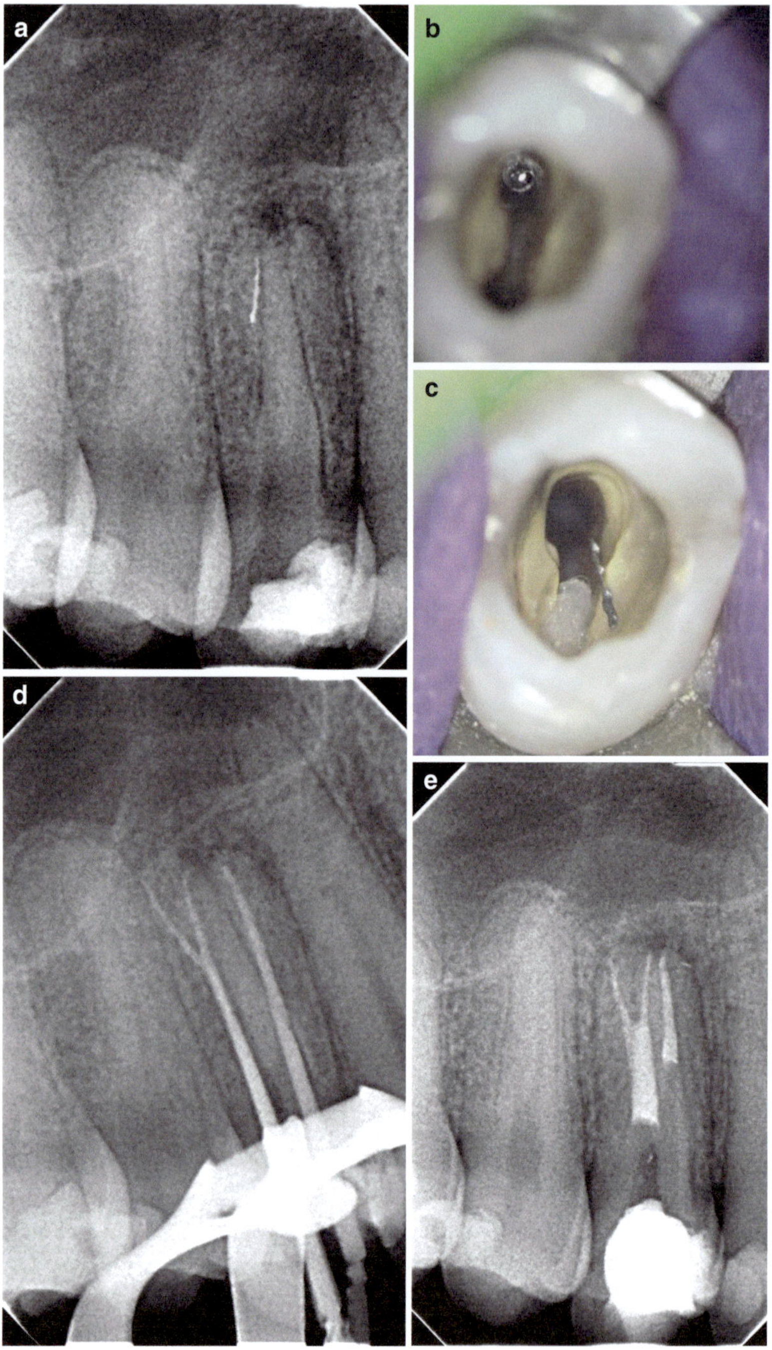

Fig. 4.26 (**a**) Immediate preoperative radiograph. (**b**) Operative microscope photography after staging platform creation and exposure of the coronal end of the fragment. (**c**) Fragment in the pulp chamber as seen through the dental operating microscope. Note the cotton pellet in orifice of the palatal canal. (**d**) Master gutta-percha cone radiograph. (**e**) Immediate postoperative radiograph (Courtesy of Dr. K. Kalogeropoulos)

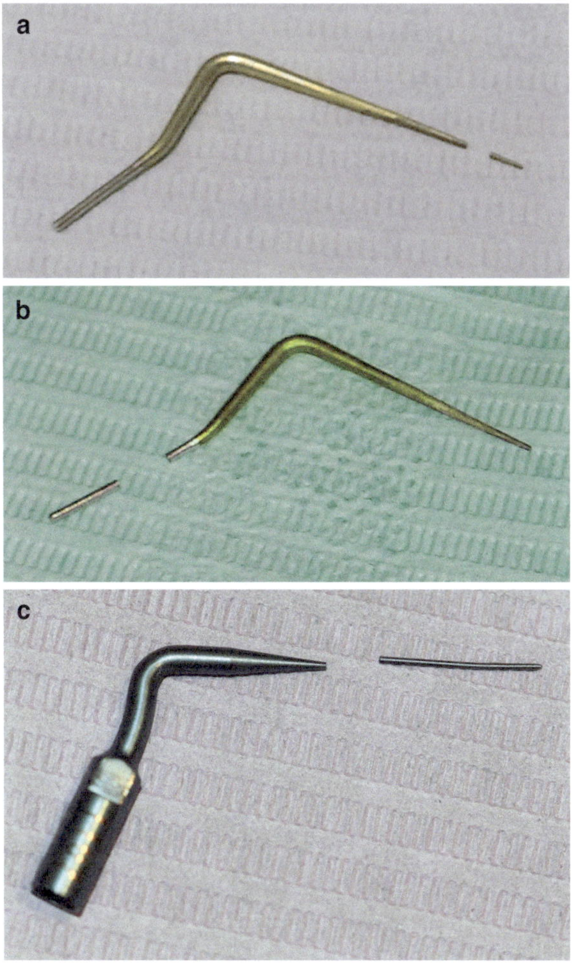

Fig. 4.27 Fractured ultrasonic tips. (**a**) Fracture of RT3 (EMS) at its tip. (**b**) Fracture of RT3 (EMS) at its shank. (**c**) Fracture of ProUltra Endo Titanium Tip

NiTi and SS instruments respond differently to ultrasonic vibration. SS fragments absorb the ultrasonic energy bodily and will show movement early on (Cohen et al. 2005). NiTi instruments are brittle and often break up into fragments (Fig. 4.28) when subjected to direct ultrasonic energy, particularly if the fragment is tightly locked. This renders the procedure considerably more difficult. Heat-generated and cyclic fatigue created by high-frequency waves of the ultrasonic tip transferring to the fragment could be contributing factors to secondary fracture (Terauchi et al. 2013). Secondary fracture of fragments appeared to be reduced when the ultrasonic tip was applied to the inner curvature of the canal (Terauchi et al. 2013).

If the fragment cannot be retrieved but is loosened and completely bypassed, vibration can be transmitted through a hand SS K-file introduced alongside the

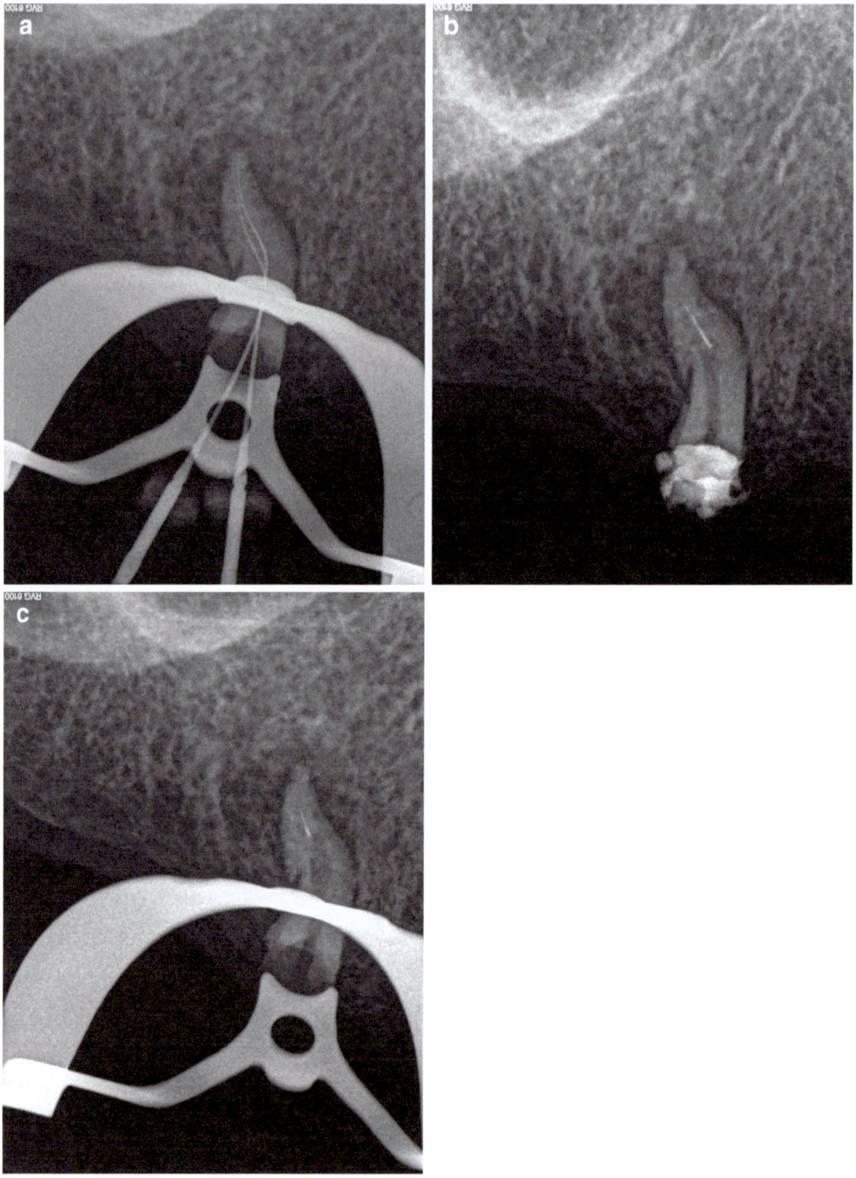

Fig. 4.28 Secondary breakage of NiTi fragment. (**a**) Working length radiograph. (**b**) Staging platform and exposure of approximately 1–2 mm of the coronal end of the NiTi fragment. (**c**) Secondary fracture of the initial fragment following the use of an RT3 tip (EMS) at a low power setting

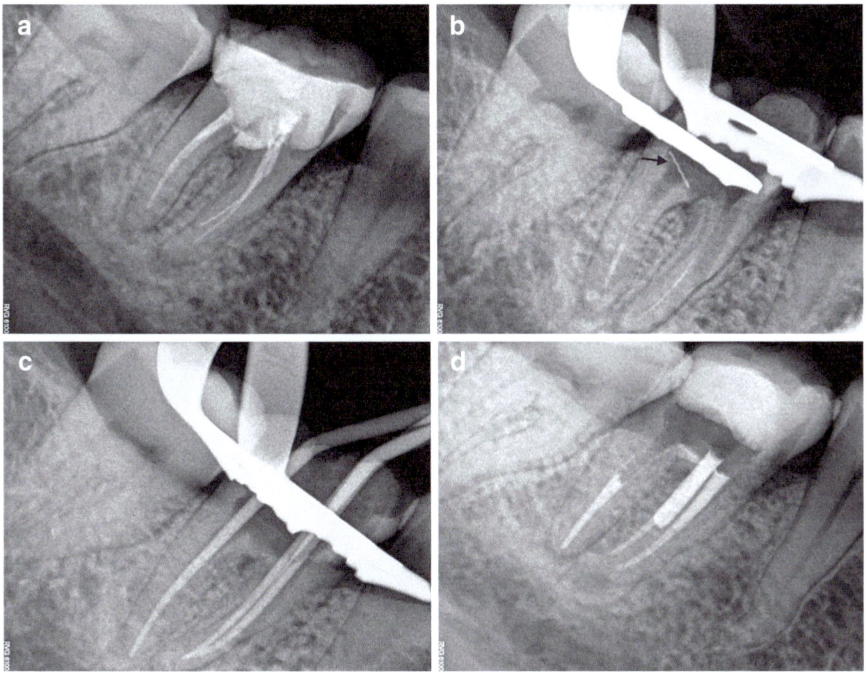

Fig. 4.29 (**a**) Preoperative radiograph showing a fractured instrument at the apical third of the mesiobuccal root canal of tooth #46 with a diagnosis of chronic apical periodontitis. (**b**) A staging platform was created around the most coronal aspects of the fragments by using modified Gates Glidden drills (#2–4). Thereafter, an RT3 (EMS) ultrasonic tip was activated at low power settings, which trephined dentin in a counterclockwise motion around the fragments. With this action and the vibration being transmitted to the fragments, the fragment began to loosen. At this stage, it was bypassed with size #10 up to size -25K-files and "washed out" (*arrow*) to the floor of the pulp chamber with the irrigant. (**c**) Master cone radiograph. (**d**) Final radiograph showing complete obturation of the root canal and temporary restoration with a cotton pellet and Cavit (Courtesy of Dr. T. Zarra)

space pre-created with hand files between the fragment and the dentin wall. This vibration, at lower power settings, of the K-file further loosens the fragment, which can eventually be washed out with the irrigant (Figs. 4.29 and 4.30). Care must be exercised to activate ultrasonically K-file(s) thinner than the last hand file used to bypass the fragment. An Ultrasonic Endo File Adapter (Fig. 4.31) needs to be threaded onto the ultrasonic handpiece so that its chuck will grasp the 0.02 SS K-file by tightening the nut with the wrench provided. It must be emphasized that K-files for the ultrasonic unit are more cost-effective and less aggressive and could be pre-bent more easily than ultrasonic tips.

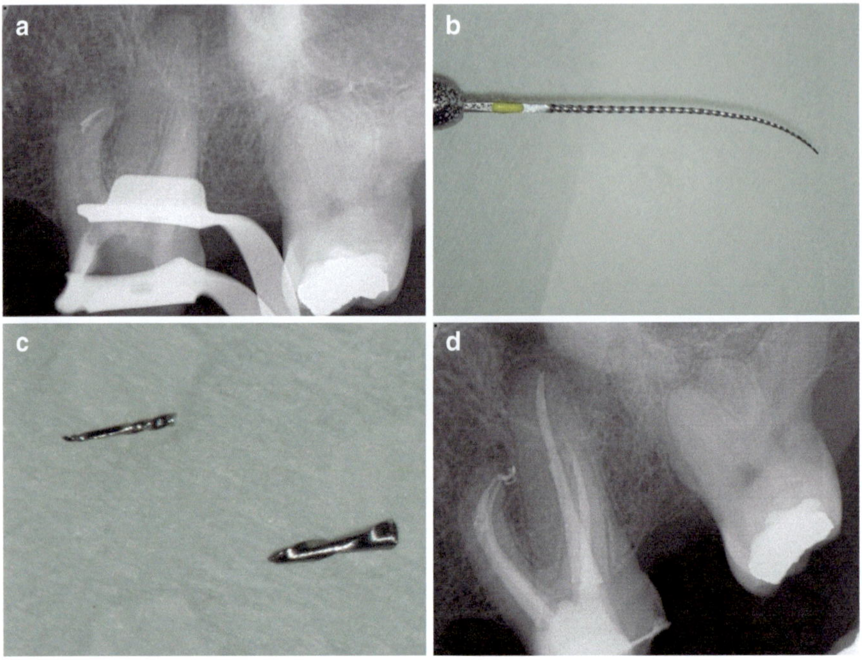

Fig. 4.30 (**a**) Preoperative radiograph showing two instrument fragments at the apical third of the mesiobuccal root canal of left maxillary first molar not visible with the operative microscope. (**b**, **c**) After coronal pre-flaring, the fragments were released and removed blindly with the U-files activated at low power settings, at the internal curvature. (**d**) Final radiograph showing complete obturation of the root canals and adhesive restoration of the access cavity with flowable composite (Courtesy of Dr. M. Leineweber)

4.3.7 Endosonic Filing

With this method proposed in the 1980s (Souyave et al. 1985; Nagai et al. 1986), the steps to be followed are:

- An endosonic file #15 or #20, attached to the handpiece and monitored under the dental operating microscope, is inserted into the root canal up to the coronal end of the fragment and energized ultrasonically to create a trough around this end of the fragment.
- A small K-file, pre-curved at its tip, is then gently pushed down to bypass the fragment.
- When the fragment can be bypassed at least to its midpoint, it may be dislodged by simultaneous irrigation and agitation with the endosonic file. A low power setting is used initially, but this can be adjusted upward depending on the fragment.

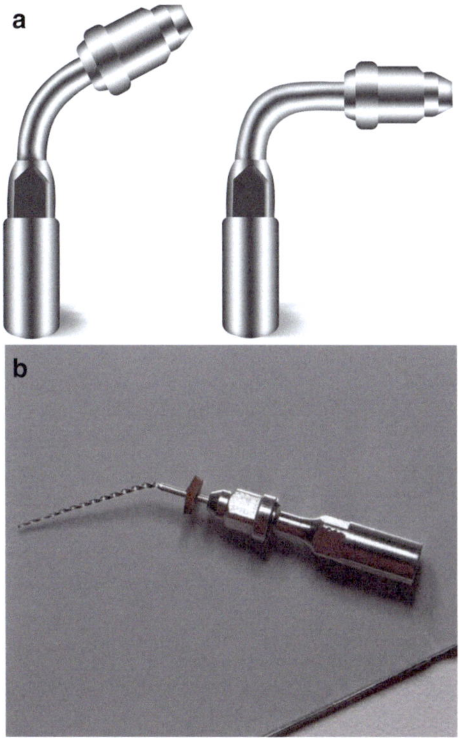

Fig. 4.31 The Ultrasonic Endo File Adapter manufactured under a variety of names and brands has been designed to function on most brands of piezoelectric-type dental ultrasonic scalers. It accepts SS or NiTi files that are between sizes 15 and 40 after the handle or latch hub has been removed

4.3.8 The File Bypass Technique

This technique does not require any special or sophisticated instrument. It utilizes endodontic instruments available in all dental practices. In this technique, an effort is made to establish patency to the apical foramen bypassing the fragment and subsequently, when the access of the instruments up to the apex is ensured, to try to retrieve the fragment by a filing motion. It is a technically challenging procedure, depending solely on the tactile sensitivity and sheer perseverance of the practitioner. The likelihood of creating another iatrogenic error such as fracture of a second file, ledge formation, perforation, or transportation is very high, and thus the whole procedure must be performed with great caution.

For this purpose (Fig. 4.32):

- The root canal is instrumented up to the fragment. Straight-line access and visualization of the coronal aspect of the instrument should be tried whenever possible.
- Copious irrigation follows to remove as much residual tissue and debris as possible.

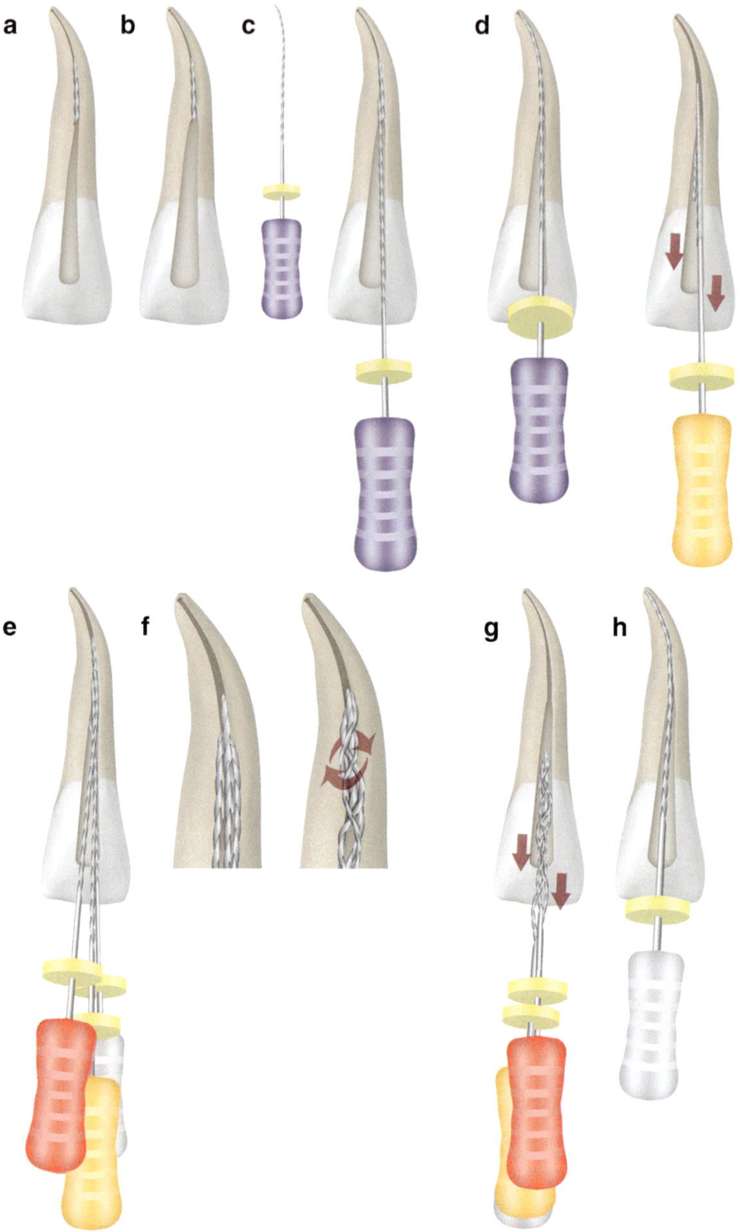

Fig. 4.32 (**a–h**) Schematic illustration of instrument fragment retrieval with the file bypass technique. (**a**) Radiographic confirmation of the presence of a fragment and recognition of its location, size, and length. (**b**) Instrumentation of the root canal up to the fragment. (**c**) Efforts to bypass it with a pre-curved size #8K-File. (**d**) After bypassing, filing continues with larger-sized instruments trying to "engage" the fragment in their flutes and to retrieve it. (**e–g**) Sometimes engagement and retrieval of the fragment are facilitated with the simultaneous insertion (braiding technique) of two and occasionally more instruments in the root canal, preferably Hedstroem files. (**h**) Once the fragment is removed, the canal is renegotiated with an ISO size 10K-file to the apical foramen, and canal instrumentation follows

- The instrumented part of the canal is flooded with EDTA to be carried with the small instrument to follow and soften root dentin.
- A small sharp bent is made to a fine hand K-file (ISO 6 or 8 and maximum 10) either with a cotton plier (Fig. 4.33) or with the SS Endo File Bender (SybronEndo, Orange, California) if available. The bent file is then inserted into the root canal and using very gentle apical pressure is rotated up to one-fourth of the turn until its tip "is blocked" in the narrow space between the fragment and the root canal wall (Fig. 4.34). The probing manipulations continue until the fragment is bypassed and the tip of the file reaches the apex. The path of the instrument is followed radiographically, and the procedure is stopped in the event of misdirection since there is an increased risk of ledge formation or root perforation. The apex locator at this stage can only verify that the tip has reached the periodontal ligament but cannot differentiate whether this is beyond the apex or at a perforation site. The file is not removed at this point. With great caution, very small in and out movements are made with copious irrigation with the file in place. Very often, it is necessary to repeat the same procedure with a new file of the same size with an identical small sharp bent.
- The remaining portion of the root canal apical to the fragment is instrumented under copious irrigation. The size 10 file is followed by careful use of the size 15 and size 20 files. Prior to the use of the size 15 file, it is suggested (Zeigler and Serene 1984) to use to full working length the size 10 file shortened by 1 mm. In this way, the cross section at the tip of the shortened file is bigger than that of the size 10 file and smaller than that of the size 15 file, with the flexibility though of the size 10 file. This eases the use of the size 15 file that will follow. The same is

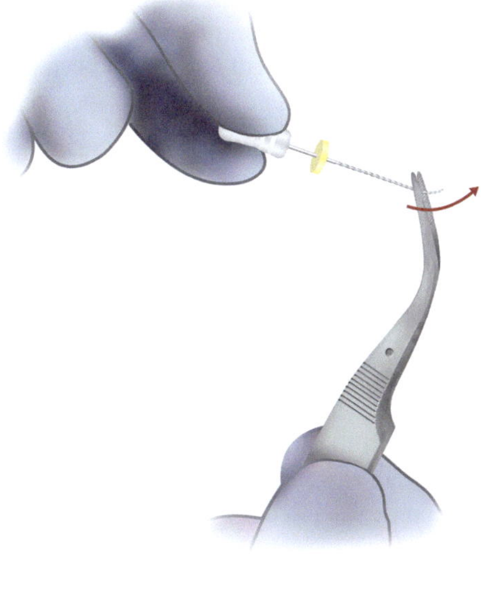

Fig. 4.33 Schematic illustration of creation of small sharp bend with cotton pliers

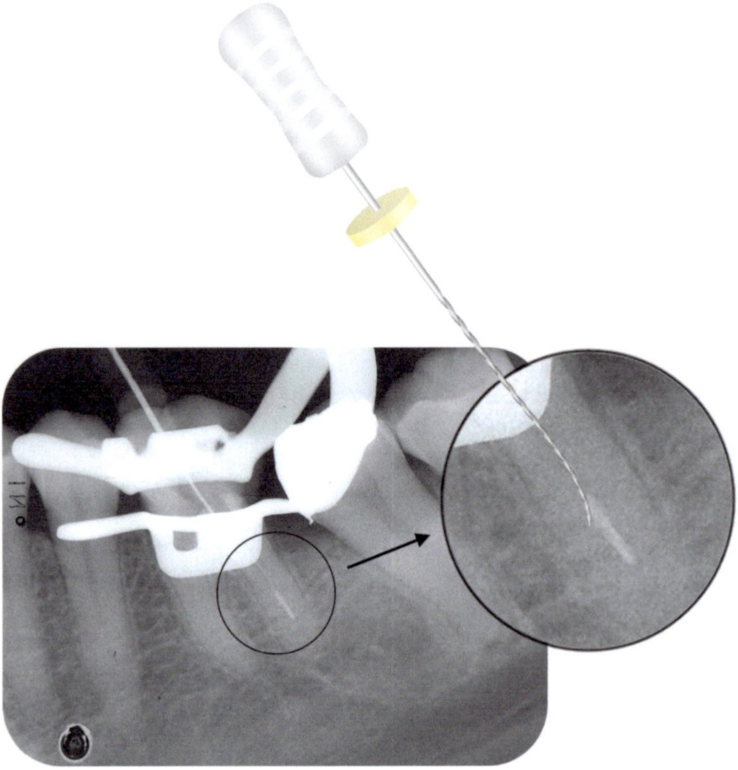

Fig. 4.34 Pre-bent K-file during the attempt to bypass a fragment in the apical third of a distal root in a mandibular first molar

repeated with file sizes 15 and 20. Golden medium sizes are mostly helpful in such cases. Care must be exercised to avoid placing any instrument directly on top of the fragment as it might push the fragment deeper into the canal and also impede the patency gained. In such cases, patency has to be regained by starting again with the initial file which, having been pre-bended, succeeded in bypassing the fragment.

Some characteristic cases of instrument fragments managed with the file bypass technique are presented (Figs. 4.35, 4.36, 4.37, and 4.38).

The objective of this procedure is to free the fragment through filing, to engage it in the flutes of the file, and to retrieve it. The capture and removal of the fragment are facilitated by the braiding technique, with which two (rarely three) files are gently screwed into the canal alongside the fragment and then wound around each other until the fragment is tightly grasped and withdrawn. Although the braiding technique was initially described using ISO size #15 files, the largest size possible should be used to decrease the risk of file fracture (Pitt Ford et al. 2002).

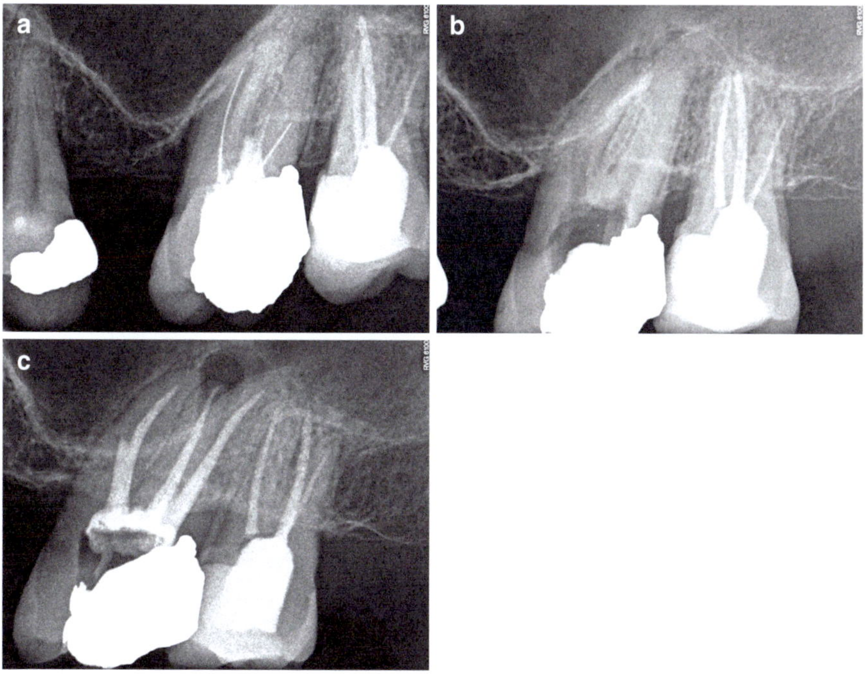

Fig. 4.35 (**a**) Preoperative radiograph of a retreatment case with two fragments, one in each buccal root of a maxillary left second molar. (**b**) Removal of the fragments with the file bypass technique. (c) Immediate post-obturation radiograph. Note the ledge formed

It is generally accepted that not all bypassed fragments are retrieved. The frequency with which bypassing but not retrieval happens in clinical practice is not substantially documented in the literature. There are many cases in the literature and in the author's archives of fragments that have been bypassed but not retrieved. In these cases if despite bypassing, the removal of the fragment is not possible, the instrumentation continues. The instrumentation technique and the master apical file that will be used for the root canal segment apical to the fragment respect all the rules of instrumentation. The obturation that follows incorporates the fragment within the filling material.

NiTi instruments are *not used at all* with this technique due to the increased risk of fracture. Bypassing efforts and cleaning and shaping of the canal accommodating the fragment are better completed by hand K-files to avoid further instrument fracture.

4.3.9 Holding Techniques

The concept of these techniques is to expose the coronal portion of the fragment (Fig. 4.39) using a range of trephine drills or ultrasonic tips prior to the use of a second instrument that will engage the coronal aspect and withdraw the fragment from the canal.

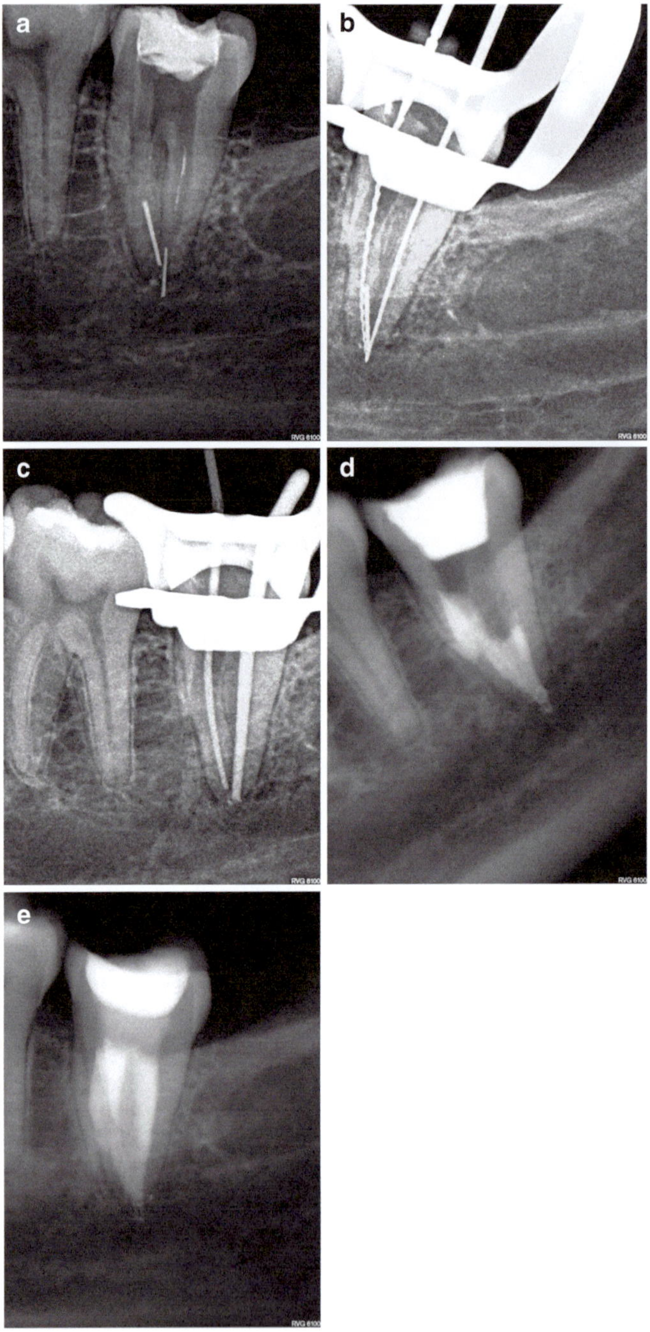

Fig. 4.36 (**a**) Preoperative radiograph of a referred case with two fractured instruments. (**b**) Bypassing of the instruments and retrieval of one of the fragments with the file bypass technique, while the other, which became loose with the technique, was suctioned during sodium hypochlorite irrigation. (**c**) Pre-final radiograph with gutta-percha cones in place. (**d**) Immediate post-obturation radiograph. (**e**) Three-month recall radiograph (Courtesy of Dr. A. Chouliara)

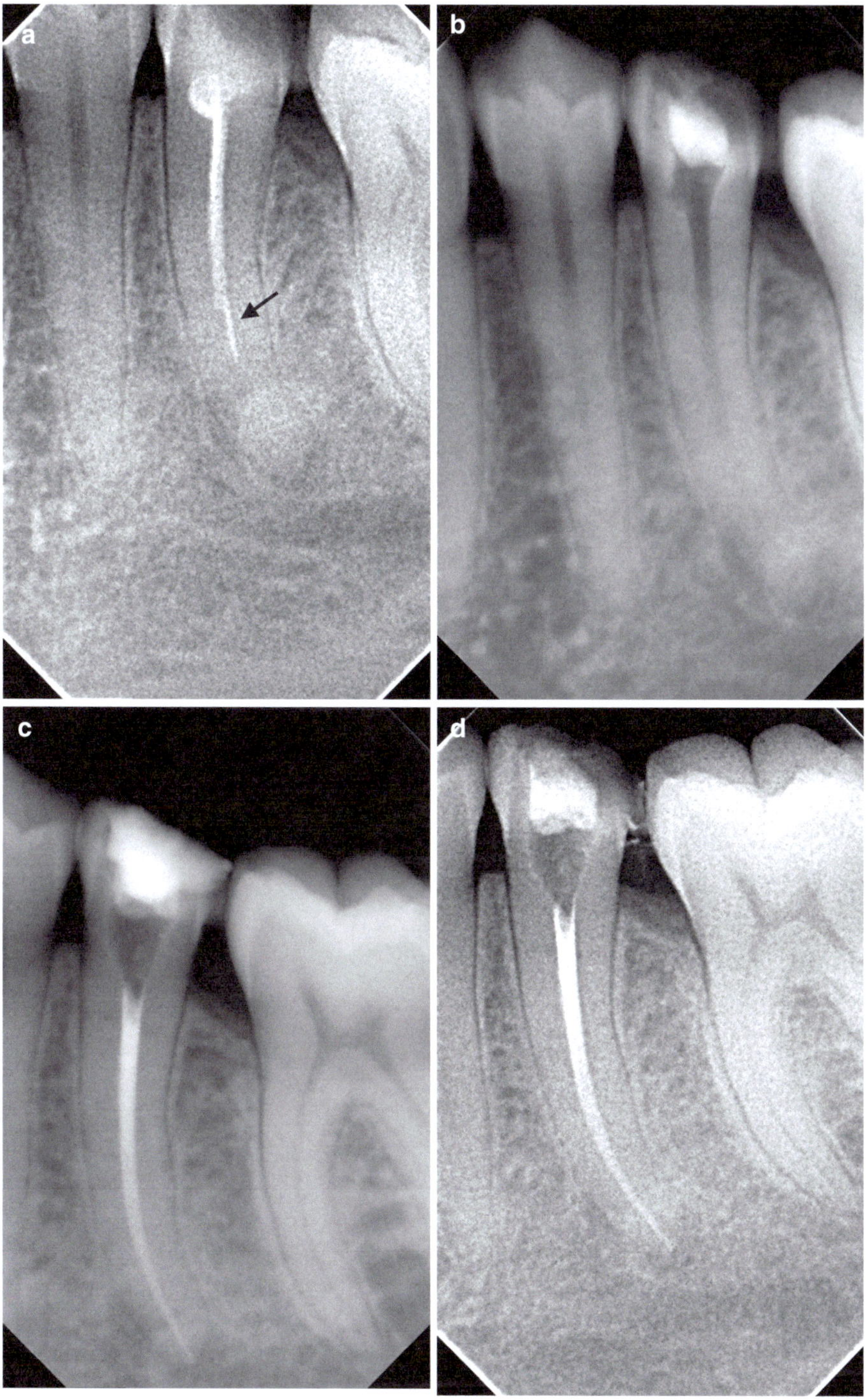

Fig. 4.37 (**a**) Preoperative radiograph. A fragment can be seen (*arrow*) apically to the obturation material of the initial RCT. (**b**) Fragment retrieved with the file bypass technique. (**c**) Immediate post-obturation radiograph. (**d**) Three-month recall radiograph

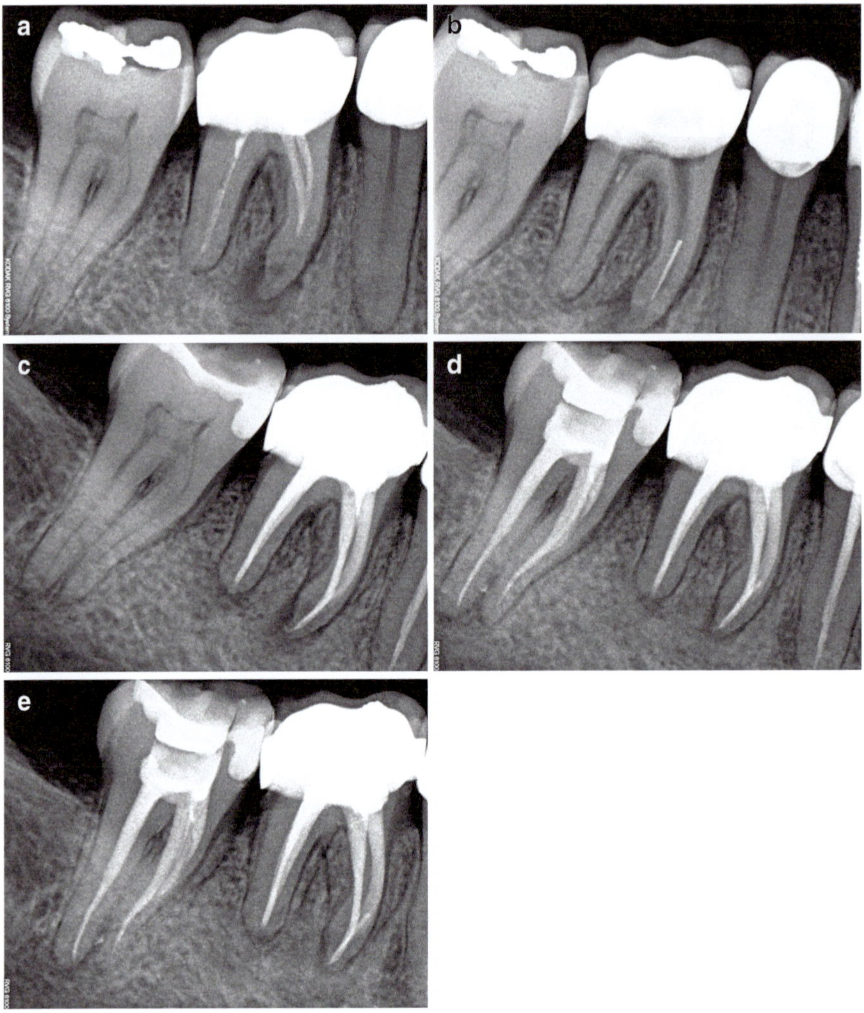

Fig. 4.38 (**a**) Preoperative radiograph of a first mandibular molar with incomplete RCT and apical periodontitis. (**b**) Radiograph with a fragment in the apical third of the mesiobuccal canal fractured during retreatment procedure. (**c**) Immediate post-obturation radiograph following bypassing of the fragment, instrumentation up to the desired length, and dressing of the root canal with $Ca(OH)_2$ for 2 weeks. (**d**, **e**) Recall radiograph at 8 and 21 months, respectively, shows healing (Courtesy of Prof. J. Molyvdas)

Among the holding techniques, the most characteristic and well known are:

- The Masserann technique
- The Feldman et al. (1974) technique
- The Meitrac Endo Safety System

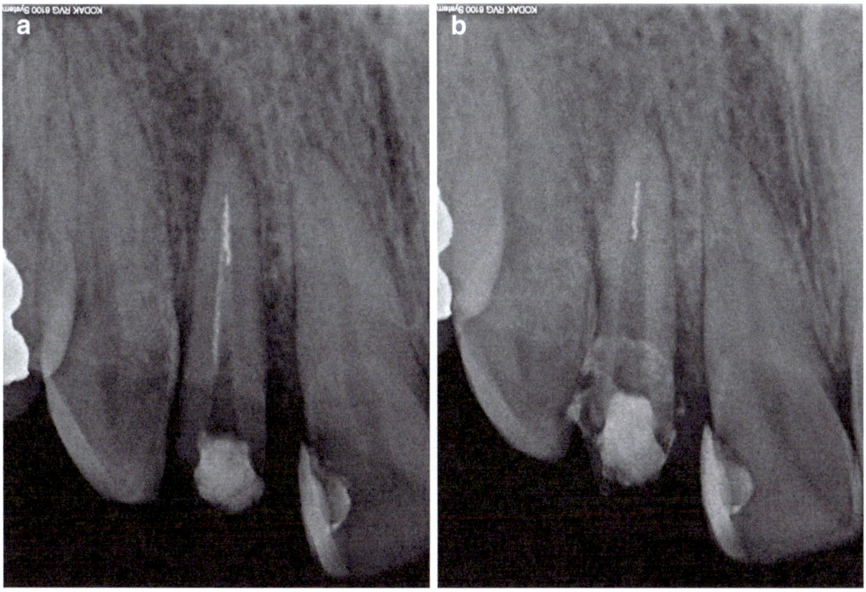

Fig. 4.39 (**a**) Preoperative radiograph in which a fragment with both ends within the root canal is visible at the apical root third. (**b**) Exposure of approximately 2 mm of the coronal segment of the fragment

- The Instrument Removal System (IRS)
- The Endo Rescue
- The Endo Extractor System

4.3.10 The Masserann Technique

The Masserann technique (Masserann 1966, 1971), being used for the removal of fractured instruments, has also been used for the retrieval from the root canal of metallic objects such as silver cones and posts. The available kit (Masserann endodontic kit, Micro-Mega, Besancon, France) consists of (Figs. 4.40 and 4.41):

- An assortment of 14 color-coded, end-cutting, tubular trepan burs of increasing size
- Two sizes of tubular extractors (1.2 and 1.5 mm)
- A gauge that assists in predicting the size of the bur and the extractor to be used

The trepan burs (Fig. 4.44) are hollow tubes with edges designed to cut dentin peripherally to the fragment. They are meant to be used with an anticlockwise rotation. During the apical movement of the drill, the coronal end of the fragment is

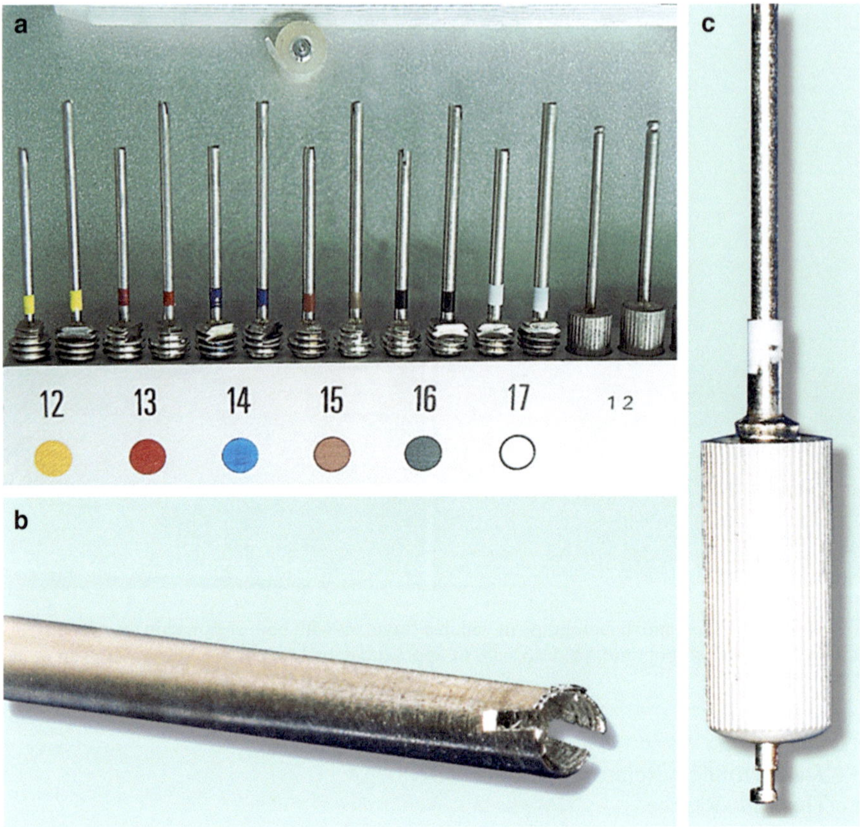

Fig. 4.40 (**a**) The Masserann kit (Masserann endodontic kit, Micro-Mega, Besancon, France). (**b**) The special trepan burs are concave. (**c**) The trepan burs may be used on a handpiece or manually

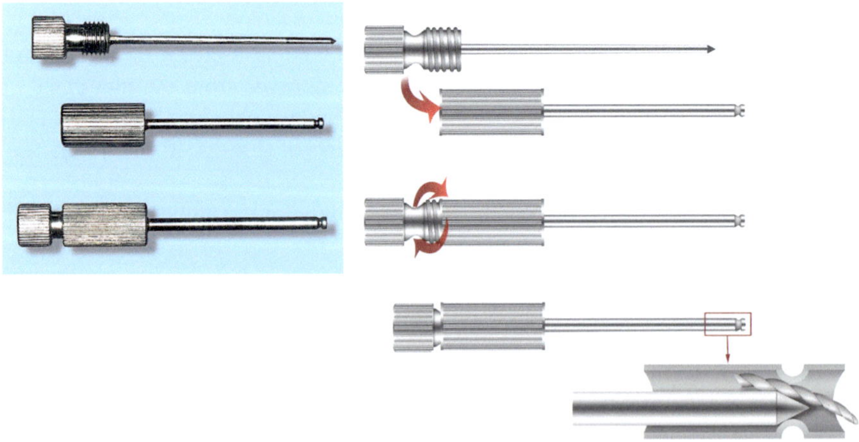

Fig. 4.41 Masserann extractor (Masserann endodontic kit, Micro-Mega, Besancon, France). Photograph and drawing of the rod, the tube, and the entire assembly. The ridge, where the fragment is gripped and removed, can be clearly seen (in the magnified area)

engulfed in the tubular portion. Trepan burs can be operated manually using the special handle provided or with a reducing contra-angled (300–600 rpm) handpiece. Manual use is preferable since it avoids a rise in temperature and offers better tactile sensation. Careful examination, preferably under magnification prior to their use, of the quality of their cutting edges is advisable.

The extractor (Fig. 4.41) is tubelike with a plunger rod (stylet) which, when screwed inside the extractor, locks the exposed coronal end of the fragment against an internal embossment just short of the end of the extractor. The smaller-sized tubular extractor (1.2 mm) is used for fragments up to size #40, while the larger (1.5 mm) is for larger instrument sizes or posts.

The rationale of this technique is first to create space in the root canal around the coronal end of the fractured instrument (or any metallic object) so that the extractor tube will pass over it. In this line, the trepan bur is rotated anticlockwise around the coronal end of the fragment cutting the surrounding root canal dentin and exposing this part of the instrument. Then the extractor plunger, a locking rod in the tube, is screwed down, locking the freed coronal end of the metallic object against a knurled ring in the tube wall. This technique provides adequate retention for the removal of most metallic objects from the root canal.

The steps to be followed are (Fig. 4.42):

- Selection of the appropriate trepan bur. The bur that can fit into the coronal segment of the fractured instrument is the ideal one.
- Root canal instrumentation up to the fragment. A cylindrical shape is prepared to allow the special bur to reach the fragment.
- Insertion of the trepan bur and, with counterclockwise rotation, creation of a trench 2–4 mm around the coronal segment of the fragment. Sometimes the fragment is pulled out incorporated in the dentin inside the groove of the special trephine drill. However, in the majority of cases, a space is simply created around the coronal segment of the fragment, which now protrudes in the groove created by the special bur.
- Removal of the fragment either with the special tubular extractor or with a trepan bur. The pre-selected extractor is gently introduced into the canal to encircle and grip the coronal end of the fragment, and the rod is rotated in a clockwise direction to snugly grip the fragment against the wall of the extractor tube. The whole assembly is then gently turned in back-and-forth motions to loosen and retrieve the fragment from the canal. In some cases, a trepan bur, a size smaller than the one initially used, can be forced over the exposed coronal end of the fragment to grip it firmly enough and retrieve it.

For the effective removal of tightly bound fragments with relatively large diameters at the coronal end and in order to avoid any additional dentin cutting and further weakening of the root, a modification of the Masserann extractor (Fig. 4.43) has been proposed (Okiji 2003). This modification ensures gripping by creating a wider space inside the tube (Okiji 2003).

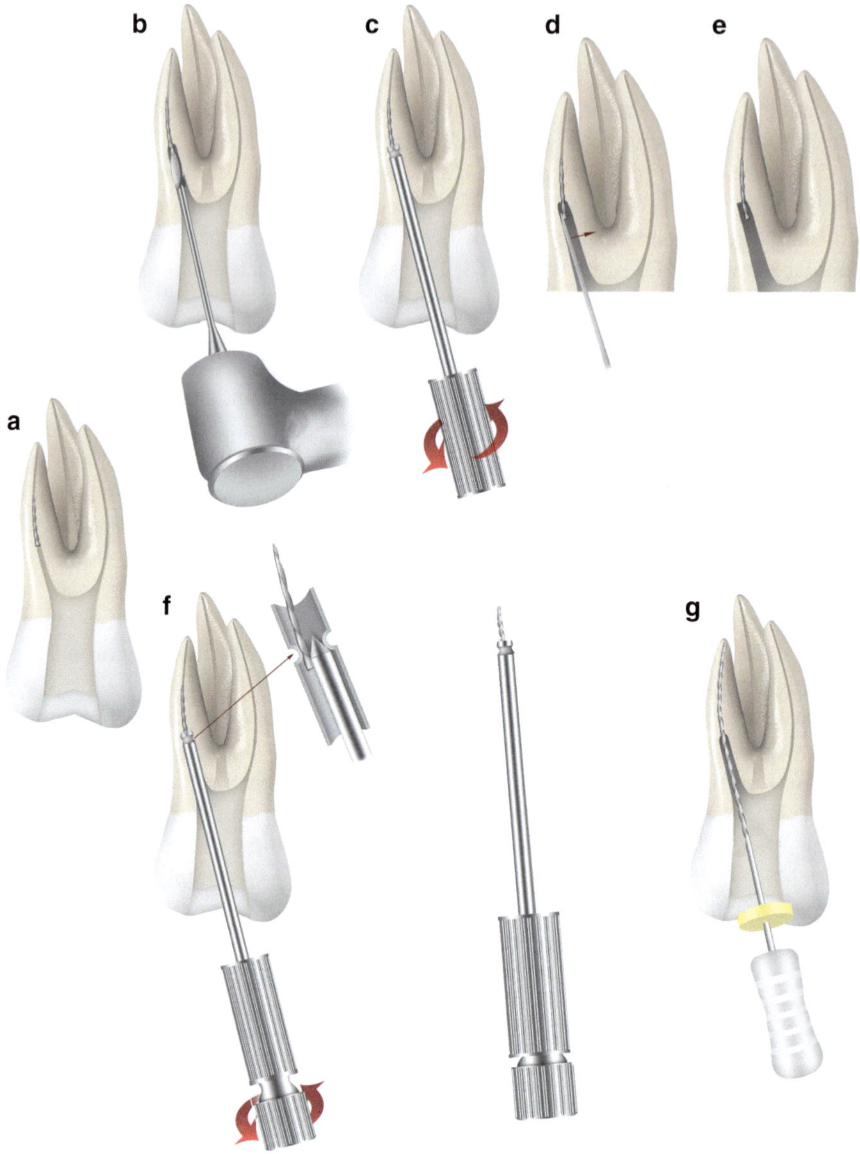

Fig. 4.42 (**a–g**) Schematic illustration of the retrieval of a fractured instrument with the Masserann technique. (**a**) Radiographic confirmation of the presence of a fragment and recognition of its location, size, and length. (**b**) Instrumentation of the root canal coronal to the fragment. A cylindrical shape is formed. (**c**) Creation of a trench around the fragment with the special trepan bur. (**d**, **e**) The exposed end of the fragment is positioned with the help of an endodontic explorer to the center of the prepared canal. (**f**) The fragment is removed with the special extractor (*arrow*). (**g**) Once the fragment is removed, the canal is renegotiated with an ISO size 10K-file to the apical foramen, and canal instrumentation follows

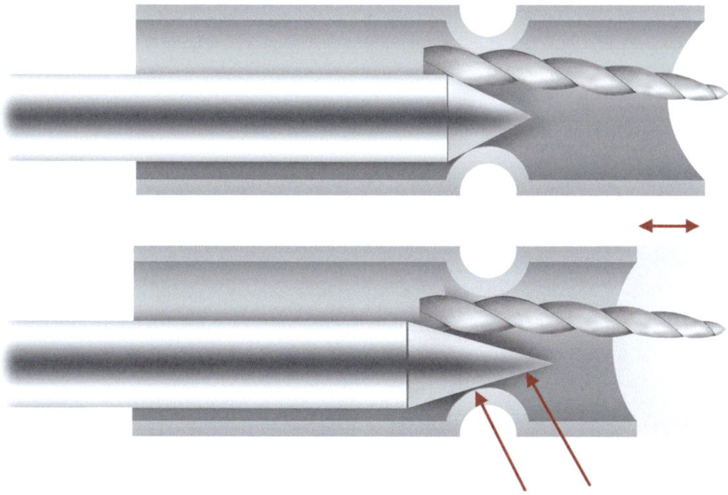

Fig. 4.43 Schematic illustration of the modification of the Masserann extractor proposed by Okiji (2003). (**a**) Before modification, the space between the tube and plunger is not sufficient to grip an instrument fragment or metallic object of relatively large cross-sectional diameter. (**b**) Modified extractor in which the tip of the tube is cut off (*arrow*) and the tip of the plunger sharpened (*double arrow*)

A characteristic case of an instrument fragment managed with the Masserann technique is presented (Fig. 4.44).

4.3.11 The Feldman and Coauthor Technique

This technique (Feldman et al. 1974) is identical to the Masserann technique with the single addition of the utilization of transilluminating light. Fiber-optic transillumination, that is, light transmission through tissues of the body, is a unanimously recognized and appreciated adjunctive diagnostic means with a broad range of clinical applications. In dentistry, it has been primarily associated with caries diagnosis (Mitropoulos 1985; Schneiderman et al. 1997; Davies et al. 2001) and in endodontics in particular with the detection of vertical root fractures (Schindler and Walker 1994; Liewehr 2001; Lubisich et al. 2010; Walton and Tamse 2015) and with the management of fractured endodontic instruments (Feldman et al. 1974). In clinical endodontics, transillumination is also useful in recognition/identification of narrow and calcified canals. Fiber-optic transillumination has also been used in surgical endodontics (Schindler and Walker 1994).

The transilluminating light (fiber optics) is used to highlight the fragment in the root canal. The light source of the dental operating microscope must be turned off, and only magnification along with the dental mirror and transilluminator must be

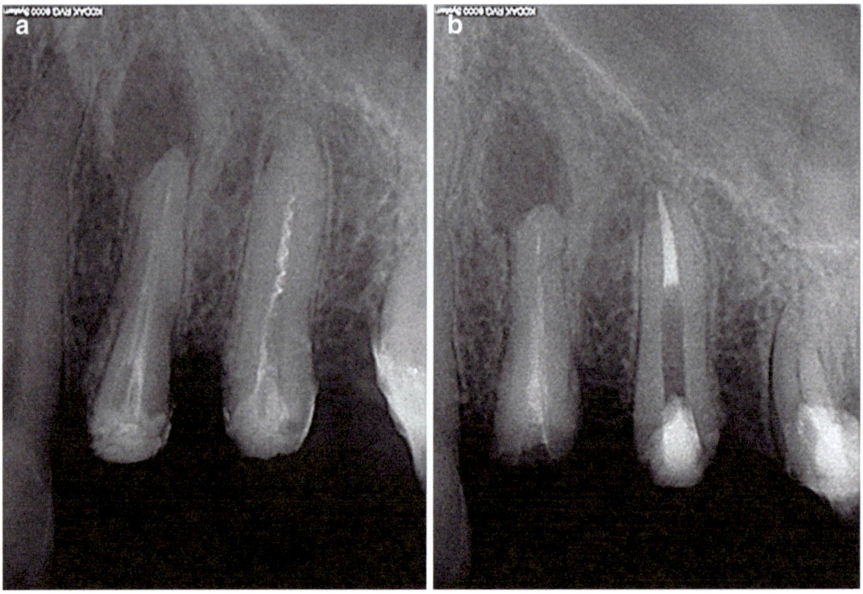

Fig. 4.44 (**a**) Preoperative radiograph of a maxillary second premolar with a fragment of a Lentulo spiral in the middle root third. (**b**) Immediate postoperative radiograph, following removal of the fragment with the Masserann technique. Note the enlargement of the canal

used. The overhead lighting should also be turned off. The fiber-optic probe can be placed perpendicular to the root on the gingiva several millimeters below the cervical area or directly on the tooth structure at the cervical area (the probe is directed into the root and inclined toward the apex). This technique ensures immediate visibility in the root canal, easing the removal and reducing the likelihood of causing new iatrogenic damage, i.e., a root perforation.

Various fiber-optic transillumination devices with distinct light output and tip diameter are commercially available. If unavailable, a fiber-optic handpiece with no bur and the water turned off, composite curing lights, and other tools as transilluminators can be used.

4.3.12 The Meitrac Endo Safety System

The Meitrac Endo Safety System (Hager & Meisinger GmbH, Neuss, Germany) is another system similar but reduced to Masserann. It is available in three kits (the Meitrac I, II, and III) designed for the removal of metallic fragments according to their diameter and type (Table 4.5). All Meitrac Endo Safety Systems are made of stainless surgical steel and thus can be sterilized and reused. These kits are designed for the removal of fractured endodontic instruments, and each consists of (Fig. 4.45):

- A trepan bur
- Two extractors

Table 4.5 Selection of the appropriate Meitrac kit in relation to the diameter of the fragment

Kit	Diameter of the fragment (mm)
Meitrac I	From 0.15 to 0.50
Meitrac II	From 0.55 to 0.90
Meitrac III	From 0.90 to 1.50

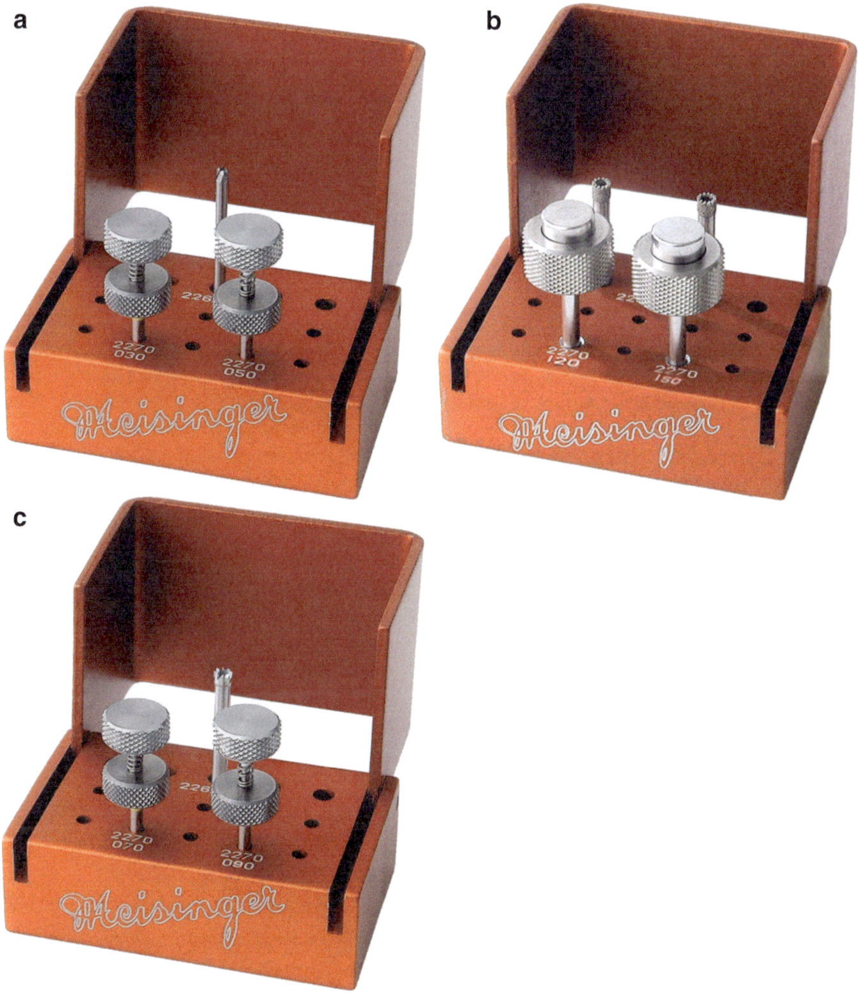

Fig. 4.45 Meitrac I, II, and III (from left to right) (Courtesy of Hager & Meisinger GmbH, Neuss, Germany)

The trephine bur resembles a typical contra-angled slow-speed round bur but is hollow throughout its length. This facilitates the drilling of dentin immediately adjacent to the fragment, leaving the fragment intact and eventually exposing its coronal end.

The extractor consists of two components: a small and a larger hollow tube. The smaller tube fits snugly into the larger one. The smaller hollow tube is attached to a finger-grip chuck at one end and has long vertical slots cut into its active end. These

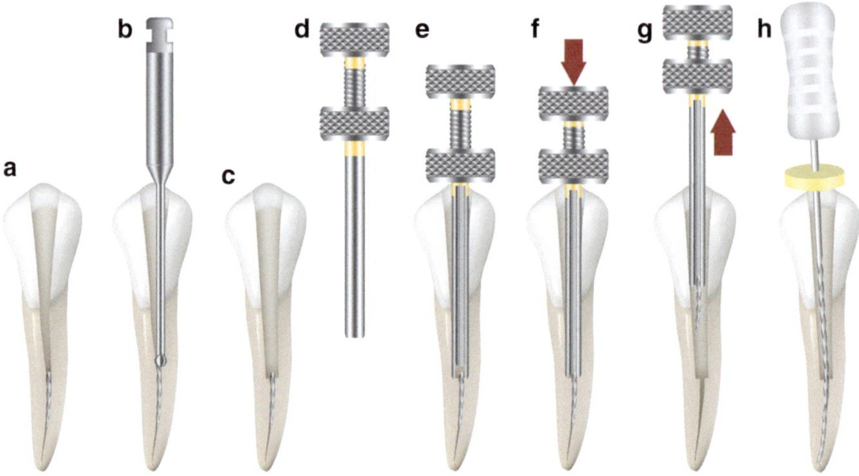

Fig. 4.46 (**a–h**) Schematic illustration of the removal of a fragment with the Meitrac Endo Safety System (Hager & Meisinger GmbH, Neuss, Germany). (**a**) Radiographic confirmation of the presence of a fragment and recognition of its location, size, and length. (**b**, **c**) Modification of the access cavity and instrumentation of the root canal up to the fragment with the trephine bur and exposure of its coronal segment. (**d**, **e**) The pre-selected extractor corresponding to the trephine bur is introduced into the canal and grasps the fragment by pressing down the upper part of the extractor. (**f**, **g**) Keeping the parts of the extractor squeezed tightly together, the fragment is removed by gently pulling the whole assembly. (**h**) Once the fragment is removed, the canal is renegotiated with an ISO size 10K-file to the apical foramen, and canal instrumentation follows

slots allow the smaller tube to be compressed, decreasing the internal lumen of the tube. The larger hollow tube is also equipped with a finger-grip chuck at one end and a slightly constricted lumen at the other end. As the smaller component of the extractor is inserted into the larger one, it is supported in a neutral position by a spring.

The steps to be followed are (Fig. 4.46):

- Selection of the appropriate trepan bur and thus the kit according to the size, length, and taper of the fragment following the steps provided by the manufacturer:
  1. *Calculate the length (in mm) of the fragment.*
  2. *Add one taper size for every millimeter of the fragment to the diameter of the file. Thus, for example, if the fragment is 3 mm in length, the diameter of the file is 0.15 and the taper is 0.02, and then the formula would look like this: 0.1 5 + 0.02 + 0.02 + 0.02 = 0.21 which falls between 0.15 and 0.50, that is, the required kit is the Meitrac I.*
- Instrumentation of the root canal up to the fragment. The trephine bur is gently inserted into the instrumented canal up to the fragment and, operating at a very slow speed, exposes 1–2 mm of the coronal segment of the fragment.
- The pre-selected extractor is guided gently into the root canal refined by the hollow trephine, until it slips over the fragment. Occasionally to achieve this, it may be necessary to rotate the extractor cautiously back and forth with light pressure as the fragment may be off to one side of the canal. It is then activated by pushing

the smaller tube further into the larger component, against the resistance of the spring. As the smaller tube exits through the larger one, the decreased lumen at the active end of the larger tube compresses the smaller tube, decreasing its internal lumen. This decrease in the internal lumen of the smaller tube firmly grasps the fragment within the slotted section of the inner tube.

– The grasped fragment is retrieved by keeping the parts of the extractor squeezed tightly together.

4.3.13 Instrument Removal System

The Instrument Removal System (Dentsply Tulsa Dental, Tulsa, OK) (Fig. 4.47) is specifically designed to assist in the removal of a variety of intracanal obstructions including fractured instruments. It has been successfully used in several cases (Chauhan et al. 2013). The "superior edition IRS" (Swiss Machining Inc., San Diego, USA), the most recent redesign kit available, can be regarded as the evolution of the Instrument Removal System which consisted of three instruments. The IRS consists of four extraction devices constructed from titanium and SS (Table 4.6), which are tubes with a 45° bevel on the end and a cutout side window. The green and black extractors are used in the coronal one-third of larger root canals. In narrower canals, the red and yellow extractors are used. Each tube has a corresponding internal stylus or screw wedge. The different screw wedges may be interchanged between each micro-tube, and this might be useful in some cases as it improves mechanics.

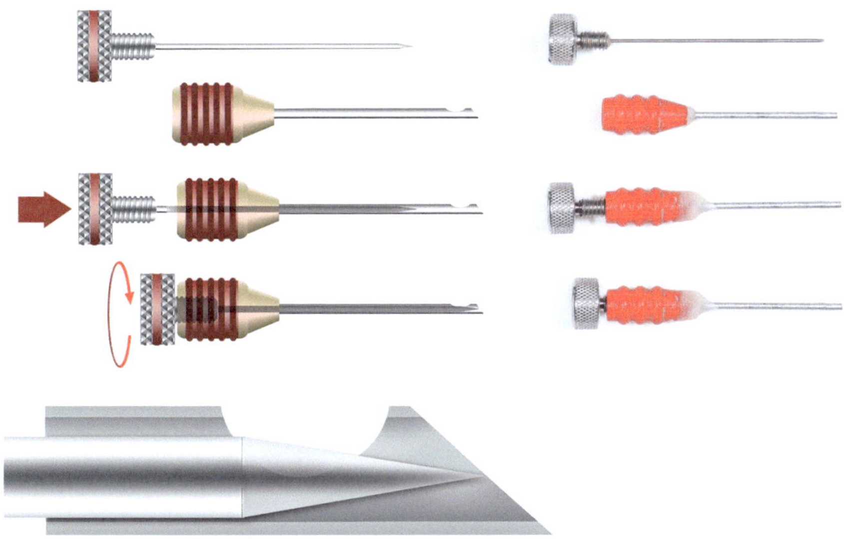

Fig. 4.47 Photograph and drawing of the parts and the whole assembly of IRS. In the magnified area, the cutout side window can be seen

Table 4.6 IRS and core drill dimensions

	External diameter (mm)		Internal diameter (mm)		Tube length (mm)	Overall length (mm)
Color	IRS	Core drill	IRS	Core drill	IRS and core drill	IRS and core drill
Green	1.6	1.7	1.3	1.4	12	21
Black	1.00	1.15	0.80	0.88	12	21
Red	0.80	0.85	0.60	0.63	16	25
Yellow	0.60	0.61	0.40	0.41	20	29

The steps to be followed are (Fig. 4.48):

- Exposure of 1.5–3 mm of the coronal segment of the fragment by troughing around it with a core drill or with an ultrasonic instrument.
- The appropriate pre-selected micro-tube is slid into place over the exposed coronal segment of the fragment. As the head of the exposed fragment lies in the vast majority of cases against the outer dentin wall, the micro-tube must be inserted into the canal with the long part of its beveled end oriented to the outer wall of the canal to "scoop up" the head of the fragment and guide it into the micro-tube.
- Once the micro-tube has been put in place, the same color-coded screw wedge is inserted and slid internally through the micro-tube's length until it makes contact with the fragment. It is then turned counterclockwise to mechanically engage and displace the head of the fragment through the side window. When engaged by rotating the micro-tube and screw wedge assembly out of the root canal, the fragment is retrieved. If difficulty is encountered when rotating the whole assembly counterclockwise, then a limited (of 3–5°) clockwise rotation should be tried in an effort to stay engaged, followed by turning the assembly counterclockwise again until snug. This repeated reciprocating handle motion would facilitate removal. In some cases, it is even necessary to place and activate an ultrasonic instrument on the engaged assembly to facilitate successful removal.

4.3.14 The Endo Rescue

The Endo Rescue Kit (Komet/Brasseler, Savannah, GA) is designed to retrieve fractured instruments from the root canal. The kit consists of:

- A cylindroconical tungsten carbide bur with a non-cutting tip
- A short Gates Glidden bur #4
- A Gates Glidden bur #3
- A centering drill
- A trepan bur that rotates in a counterclockwise direction
- A manual screw available for clinicians who want to avoid using a handpiece

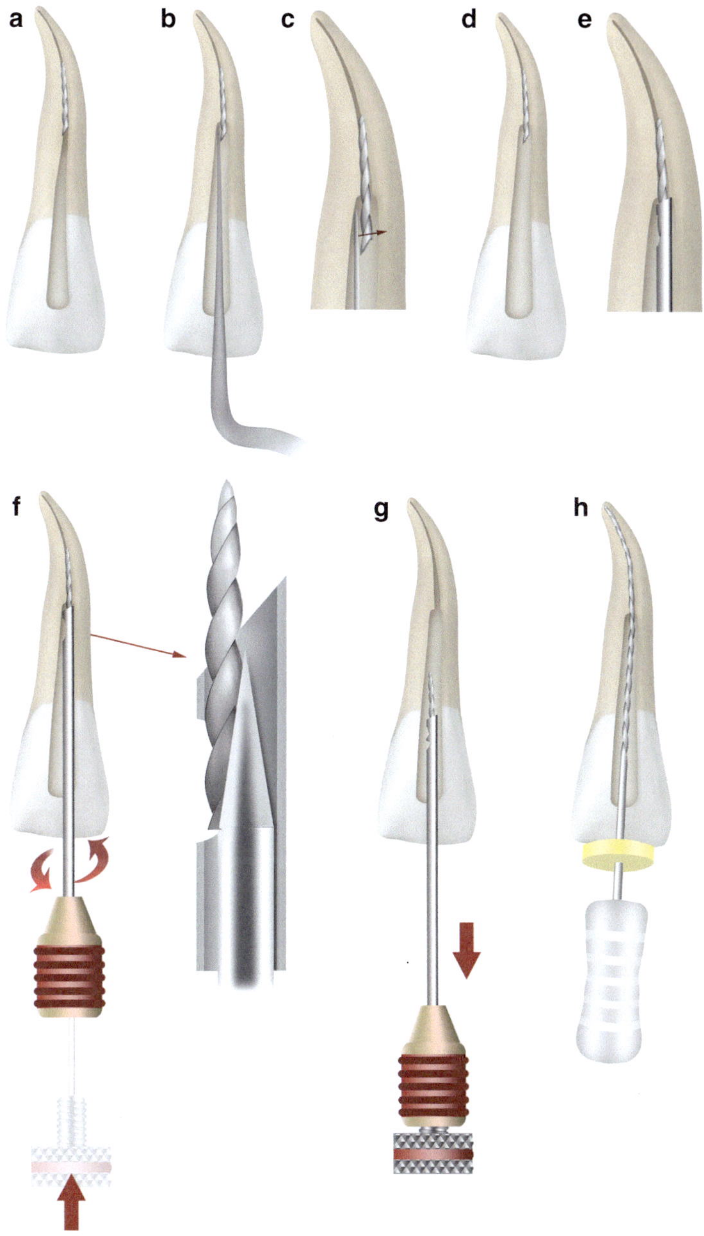

Fig. 4.48 (**a–h**) Schematic illustration of the retrieval of fractured instrument with the IRS (Dentsply Tulsa Dental, Tulsa, OK). (**a**) Radiographic confirmation of the presence of a fragment and recognition of its location, size, and length. (**b–d**) Exposure of the coronal segment of the fragment and its positioning in the center of the canal. (**e**) The exposed segment of the fragment is guided into the micro-tube inserted into the canal. (**f**) The same color-coded screw wedge is inserted into the micro-tube until it makes contact with the fragment and is turned counterclockwise to mechanically engage and displace the head of the fragment through the side window. (**g**) The fragment is retrieved by rotating and pulling the whole assembly out of the canal. (**h**) Once the fragment is removed, the canal is renegotiated with an ISO size #10K-file to the apical foramen, and canal instrumentation follows

Table 4.7 Internal and external diameter of the three sizes of Endo Rescue instruments

Color	Internal diameter (mm)	External diameter (mm)
Blue	0.7	1.1
Red	0.5	0.9
Yellow	0.4	0.7

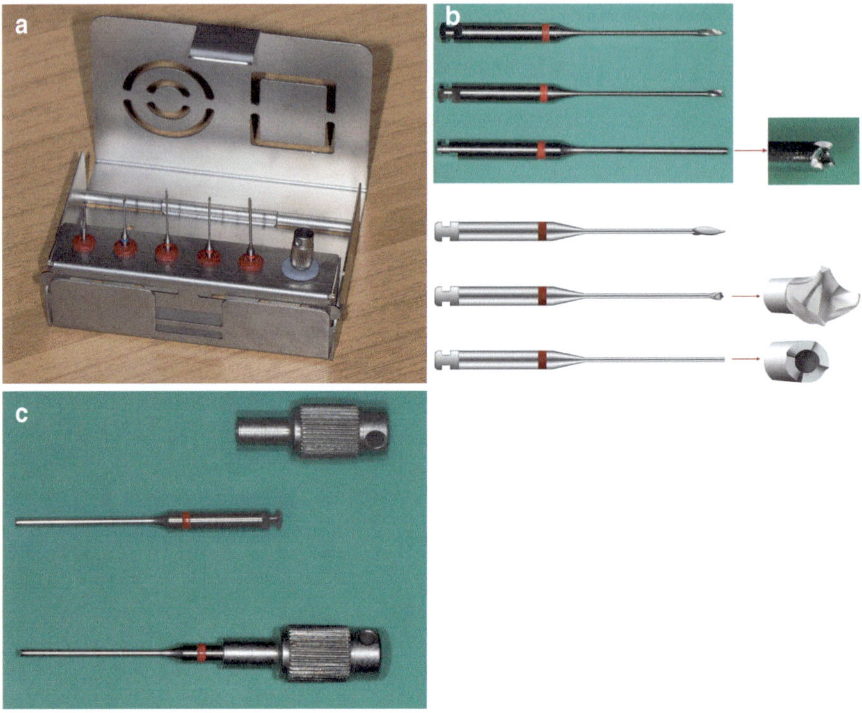

Fig. 4.49 (**a**) The Endo Rescue Kit (Komet/Brasseler, Savannah, GA). (**b**) The centering drill and the trepan bur have the same external diameter as the Gates Glidden size #3. The tip of the centering drill at its active part has a tapered concave shape. The internal part of the trepan bur has a diameter of 0.5 mm and a length of 5 mm. (**c**) The instruments can also be used with the available manual screw

These instruments are available in three sizes (Table 4.7, Fig. 4.49). The centering drill has the same external diameter as the Gates Glidden #3 (0.9 mm), but the active part at its end has a tapered, concave shape. The outer blades cut into the dentin surrounding the fragment, and the concave, tapered area that encounters the coronal part of the fragment allows centering of the preparation by advancing the drill apically.

The procedures to be followed are (Fig. 4.50):

- Creation of an unobstructed straight-line access to the coronal portion of the fragment. The specially designed cylindroconical bur with a non-cutting tip is used to improve visibility. The short Gates Glidden bur size #4 follows to relocate the canal entrance. It is moved along the wall opposite the coronal curve with vertical back-and-forth movements. Direct access to the fragment is then created with a

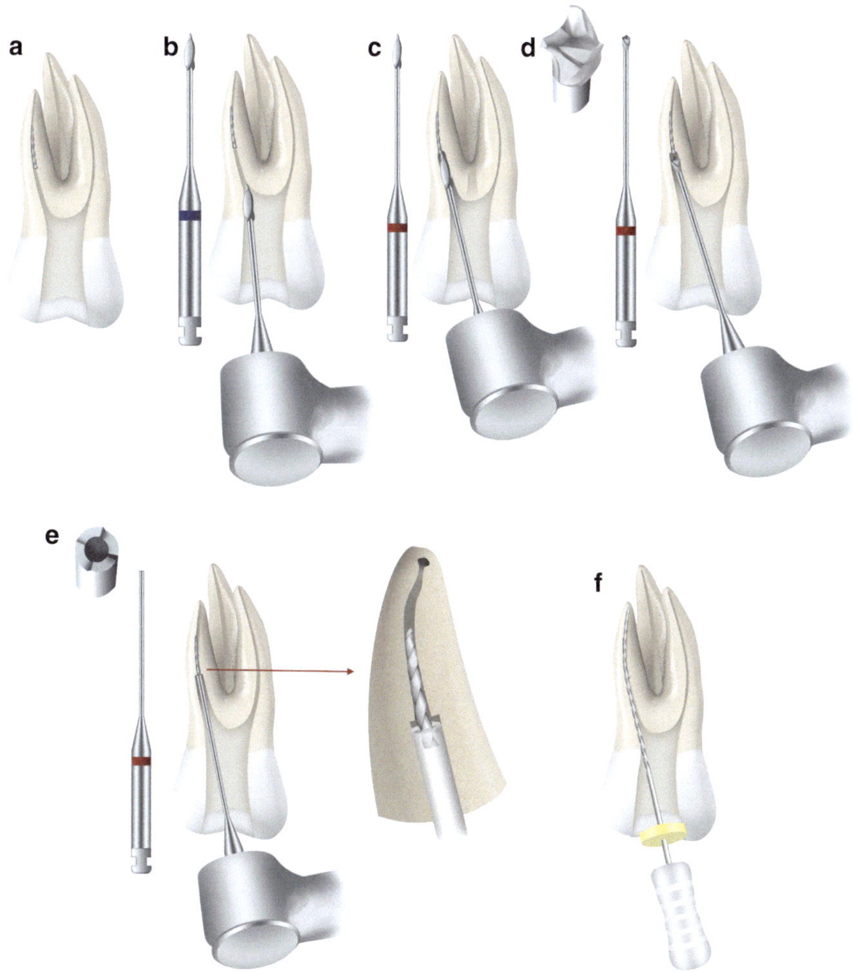

Fig. 4.50 (**a–g**) Schematic illustration of the retrieval of a fractured instrument with the Endo Rescue Kit. (**a**) Radiographic confirmation of the presence of a fragment and recognition of its location, size, and length. (**b**) The specially designed cylindroconical bur with a non-cutting tip and the short Gates Glidden bur size #4 are used to improve visibility and relocate the canal entrance. (**c**) Direct access to the fragment is then created with a Gates Glidden bur size #2 or 3, depending on the size of the canal and the location of the fragment. (**d**) Excavation with the corresponding centering drill of the last few millimeters of dentin coronal to the fragment and providing access to it. (**e**, **f**) The corresponding trepan bur, rotated in a counterclockwise direction, surrounds the fragment and removes it firmly held in the trepan bur by the residues of dentin. (**g**) Once the fragment is removed, the canal is renegotiated with an ISO size #10K-file to the apical foramen, and canal instrumentation follows

Gates Glidden bur size #2 or #3, depending on the size of the canal and the location of the fragment.

- Excavation with the centering drill, whose external diameter precisely matches the size of the previously used Gates Glidden bur, of the last few millimeters of dentin coronal to the fragment, providing access to it.

4.3.15 The Endo Extractor System

The Endo Extractor System (Roydent Dental Products, Johnson City) consists of the following SS sterilizable components (Fig. 4.51):

- A hollow trepan drill with an internal diameter of 0.80 mm and an external diameter of 1.6 mm
- Three extraction devices all with a 1.5 mm external diameter:
  - The white corresponding to ISO size #0.30
  - The yellow corresponding to ISO size #0.50
  - The red corresponding to ISO size #0.80

The steps to be followed are (Fig. 4.52):

- Exposure of the coronal segment of the fragment with the trepan drill.
- The pre-selected extractor is carefully slid over the exposed coronal segment of the fragment while turning the knurled ring counterclockwise to open its jaw. Then, holding the extractor on the fragment, the knurled ring is rotated clockwise

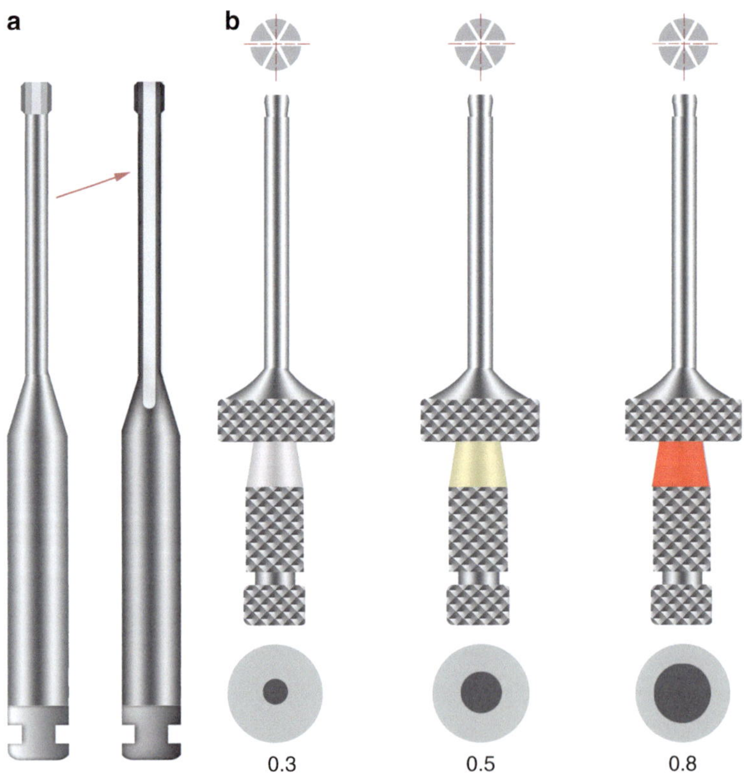

Fig. 4.51 (**a**) Hollow trepan drill. (**b**) Endo Extractor seen in the close-up view of the Roydent Endo Extractor System (Roydent Dental Products, Johnson City)

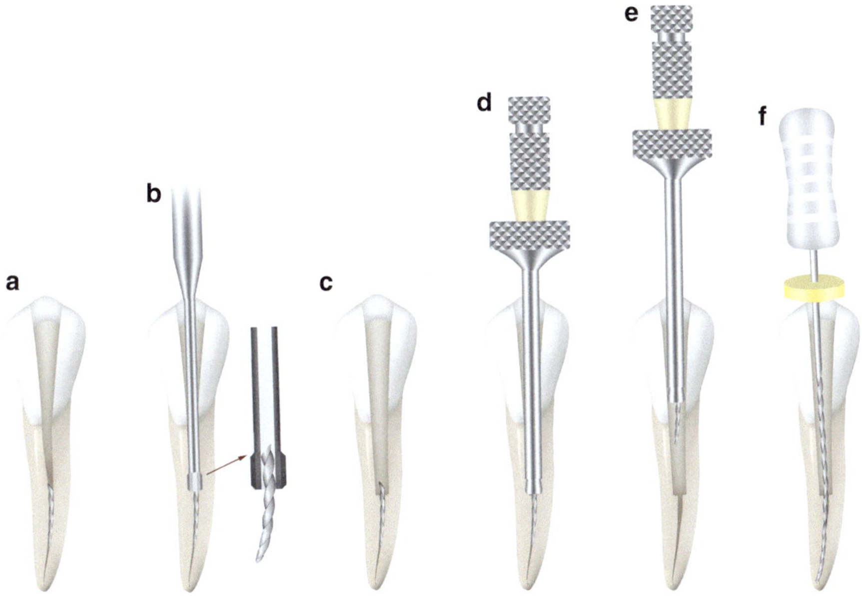

Fig. 4.52 (**a–f**) Schematic illustration of the removal of an instrument fragment with the Endo Extractor (Johnson and Beatty 1988 method). (**a**) Radiographic confirmation of the presence of a fragment and recognition of its location, size, and length. (**b**, **c**) Instrumentation of the canal coronal to the fragment and exposure of its coronal end with the trepan drill. (**d**, **e**) The pre-selected extractor is slid over the exposed coronal segment of the fragment while turning the knurled ring counterclockwise to open its jaw. Then, by turning the knurled ring clockwise, the extractor engages/grips the freed segment of the fragment and retrieves it. (**f**) Once the fragment is removed, the canal is renegotiated with an ISO size #10K-file to the apical foramen, and canal instrumentation follows

so that the six prongs existing in every extractor engage/grip the exposed coronal segment of the fragment with equal force all the way round and retrieve it by applying strict tensile force during removal.

The major disadvantages of the Endo Extractor System are the limited number of instrument sizes and the possibility of breaking the prongs on the extractor if a bending rather than strict tensile force is applied during removal.

4.3.16 The Endo Removal System

The Endo Removal System (Cerkamed Medical Company) consists of the following SS sterilizable components (Fig. 4.53):

- Endodontic micro-tweezers with a total length of 130 mm, length of tips 25 mm, length of serrated working part 5 mm, diameter of working part with tips closed 0.6–0.8 mm, and force of pressure 100–150 g

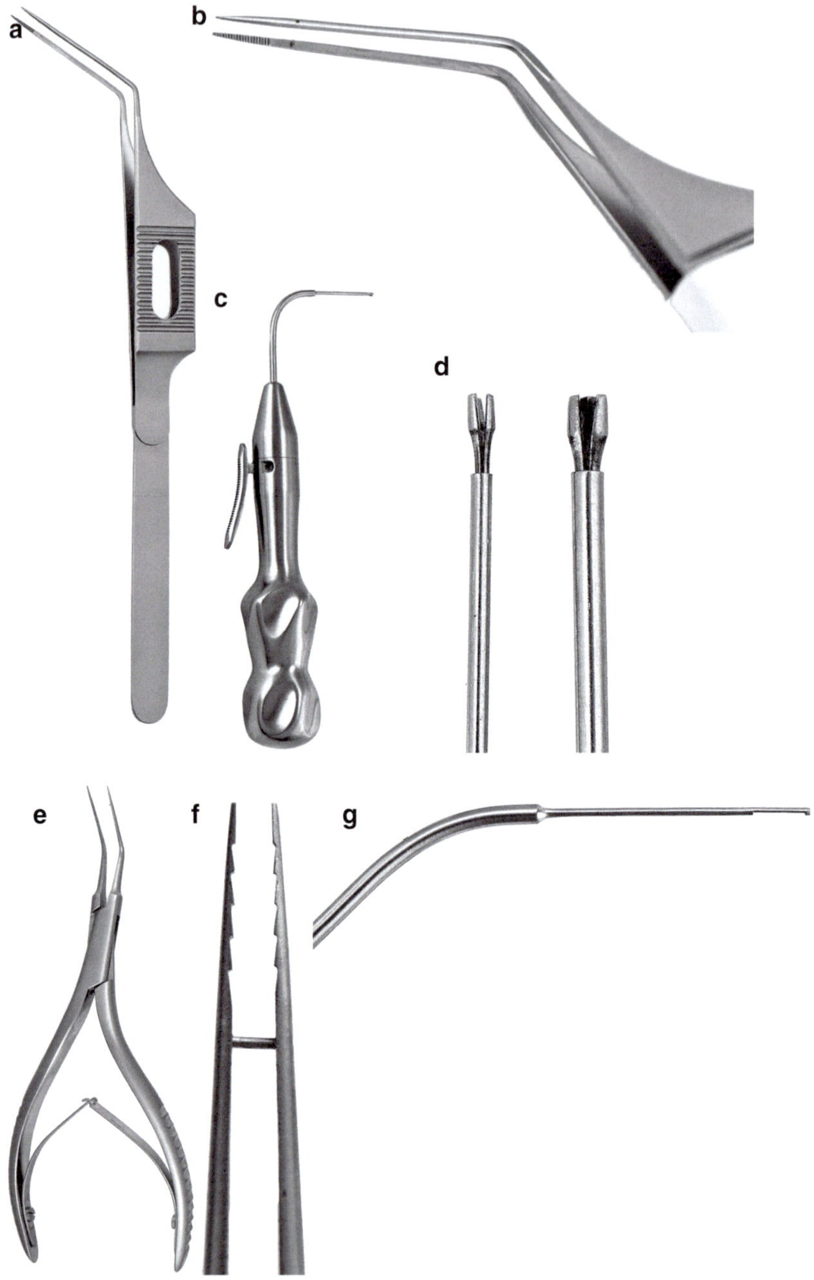

Fig. 4.53 (**a–g**) Endo Removal System (Cerkamed Medical Company). (**a**) Endodontic micro-tweezers. (**b**) The long thin tips are bent at a 60° angle to the handle. (**c**) Endodontic micro-forceps. The long thin tip is bent at a 90° angle to the handle. (**d**) The working part of the tip comprises of three movable and serrated jaws clamped by means of a tube sliding over them. (**e**) Endodontic forceps. Its long thin tips are bent at a 60° angle to the handle. (**f**) The teeth at the tip are positioned stepwise to the long axis instead of the classic right angle serration. (**g**) Endodontic micro-lever. Its working part has the shape of a semi-open tube with a sharp cutting edge at the top

- Endodontic micro-forceps with a total length of 170 mm, length of tip 30 mm, diameter of working part with tips closed 0.8 mm, and force of pressure 200–300 g
- Endodontic forceps with a total length of 125 mm, length of tips 20 mm, length of serrated working part 5 mm, diameter of working part with tips closed 0.8 mm, and a force of pressure 150–200 g
- Endodontic microprobe bent and straight with total a length of 195 mm (bent) and 205 mm (straight), length of working part 30 mm, and diameter of working part 0.5 mm
- Endodontic inward and outward micro-chisel with a total length of 205 mm, length of working part 7 mm, and width of working part 0.6 mm
- Endodontic micro-lever with a total length of 205 mm, length of working part 7.5 mm, diameter of working part (rounded cutting edge) 0.6 mm, and exit diameter of cone blocking the broken instrument 0.8 mm

The steps to be followed are:

- Exposure and/or some movement of the coronal segment of the fragment with an ultrasonic tip or with the appropriate endodontic micro-chisel. With the latter, the working part is introduced with its concave surface toward the fragment between the fragment and the dentin root canal wall.
- Ensure free access to the fragment with an endodontic microprobe.
- The fragment is then seized and removed with endodontic micro-forceps, endodontic forceps, or an endodontic micro-lever depending on its location, the width of the instrumented canal, and the blocking strength of the fragment. Only loose fragments can be removed with micro-tweezers. Endodontic micro-forceps with their three moving jaws locked by a sliding-over tube can seize the fragment strongly and firmly either centrally between their three jaws or laterally in a slit between any two jaws and retrieve it. An endodontic micro-lever is used with a retention material applied to its cutting end to bond the fragment. Wax or glass ionomer can be used as proposed by the manufacturers.

4.3.17 Tube Techniques

With this technique, the coronal segment of the fragment is exposed and positioned in the center of the root canal, and then a hollow tube device with an adhesive is slid into it. In most of the proposed tube techniques, cyanoacrylate is used as an adhesive. The alternative to cyanoacrylate is resin (Fig. 4.54). The tube with the adhesive must fit the external diameter of the instrument exactly. Use of a tube with adhesive has been found to be effective in the removal of fragments of instruments (Gettleman et al. 1991; Andrabi et al. 2013; Brito-Junior et al. 2015), silver cones (Spriggs et al. 1990), and a McSpadden compactor extruding the foramen about 4 mm (Filho et al. 1998).

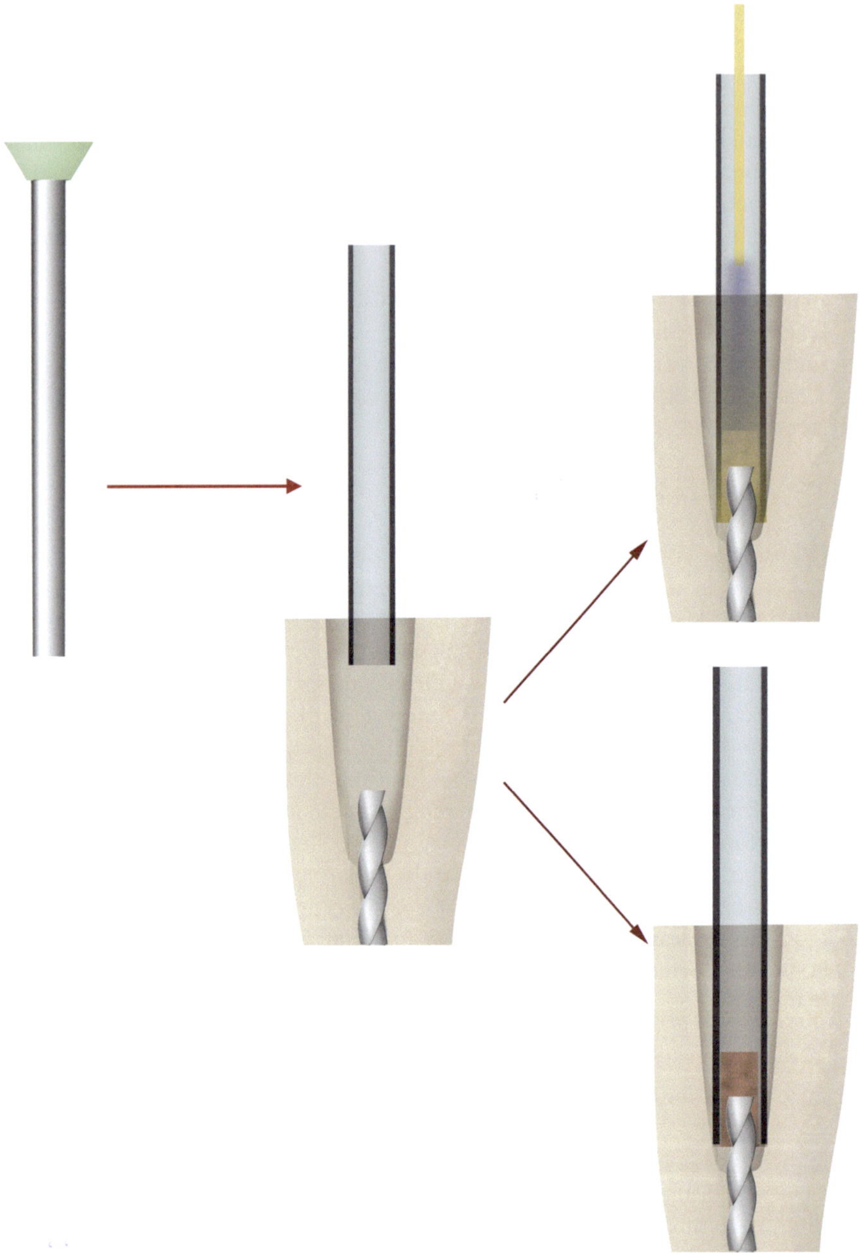

Fig. 4.54 A schematic illustration showing the adhesion of the fragment to the tube either with a self- or light (*top*)-curing composite resin or with cyanoacrylate (*bottom*)

In a pullout in vitro comparison of dual- and light-curing composite resin polymerized with optical fiber inserted into the micro-tube and pushed forward until the fiber came into contact with the endodontic instrument, the light-curing composite resin was found to be superior compared with the use of cyanoacrylate or chemically cured composite (Wefelmeier et al. 2015).

The most characteristic and well-known systems for this technique are:

1. The Endo Extractor
2. The Cancellier Extractor Kit
3. Hypodermic surgical needles
4. The separated instrument removal system
5. The Micro-Retrieve & Repair System

4.3.17.1 The Endo Extractor

The Endo Extractor kit (Brasseler USA Inc., Savannah, GA) consists of:

- Four extractors of different sizes and colors
- Four trephine burs corresponding to each extractor
- A cyanoacrylate adhesive
- A debonding agent

The steps to be followed in this technique proposed by Johnson and Beatty (1988) include (Fig. 4.55):

- Exposure of approximately 2 mm of the coronal segment of the fragment by troughing around it with the appropriate trephine bur. It should be noted, however, that care must be exercised during their use as their aggressive cutting when new may weaken the root or cause root perforation. The manufacturer has developed a separate smaller trephine bur not included in the kit, which corresponds better to the smaller extractors and removes less dentin.
- The appropriate pre-selected micro-tube extractor with cyanoacrylate adhesive is slid into place over the exposed coronal segment of the fragment. The adhesive is used to bond the hollow tube to the exposed end of the file. Care must be exercised to use only a few drops of adhesive and not too much in order to avoid inadvertently blocking the canal.
- Additionally, to prevent leakage of the adhesive to the outside surface of the extractor, isolation with glycerol or petroleum jelly is advisable. Even though the suggested overlap between the extractor tube and the fragment is 2 mm, the bond created between them with a 1 mm snug fit overlap is strong enough to retrieve the majority of fragments. The time required for the adhesive to set to ensure sufficient bond strength for retrieval is 5 min for a snug fit and 10 min for a loose fit (Spriggs et al. 1990; Gettleman et al. 1991). The extractors may be reused, either by removing the embedded instrument from the extractor tube using the debonding agent included in the kit or by cutting the extraction device with a bur beyond the extent that the fragment has penetrated.

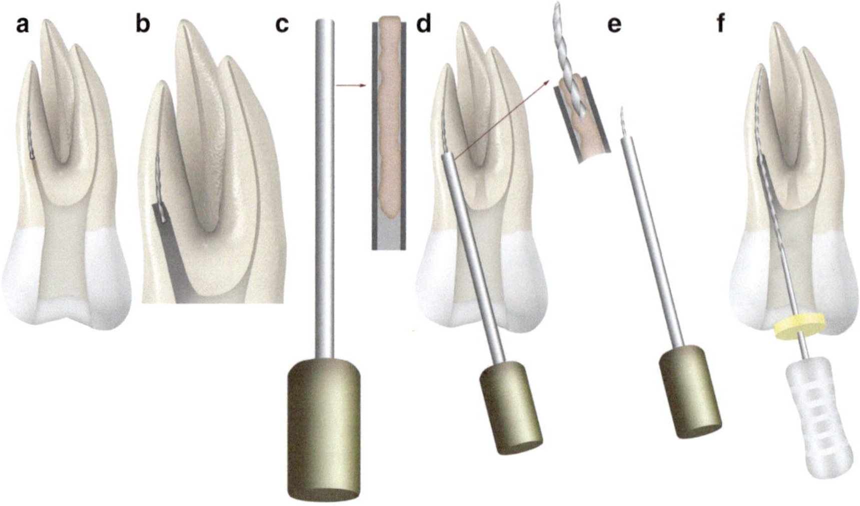

Fig. 4.55 (**a–f**) Schematic illustration of the removal of an instrument fragment with the Endo Extractor (Johnson and Beatty 1988 method). (**a**) Radiographic confirmation of the presence of a fragment and recognition of its location, size, and length. (**b**) Instrumentation of the canal coronal to the fragment and exposure of its coronal end. (**c–e**) The pre-selected extractor with adhesive is slid into place over the exposed coronal segment of the fragment, and the fragment is retrieved bonded to the extractor. (**f**) Once the fragment is removed, the canal is renegotiated with an ISO size #10K-file to the apical foramen, and canal instrumentation follows

4.3.17.2 The Cancellier Extractor

The Cancellier Extractor Kit (SybronEndo, Orange, California) consists of:

- One handle
- Four assorted extractors (disposable tubes) with outside diameters of 0.50, 0.60, 0.70, and 0.80 mm.

  There are no trephine burs in the Cancellier kit.
  The steps to be followed are:

- Exposure of 2–3 mm of the coronal segment of the fragment with ultrasonics.
- The appropriate pre-selected extractor is then used in conjunction with an adhesive (usually cyanoacrylate) to bond onto the exposed coronal end of the fragment and eventually retrieve it. The handle enables Cancellier extractors to be used without blocking visibility when using the dental operating microscope. The Cancellier extractors can be cleaned and reused.

4.3.17.3 Hypodermic Surgical Needle

This is a simple cost-effective method in which no special sophisticated equipment is needed, which can still result in predictable success (Andrabi et al. 2013). Cut hypodermic surgical needles, transformed into micro-tubes, are used in this technique either as:

1. A hypodermic surgical needle with an adhesive
2. A hypodermic surgical needle with a Hedstroem file

Hypodermic Surgical Needle with an Adhesive

The armamentarium used in this technique consists of:

- Hypodermic surgical needles of various sizes cut as micro-tubes 5–10 mm long
- Adhesive

The steps to be followed (Fig. 4.56) and a characteristic case (Fig. 4.57) managed with this technique are presented:

- Exposure of approximately 1.5–2 mm of the coronal segment of the fragment by troughing around it with a trephine bur, by ultrasonic means, or even with a shortened hypodermic needle rotated under light pressure to groove around the coronal part of the fragment.
- Selection of the appropriate needle, based mainly on its external diameter as this dictates how deeply it can be introduced into the canal (Table 4.8). The pre-selected hypodermic needle is cut with a disk and converted into a micro-tube. The modified needle micro-tube is then inserted into the canal in order to check whether it can engulf the exposed coronal segment of the fragment.
- A few drops of cyanoacrylate glue or strong dental cement (i.e., polycarboxylate) are dropped into the cut hypodermic needle, and the needle, coated externally with glycerol or petroleum jelly, is reinserted over the exposed coronal segment of the fragment.
- When set, the whole assembly (needle-adhesive-fragment) as a single unit is pulled out of the canal through gentle slight counterclockwise rotation and a simultaneous pullout motion.

Hypodermic Surgical Needle with Hedstroem File

An alternative to the use of adhesive in connection with the piece of hypodermic needle converted into a micro-tube has also been proposed (Suter 1998) and used (Monteiro et al. 2014). The armamentarium of this technique consists of:

- Hypodermic surgical needles of various sizes cut as micro-tubes 5–10 mm long.
- Hedstroem files because of their unique ability to engage. The size of the file to be used is related to the size of the needle micro-tube selected as its taper might hamper its placement through a smaller-sized parallel micro-tube.

The steps to be followed are (Fig. 4.56):

- Exposure of approximately 1.5–2 mm of the coronal segment of the fragment.
- Insertion of the needle micro-tube over the exposed 1–2 mm of the coronal segment of the fragment.

- A correctly pre-selected Hedstroem file is pushed in a clockwise motion through the needle to wedge the upper part of the fragment and the needle's inner wall tightly together.
- With good interlocking between the fragment and the Hedstroem file, the three connected objects can then be gently pulled out of the root canal.

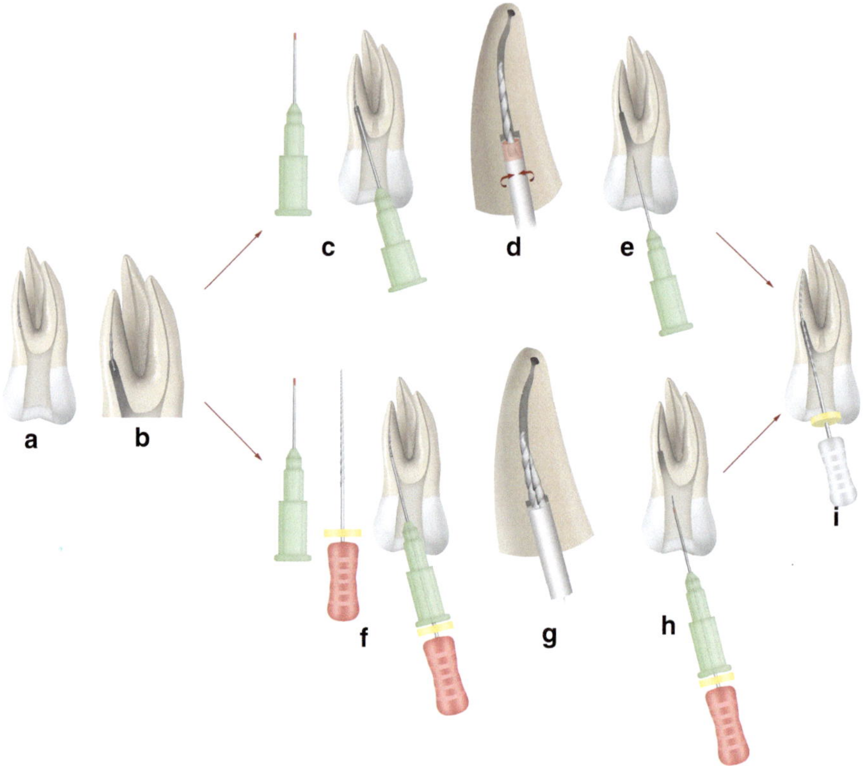

Fig. 4.56 (**a–i**) Schematic illustration of the removal of a fractured instrument with the hypodermic surgical needle micro-tube method either with an adhesive (*top row*) or with a Hedstroem file (*bottom row*). (**a**) Radiographic confirmation of the presence of the fragment and recognition of its location, size, and length. (**b**) Instrumentation of the root canal coronal to the fragment and exposure of its coronal segment. (**c**) Insertion of the pre-selected and modified needle micro-tube into the 1–2 mm exposed coronal segment of the fragment immediately after a few drops of cyanoacrylate glue or strong dental cement were dropped into the cut hypodermic needle. (**d**, **e**) Through gentle, slight counterclockwise rotation and a simultaneous pullout motion, the fragment, which has adhered to the needle tube, is pulled out of the canal. (**f**, **g**) In the hypodermic surgical needle and the Hedstroem file technique, the pre-selected file is introduced into the canal through the already inserted needle—micro-tube—over the exposed 1–2 mm coronal segment of the fragment. The Hedstroem file is introduced until it is tightly engaged between the fragment and the internal lumen of the micro-tube. (**h**) The three connected objects are then withdrawn from the canal by pulling the tube and the Hedstroem file. (**i**) Once the fragment is removed, the canal is renegotiated with an ISO size #10K-file to the apical foramen, and canal instrumentation follows

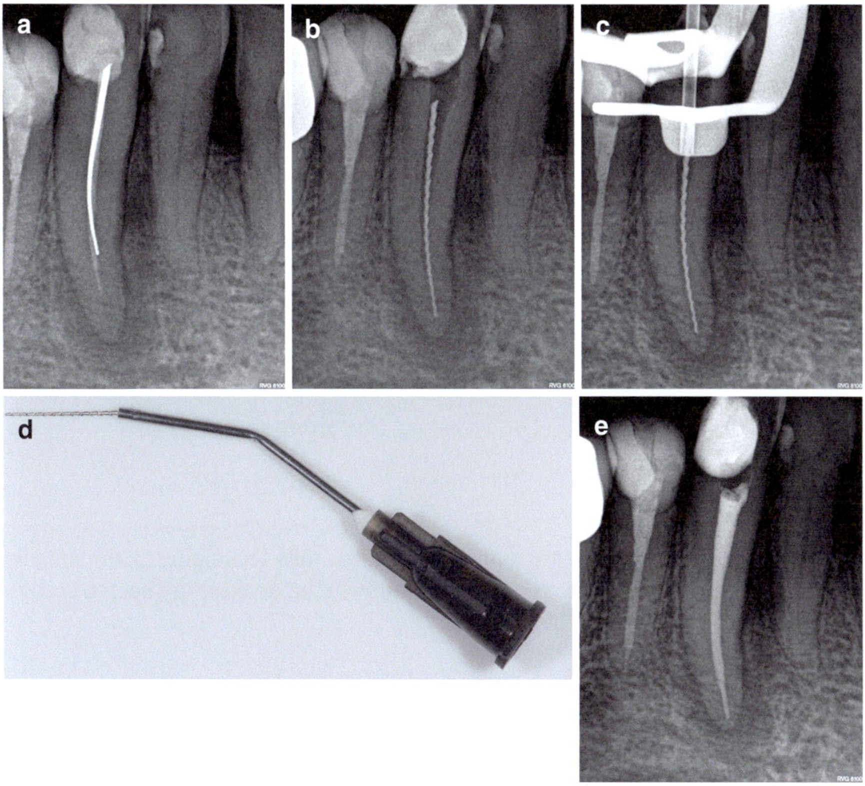

Fig. 4.57 (**a**) Preoperative radiograph of a left mandibular canine with an incomplete RCT with silver points. (**b**) Exposure of 2–3 mm of the coronal segment of the 7 mm GiroFile #30 fragment extending from the coronal to the apical third that fractured during retreatment. (**c**) Pre-selected needle—tube was inserted into the canal over the exposed coronal segment of the fragment, and a radiograph was obtained to check its placement. (**d**) A few drops of cyanoacrylate were then dropped into the needle micro-tube coated externally with glycerol, and the tube was reinserted in the previous position. The whole assembly was removed after 6 min in place, a sufficient period for the setting of the cyanoacrylate. (**e**) The canal was instrumented and obturated up to the desired length (Courtesy of Prof. J. Molyvdas)

4.3.17.4 The Separated Instrument Removal System

This kit (Vista Dental Products, Wisconsin, USA) contains:

- 100 dead-soft bondable tubes in five internal diameters (18 ga, 19 ga, 20 ga, 22 ga, and 25 ga). These soft tubes allow easy access, even in cases of curved canals.
- A bottle of bonding agent.
- A bottle of accelerator to be combined with the bonding agent and create a speedy, durable bond.
- Assorted instrument fulcrum props.
- A curved hemostat.

Table 4.8 Range of diameters of tubing with gauge size from 27 to 16 (ISO 9626:1991/Amd.1:2001)

Gauge size	Range of external diameters (mm)		Internal diameter of tubing (mm)		
	Minimum	Maximum	Normal-walled minimum	Thin-walled minimum	Extra-thin-walled minimum
27	0.400	0.420	0.184	0.241	–
26	0.440	0.470	0.232	0.292	–
25	0.500	0.530	0.232	0.292	–
24	0.550	0.580	0.280	0.343	–
23	0.600	0.673	0.317	0.370	0.460
22	0.698	0.730	0.390	0.440	0.522
21	0.800	0.830	0.490	0.547	0.610
20	0.860	0.920	0.560	0.635	0.687
19	1.030	1.100	0.648	0.750	0.850
18	1.200	1.300	0.790	0.910	1.041
17	1.400	1.510	0.950	1.156	1.244
16	1.600	1.690	1.100	1.283	1.390

The steps to be followed are quite similar to all tube techniques with the main difference that the dead softness of the tubes allows them to be easily bent to accommodate any insertion path. They include:

- Exposure of approximately 1.5–2 mm of the coronal segment of the fragment.
- Trial insertion of the pre-selected pre-bent tube over the exposed portion of the fragment. Several trial insertions at this stage and adjustments are made until a trouble-free final insertion is ensured.
- A second dead-soft tube of the same size as the first one is selected.
- With the aid of the second tube, a highly active accelerator (Vista's Prime-Set, Agent A) is discretely applied to the fragment by placing the tip of the tube over its exposed portion. This tube is then left in place until the tube with Quick-Set (Agent B) is ready to be placed.
- The specially formulated metal-to-metal bonding agent (Vista's Quick-Set, Agent B) is introduced into the pre-selected tube and slid over the exposed segment of the fragment to replace the tube left there. The accelerated bond starts immediately. The maturation of the bond may take several minutes, during which time the "bonding system" must remain undisturbed to avoid interruption of the reaction.
- The bonded assembly is grasped with the curved hemostat and is removed using a fulcrum on the next anterior tooth, which is protected by the available instrument prop inserted over it.

4.3.17.5 The Micro-Retrieve & Repair System

This small diameter trepan bur technique, comparatively evaluated (Yang et al. 2017) in vitro with the ultrasonic technique regarding the amount of dentin removal and the time required for the retrieval of intentionally fractured K3-files, utilizes the Micro-Retrieve & Repair System (Superline NIC Dental, Shenzhen, China). This system consists of:

- Trepan burs in five different sizes (Table 4.9 and Fig. 4.58)
- Needle cannulas with side oval window at the working length in corresponding sizes (Fig. 4.59)

The length of the trepan bur and needle cannulas can be individually adjusted to improve access to posterior teeth.

Table 4.9 Trepan bur symbols and sizes of the Micro-Retrieve & Repair System (Superline NIC Dental, Shenzhen, China)

Symbol		External diameter (mm)	Internal diameter (mm)
18G	5 circles	1.26	0.86
19G	4 circles	1.10	0.70
20G	3 circles	0.90	0.60
21G	2 circles	0.80	0.50
22G	1 circle	0.70	0.40

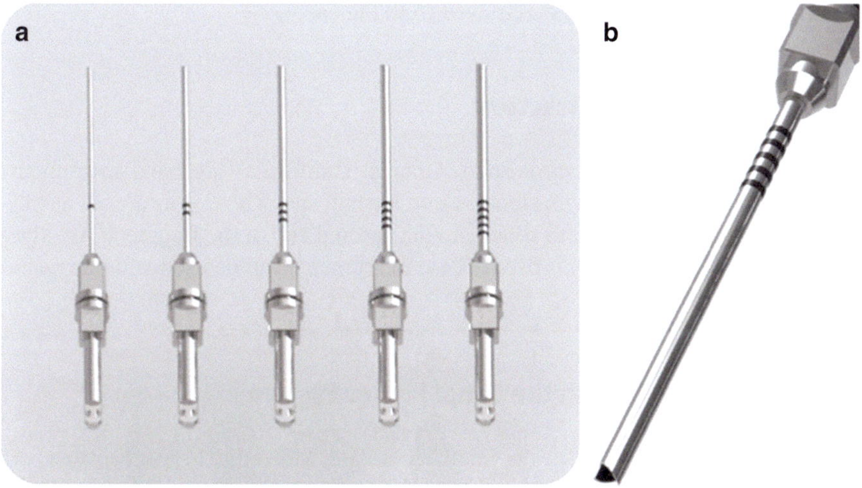

Fig. 4.58 (**a**) The five trepan bur sizes of the Micro-Retrieve & Repair System (Superline NIC Dental, Shenzhen, China). (**b**) Magnification of size 5

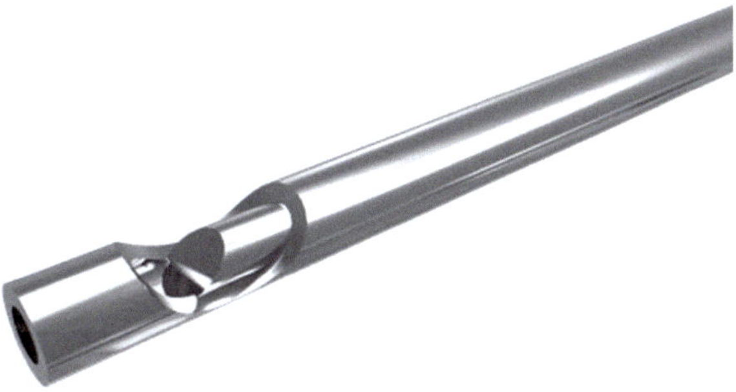

Fig. 4.59 Needle cannula with side oval window of the Micro-Retrieve & Repair System (Superline NIC Dental, Shenzhen, China)

The steps to be followed with this technique are:

- The root canal is instrumented up to the fragment. Straight-line access and visualization of the most coronal aspect of the fragment are tried whenever possible.
- Under direct microscopic vision, a staging platform is prepared at the most coronal aspect of the fragment using modified pre-selected Gates Glidden burs sizes #1–#3.
- A trepan bur operated with an endodontic motor in a counterclockwise direction (it) is used to expose the coronal 1 to 1.5 mm length of the fragment.
- The fragment might become loose and retrieved just by exposing it with the trepan bur. If it is retrieved, the needle cannula is used. The needle cannula, with dimensions corresponding to the trepan bur used, is inserted into the canal and placed over the exposed portion of the fragment. By pushing the sliding push bottom on the handle, the fragment is gripped and locked in the needle cannula with an insert wedge. The curved and beveled surface at the end of the insert wedge set opposite to the side oval window in the needle cannula improves the engagement and thus ensures firm grip. Once the fragment is grasped mechanically, the whole assembly is retrieved from the canal.

4.3.18 The Mounce Extractors

The Mounce extractors (SybronEndo, Orange, California) are hand instruments similar to a ball burnisher with slots cut into the ball end. These slots are cut at various angles and are designed to slide onto the coronal end of the fragment. An adhesive (usually cyanoacrylate) is used. These instruments can be used with the dental operating microscope.

4.3.19 Technique Using the Canal Finder System

The Canal Finder System (Societe Endo Technique, Marseille, France) consists of:

- A special handpiece. The system produces an up-and-down pecking motion and a quarter of a turn rotation that guides the instrument into the path of the root canal.
- Exclusively designed for the system engine-driven instruments.

The system has been used effectively in the removal of fractured instruments and silver cones (Hülsmann 1990a, b).

In this technique, starting with a size #8 and size #10 path-finding file, an attempt is made to work along the obstruction and to loosen the fragment by circumferential filing under copious irrigation. The files are initially moved at an amplitude of 1–2 mm and subsequently at a smaller amplitude with a higher speed. The flutes of the files are mechanically engaged with the fragment, and through the vertical vibration of the file, the fragment is loosened and eventually retrieved in the majority of cases (Fig. 4.60). Care must be exercised to avoid extruding the fragment apically and in cases of curved canals to avoid root perforations.

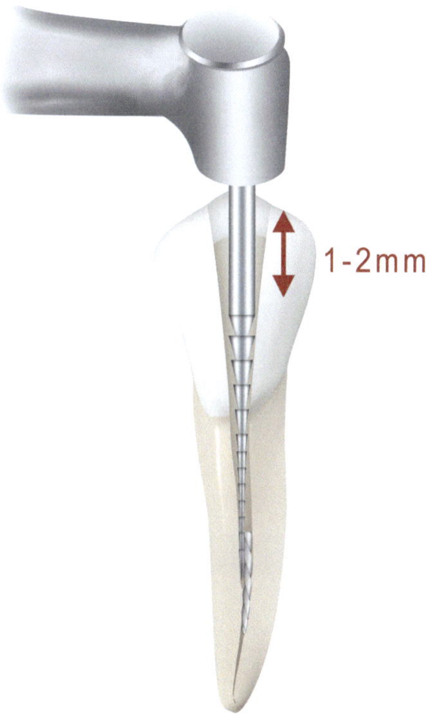

Fig. 4.60 The Canal Finder System (a handpiece and specially designed files) produces a 1–2 mm up-and-down movement. When bypassing the fragment, the file flutes can engage it, and with the up-and-down motion, the fragment can be loosened or even retrieved

In very difficult cases, a combined use of the Canal Finder System and ultrasound devices is recommended (Hülsmann and Schinkel 1999).

This system has been replaced by the EndoPulse system (EndoTechnic, San Diego, CA, USA) in which SS files are used in vertical reciprocation and a passive ¼ turn motion. To our knowledge, there is no report in peer-reviewed journals on the application of the new system for managing fractured endodontic instruments.

4.3.20 File Retrieval System

This system, which was developed in 2006, has been found effective in laboratory studies and in clinical cases of instruments fractured at the apical third of the canal in a relatively short retrieval time with the removal of a minimal amount of root dentin (Terauchi et al. 2006, 2007; Terauchi 2012).

The Terauchi File Retrieval Kit (TFRK, Dental Care, Santa Barbara, California, USA) in its autoclavable cassette (Fig. 4.61) contains:

- A modified Gates Glidden #3 bur
- A microtrephine bur
- A microexplorer instrument
- A loop device
- Gutta-percha removal instrument
- Four customized ultrasonic tips that can be bent to accommodate canal curvature
- A tooth replica with three broken files for practice.

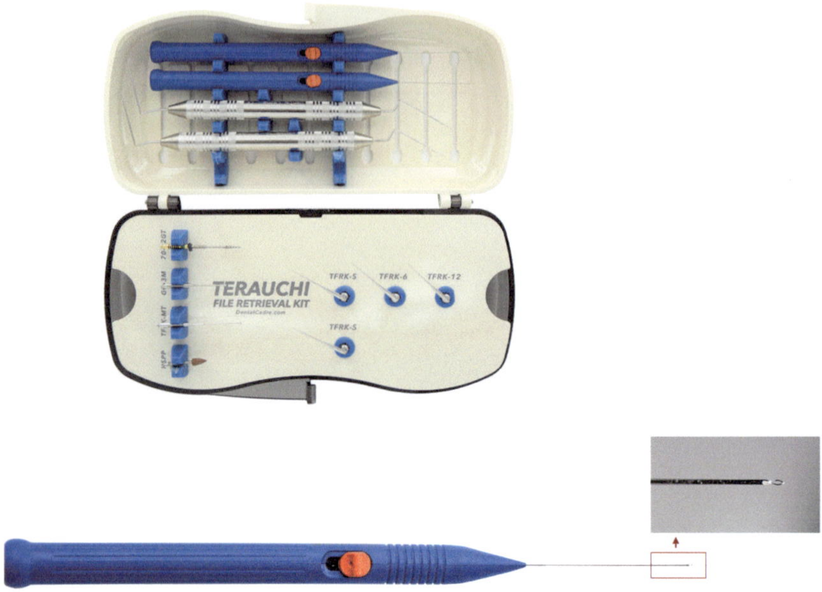

Fig. 4.61 Terauchi File Retrieval Kit (TFRK, Dental Care, Santa Barbara, California, USA)

The stages to be followed (Fig. 4.62) start as in all techniques with a radiographic interpretation to confirm the presence of the fragment, to reveal its location in relation to the root canal curvature if present, and to estimate its size and radiographic length. Three sequential steps that use especially newly designed instruments then follow (Terauchi et al. 2006, 2007; Terauchi 2012).

Step 1
Enlargement of the canal and thus creation of an unobstructed straight-line access to the coronal portion of the fragment. For this purpose, Terauchi et al. (2006) originally proposed the use of two newly developed low-speed cutting burs (28 mm long) flexible enough in the shanks to be able to go around a curved canal. They were used in a counterclockwise motion, and they loosened or even removed the fragment. In a later article, Terauchi (2012) proposed the creation of straight-line access and enlargement of the canal up to the fragment with a Gates Glidden bur size #2 or a maximum Gates Glidden bur size #3.

Step 2
With the ultrasonic tip (30 mm long with a diameter of 0.2 mm), a small pocket (1 mm) is created on the dentin wall in the inner curvature, and a shallow groove is cut on the outer curvature. The root canal is then filled with EDTA to enhance the ultrasonic cavitation effect and acoustic streaming and at the same time reduce the thermal effect. Ultrasonics with the specially designed ultrasonic tip is applied to the fragment in the space created between the fragment and the inner curve of the root canal. This continues until the fragment is retrieved. If no release of the fragment is seen for more than 1 min, more tooth structure needs

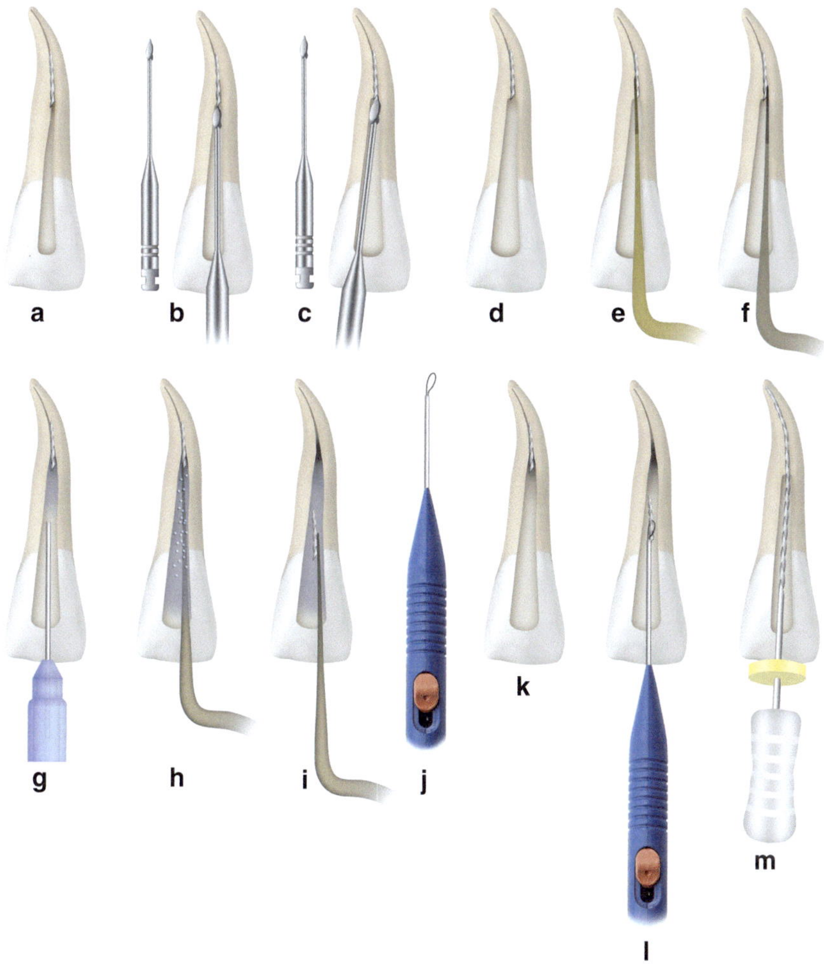

Fig. 4.62 (**a–l**) Schematic illustration of the retrieval of an instrument fragment with the File Retrieval System (Terauchi technique). (**a**) Radiographic confirmation of the presence of a fragment and recognition of its location, size, and length. (**b–d**) Enlargement of the canal and creation of straight-line access to the canal with Gates Glidden burs #2 and 3. (**e**, **f**) With the ultrasonic tip, a small pocket is created on the dentin wall in the inner curvature, and a shallow groove is cut on the outer curvature. (**g**) The canal is then filled with EDTA. (**h**, **i**) The ultrasonic tip is activated with its tip in "push-and-pull" motions until the fragment is removed. In unsuccessful attempts with no sign of fragment disengagement for 5 min despite removal of more dentin apically along the inside wall of the fragment, the wire loop technique follows. (**j–l**) With the specially designed loop device, the NiTi wire loop is placed over the fragment, and the loop is pulled in all directions to retrieve the fragment. (**m**) Once the fragment is removed, the canal is renegotiated with an ISO size #10K-file to the apical foramen, and canal instrumentation follows

to be removed apically along the inside wall of the fragment. If after 5 min efforts have produced no sign of disengagement, the next step follows.

Step 3

In this step, a loop device with a NiTi wire (0.08 mm) is used to mechanically engage the peripherally exposed (by at least 0.7 mm) fragment and retrieve it.

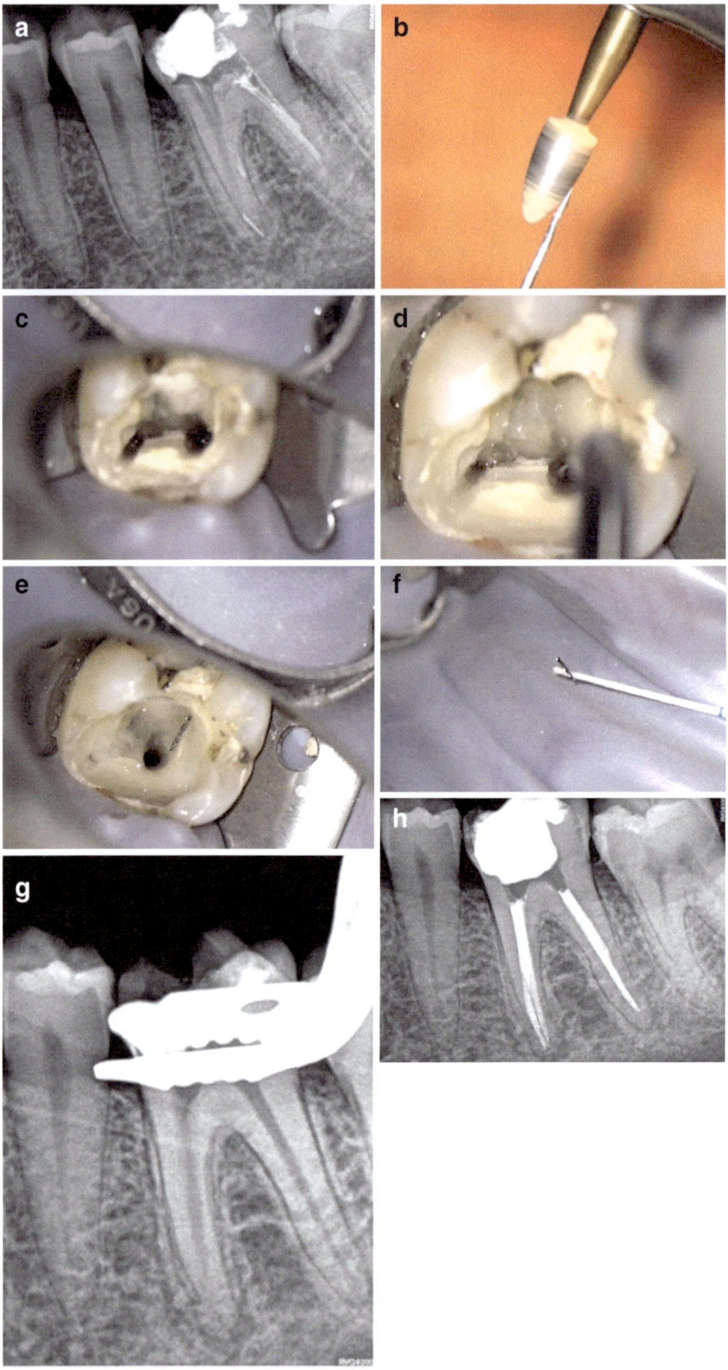

Fig. 4.63 (**a**) Preoperative radiograph. (**b**) Fragment visible with the microscope on the mesiolingual canal. (**c**) Sharpening of the FRK S tip. (**d**) Sharpened FRK S tip preparing space next to the fragment. (**e–g**) Fragment removed with the TFRK. (**h**) Postoperative radiograph. Note the minimal amount of root dentin removed (Courtesy of Dr. S. Floratos)

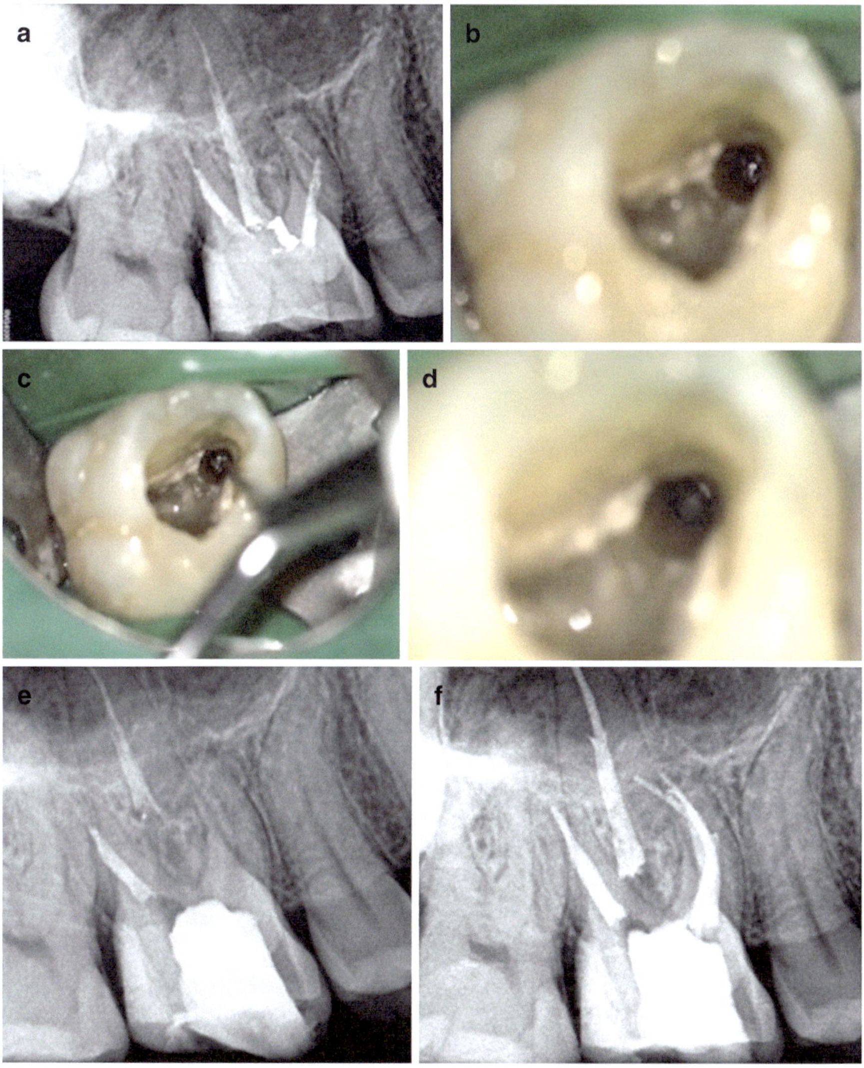

Fig. 4.64 (**a**) Preoperative radiograph of a maxillary first molar with incomplete RCT and a fractured file beyond the curvature on the mesiobuccal canal. (**b**) File visible after removing a dentin overhang. (**c**) Space created next to the file with the FRK S tip. (**d**, **e**) Fragment removed with a minimal sacrifice of root dentin. (**f**) Immediate post-obturation radiograph (Courtesy of Dr. S. Floratos)

Characteristic cases of fragments removed with the File Retrieval System (Terauchi technique) are presented (Figs. 4.63 and 4.64).

4.3.21 The Micro-forceps Grasping Technique

The armamentarium of the micro-forceps grasping technique (Fors and Berg 1983) consists of (Fig. 4.65):

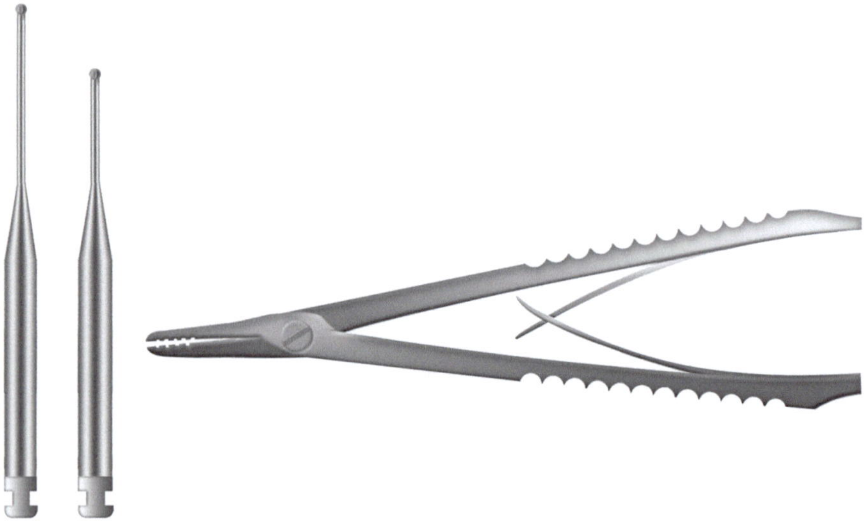

Fig. 4.65 A long round bur, an ordinary bur, and a Castroviejo needle holder

- Round burs with extra-long and very thin shanks (pulp chamber bur "Muller," Hager & Meisinger GmbH, Dusseldorf, Germany).
- A special bur (Maillefer, Ballaigues, Switzerland).
- A needle holder used in microsurgery by ophthalmologists (Castroviejo needle holder, Stiwernom164-96448-5, Stille-Werner, Stockholm, Sweden). The needle holder is modified by repositioning the springs from the back of the handles to a position between the handles, thus shortening the instrument considerably, and by cutting grooves into the jaws to ensure a stronger grip.

The steps to be followed are (Fig. 4.66):

- Creation of access to the fragment by careful instrumentation with the long round burs. The pulp chamber and the root canal are illuminated with fiber optics.
- Exposure of the coronal 1.5–2 mm of the fragment by careful drilling followed by gentle loosening from the canal walls with a K-file. Loosening continues until approximately one-fourth of the fragment is freed.
- Grasping of the visible, exposed portion of the fragment with the modified Castroviejo needle holder and through gentle movements and retrieval of the fragment.

4.3.22 The Wire Loop Technique

This technique (Roig-Greene 1983) aims at removing the segment by circling it with a wire loop. It employs a disposable 25-gauge dental injection needle with an external diameter of 0.46 mm; a 12–15 cm piece of steel wire, 0.14 mm in diameter; and a small hemostatic forceps (Fig. 4.67).

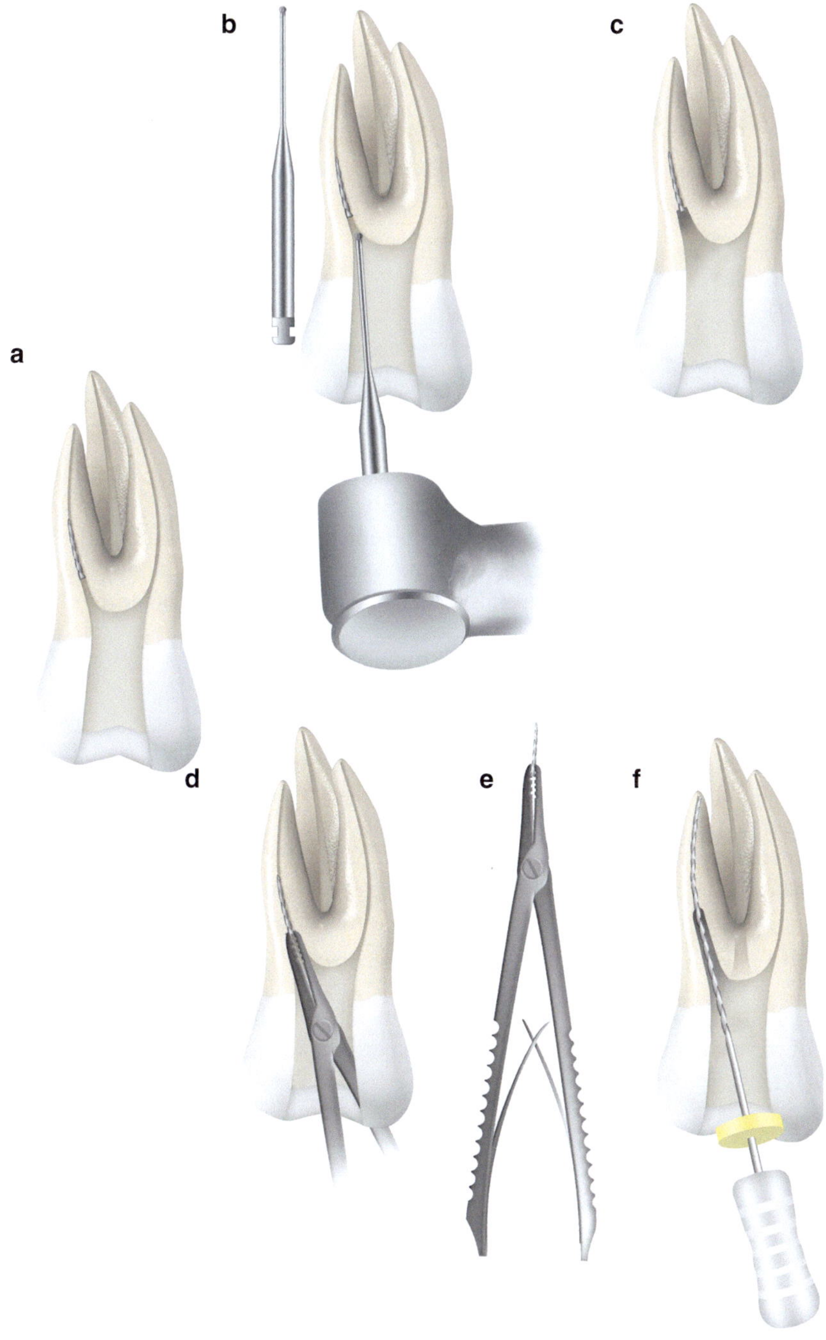

Fig. 4.66 (**a–f**) Schematic illustration of the removal of a fragment with the micro-forceps grasping technique. (**a**) Radiographic confirmation of the presence of a fragment and recognition of its location, size, and length. (**b**, **c**) Instrumentation of the canal coronal to the fragment and careful drilling with a fine elongated round bur to expose its coronal end. (**d**, **e**) Retrieval of the fragment with the modified Castroviejo needle holder. (**f**) Once the fragment is removed, the canal is renegotiated with an ISO size #10K-file to the apical foramen, and canal instrumentation follows

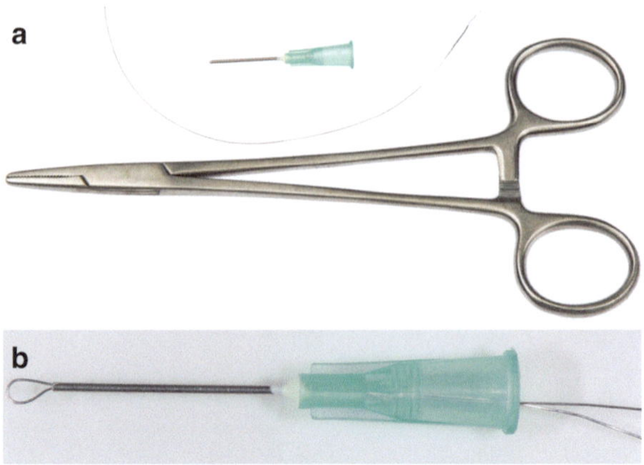

Fig. 4.67 (**a**) The armamentarium required in the wire loop technique (Roig-Greene 1983) includes a cut disposable needle, an orthodontic wire, and small hemostatic forceps. (**b**, **c**) A loop formed with the help of an instrument whose size is larger than that of the fragment

The needle is prepared by cutting it twice, once at about 5 mm from the bevel end, and then flush with the hub at the opposite end. Both free ends of the wire are inserted into the needle through the injection end until they slide out of the hub end. A small mosquito hemostat is used to tighten the wire loop around the object to be retrieved by clamping both free ends of the wire and rotating the hemostat about an axis perpendicular to the needle.

The steps to be followed are (Fig. 4.68):

- Root canal instrumentation up to the fragment.
- Exposure of the coronal 1.5–2 mm of the fragment.
- Radiographic control to confirm that the loop surrounds the instrument. This is required only in cases of difficulty or doubt.
- Tightening of the loop around the exposed portion of the fragment with the help of hemostatic forceps. By pulling the complete assembly out of the canal in various directions to dislocate the fragment from the dentine walls, the fragment is retrieved.

The effectiveness of this technique may increase if some tips cited by the inventor of the technique gained from clinical experience of the technique (Roig-Greene 1983) are considered:

Fig. 4.68 (**a–h**) Schematic illustration of the retrieval of an instrument fragment with the wire loop technique. (**a**) Radiographic confirmation of the presence of a fragment and recognition of its location, size, and length. (**b–d**) Instrumentation of the root canal coronal to the fragment and exposure of its coronal end. (**e**, **f**) The pre-prepared loop is oriented according to the existing space and tightened around the fragment. (**g**) Once positioned, the hub of the needle is held with the other hand. Both free ends of the wire are clamped with the hemostatic forceps and tightened, and the complete assembly is moved back and forth until the segment is loosened and can be removed. (**h**) Once the fragment is removed, the canal is renegotiated with an ISO size #10K-file to the apical foramen, and canal instrumentation follows

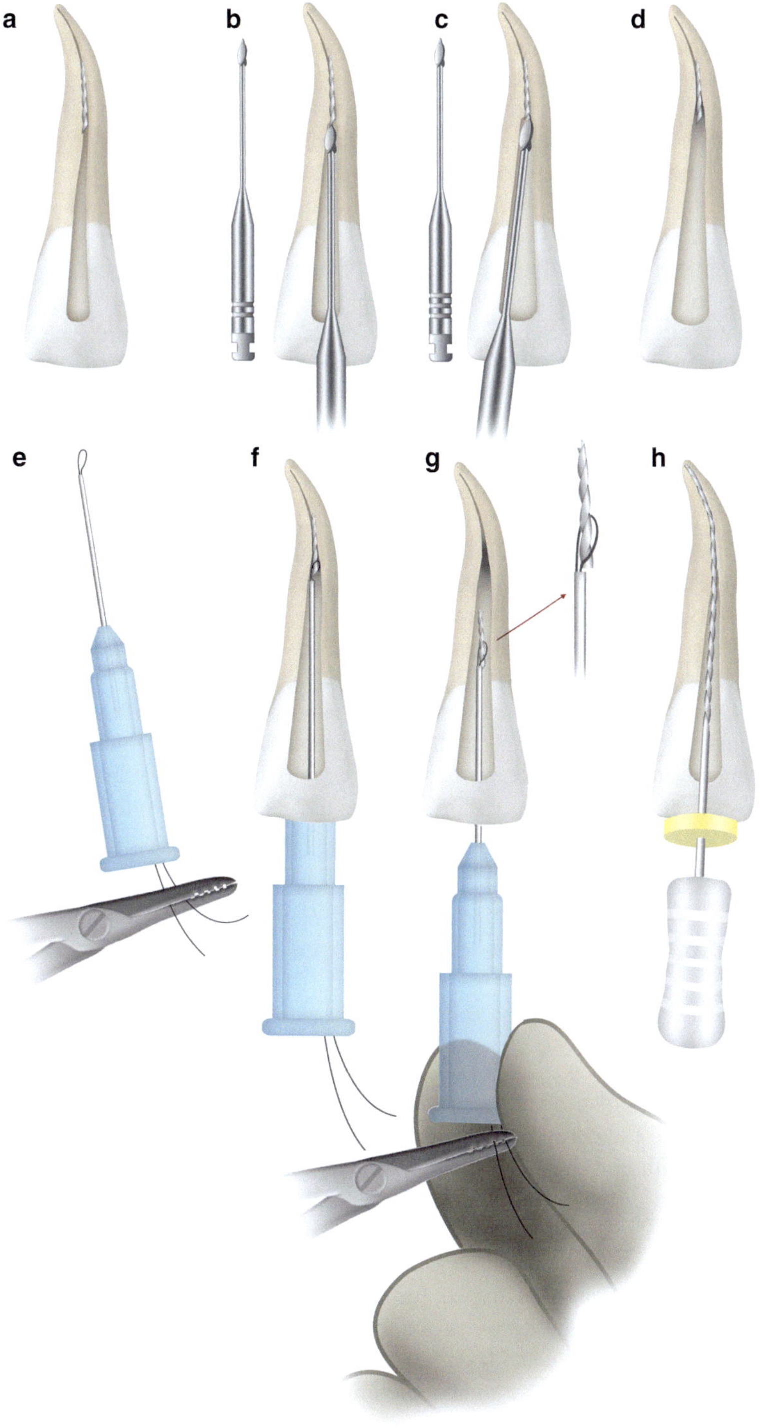
a
b
c
d
e
f
g
h

1. If the coronal segment of the fractured instrument is resting against a wall of the root canal, it must be freed with an endodontic explorer in order to position it toward the center of the canal.
2. The loop is oriented according to the existing space. Thus, for instance, if there is greater space along the distal wall of the root canal, the loop is oriented mesially in order for the needle to be accommodated on the distal.
3. The complete assembly of the needle and loop can be placed more easily into position with the help of a small hemostatic forceps. If problems of visibility emerge or if the manipulations are hindered, then the hub is bent in whatever position is desired to overcome the problem.
4. Once positioned, the hub of the needle is held with the other hand. The needle is then unclamped, and both free ends of the wire are clamped with the hemostatic forceps and tightened.
5. If the instrument is not easily dislodged, despite the fact that the loop has been tightened around it, the complete assembly is moved back and forth until the segment is loosened and can be removed.

The latest developments of this technique include the loop device available in the Terauchi File Retrieval Kit (TFRK, Dental Care, Santa Barbara, California, USA) comprised of a tiny titanium wire loop at the end of an SS cannula with a sliding handle (Fig. 4.61) and the Frag Remover (HanCha-Dental, Zwenkau, Germany) with any Luer fitting cannula or the single or double cannula proposed by the inventors (Figs. 4.69 and 4.70). With the Frag Remover, wires made of SS alloy of four different diameters (0.075, 0.1, 0.15, and 0.2 mm) can be used. The stronger wires, according to the inventors/manufacturers, are used for retrieving highly retentive fragments and posts from the coronal root third. Shaping and adjustment of the loop is a simple one-handed operation that facilitates easy use of the dental operating microscope.

Characteristic cases with the Frag Remover are presented (Figs. 4.71 and 4.72).

4.3.23 Softened Gutta-Percha Technique

A simple novel technique using softened gutta-percha has been reported (Rahimi and Parashos 2009) to remove loosely bound fragments located in hard-to-reach areas inhibiting straight-line access and thus not allowing direct vision. With this technique:

- A periapical radiograph located the known in size and type fragment (approximately 3 mm of a size #25/0.02 RaCe rotary instrument).
- Instrumentation of the remaining canals continued.
- With small-sized SS Hedstroem files (#8, #10, and #15), the fragment was partially bypassed and loosened.
- A gutta-percha point was dipped, for about 30 s, in chloroform and then inserted into the canal and allowed to harden for roughly 3 min.
- The gutta-percha point and fragment were then successfully removed using careful and delicate clockwise and counterclockwise pulling actions.

Characteristic cases of fragments protruding into the periapical tissues managed with this technique (Fig. 4.73) and with an inadvertently successfully used slight modification of this technique (Fig. 4.74) are presented. In the case with the

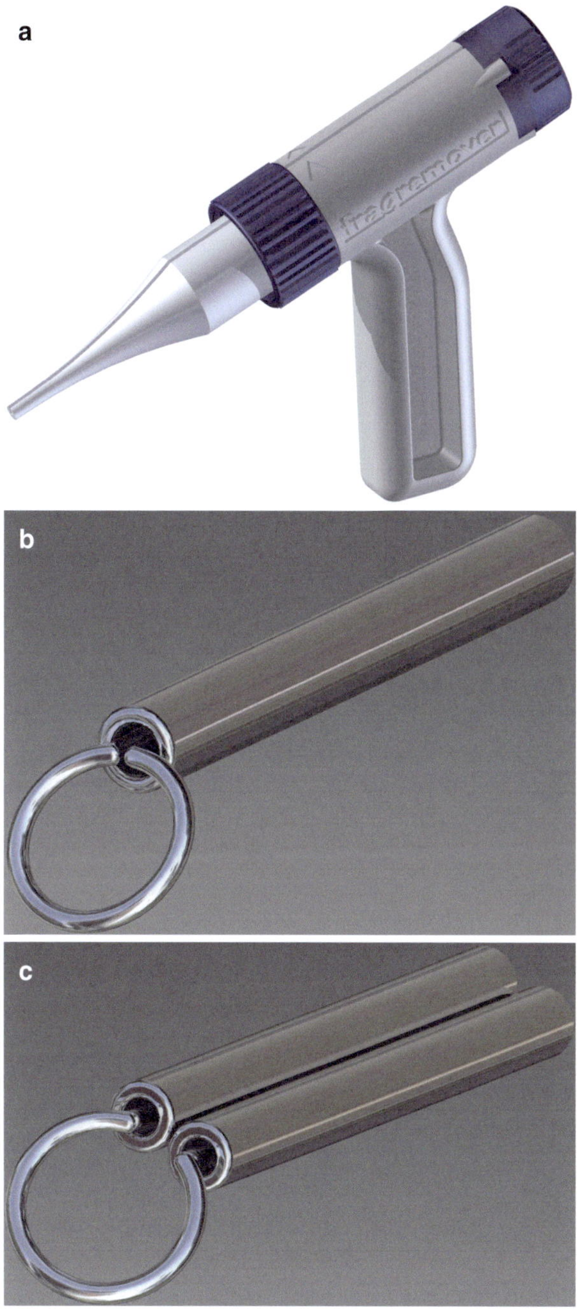

Fig. 4.69 Frag Remover (Frag Remover HanCha-Dental, Zwenkau, Germany) with the single and double fitting cannula (Courtesy of Dr. M. Leineweber)

modified technique, the instrumented canal was obturated with laterally compacted gutta-percha and 811 sealer (Roth International Ltd., Chicago, IL, USA), and immediately the filling material was removed as the clinician was not satisfied with the condensation of gutta-percha in the middle third of the distal canal. The fragment was retrieved attached to the mass of gutta-percha, and the distal canal was re-instrumented and re-obturated (Fig. 4.74).

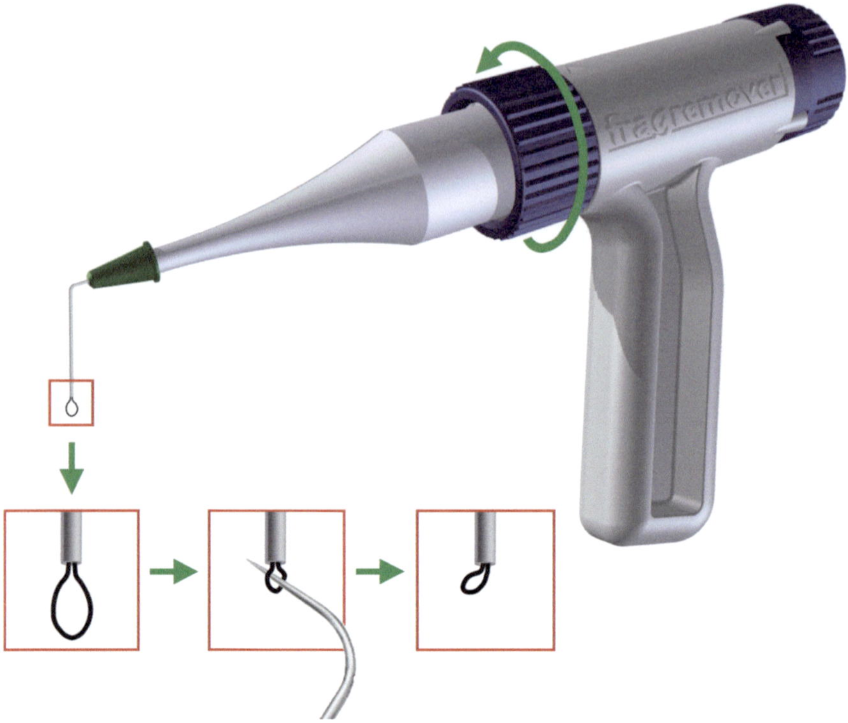

Fig. 4.70 Shaping and adjustment of the loop with the Frag Remover (Frag Remover HanCha-Dental, Zwenkau, Germany). The wire loop is controlled by twisting the adjustment ring (*arrow*). This clockwise twisting pushes the Luer fitting forward and tightens the wire loop. The desired loop size is then created with a special tip, and the wire loop is angled at a degree of approximately 45° (Courtesy of Dr. M. Leineweber)

4.3.24 Multisonic Ultracleaning System

The GentleWave® System, a Multisonic Ultracleaning System (Sonendo Inc., Laguna Hills, Orange County, CA, USA), consists of:

- A console
- A handpiece resembling externally the dental handpiece

This system continuously delivers an irrigating solution throughout the root canal system via its handpiece positioned on an accessed occlusal tooth surface. The system is designed to produce a broad spectrum of sound waves within the irrigation solution to facilitate the cleaning of the root canal system with minimal preceding instrumentation, while the built-in vented suction removes into a waste canister inside the console the outflowing fluid, creating negative pressure within the root canal. The manufacturer suggests that canals do not need to be enlarged beyond ISO

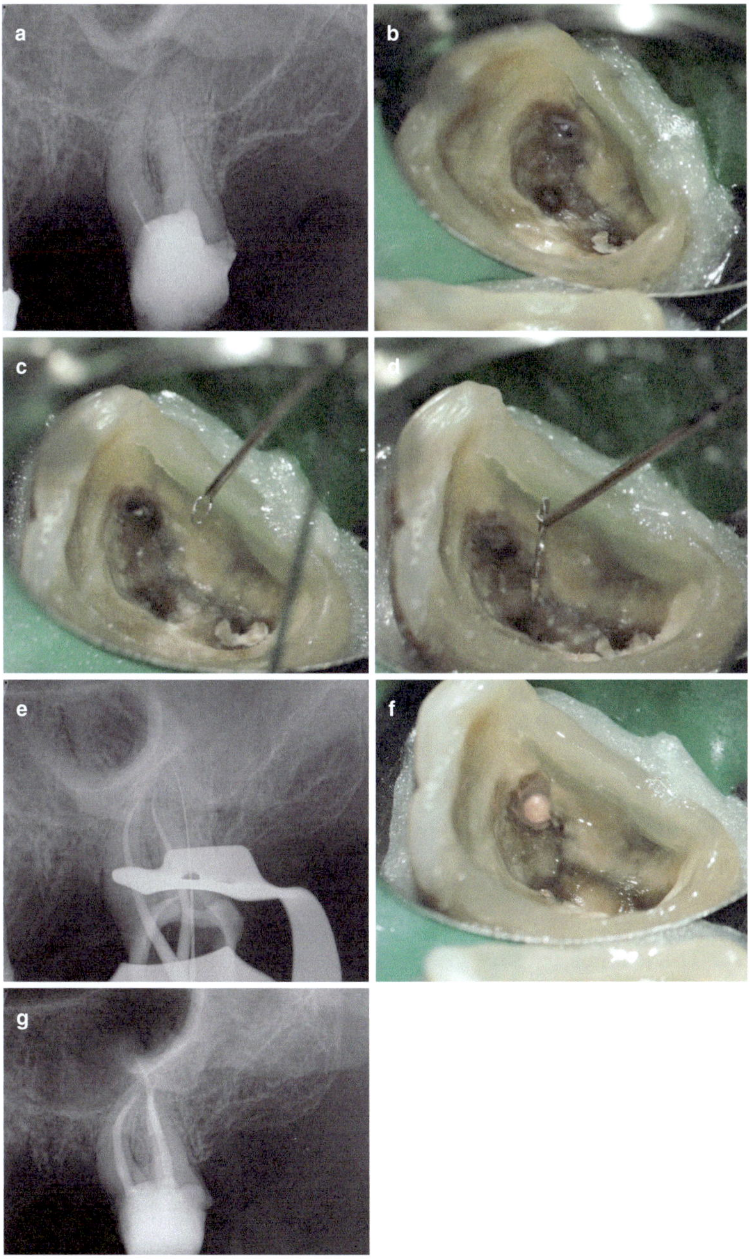

Fig. 4.71 (**a**) Initial radiograph of a maxillary second left molar with a fragment in the coronal third of the mesiobuccal canal. (**b**) Exposure of the coronal segment of the fragment. (**c**) Creation of a wire loop to attach the fragment. (**d**) Removal of the fragment with the wire loop technique using the Frag Remover (Frag Remover HanCha-Dental, Zwenkau, Germany). (**e**) Working length determination radiograph of the mesiobuccal canal. (**f**) Immediate post-obturation clinical image of the pulp cavity. (**g**) Final radiograph (Courtesy of Dr. M. Leineweber)

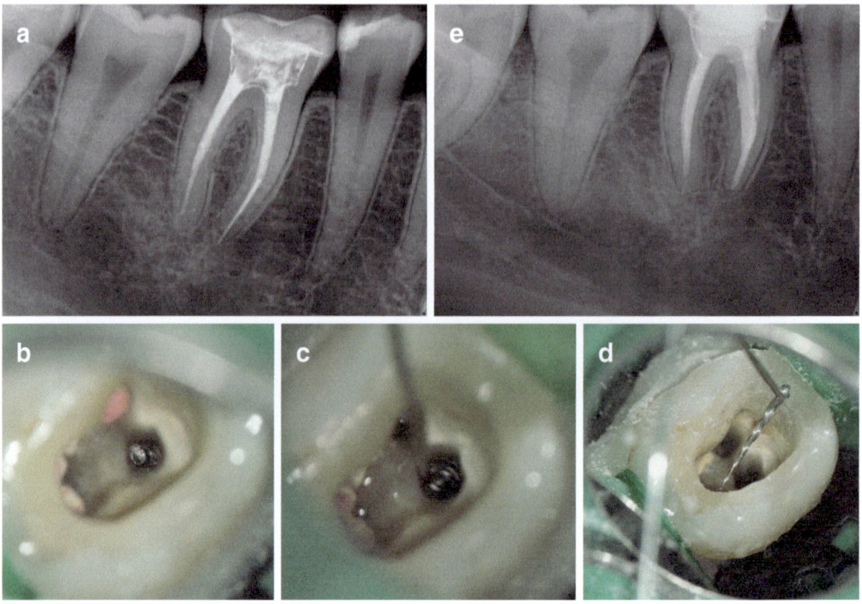

Fig. 4.72 (**a**) Initial radiograph of a mandibular right first molar with existing RCT and a fragment in the apical third of the mesial root. (**b**, **c**) Exposure of the coronal segment of the fragment. (**d**) Wire loop to attach and removal of the fragment with the wire loop technique using the Frag Remover (Frag Remover HanCha-Dental, Zwenkau, Germany). (**e**) Final radiograph (Courtesy of Dr. M. Leineweber)

size 15 for the GentleWave System to work effectively. The technology and its mechanism of action have been described in studies measuring the apical pressure created during its use (Haapasalo et al. 2016), evaluating its tissue-dissolving effectiveness (Haapasalo et al. 2014), the apical extrusion of the solution (Charara et al. 2016), its efficiency in debris removal (Molina et al. 2015) or $Ca(OH)_2$ (Ma et al. 2015), and the retrieval of fractured instruments from the root canal (Wohlgemuth et al. 2015). Also, a multicentered clinical study was conducted to evaluate the healing rates for molars after RCT employing the GentleWave® System and reported a 97.4% success rate of healing (Sigurdsson et al. 2016).

Caries, when present, must be removed, and missing coronal tooth structure must be restored prior to the initiation of this technique.

During use, the tip of the handpiece is held within the pulp chamber of an accessed tooth, 1 mm above the pulp chamber floor. No part of the handpiece should enter the root canal at any point of the procedure. The system is operated from a touch screen control panel that regulates the high-speed flow of the irrigating solution from the central unit to the handpiece, where it hits a metal impingement plate at the end of the tip and creates a spray that is released from the tip at approximately 45 mL/min at a temperature of approximately 40 °C. The strong hydrodynamic cavitation cloud generates a broad spectrum of sound waves within the degassed

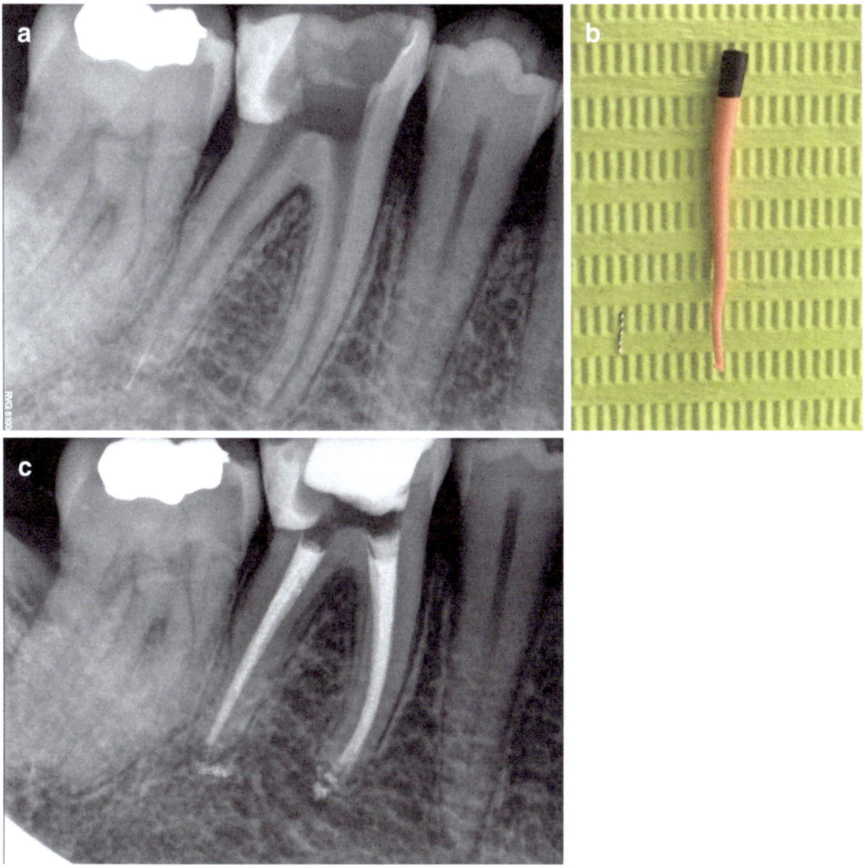

Fig. 4.73 (**a**) Preoperative radiograph of a mandibular molar with a fragment in the distal root protruding to the periapical tissues. (**b**) Removal of the loose fragment attached to the softened gutta-percha. (**c**) Immediate post-obturation radiograph (Courtesy of Dr. K. Mastoras)

fluid inside the tooth. The built-in suction via small suction holes in the sealing lid of the handpiece removes the outflowing irrigant, creating negative pressure within the root canal system.

4.3.25 Electrolytic Technique

The removal of fractured instruments by mechanical means requires the removal of dentin, which may weaken the root and increase the risk of perforation particularly when the fragment is beyond the root curvature. The electrolytic technique aims to partially or even totally dissolve the fragment through electrolysis, thus enabling the recovery of the original canal path to the apex. For this purpose, a system of electrodes is inserted into the root canal so that the anode comes into contact with the fragment

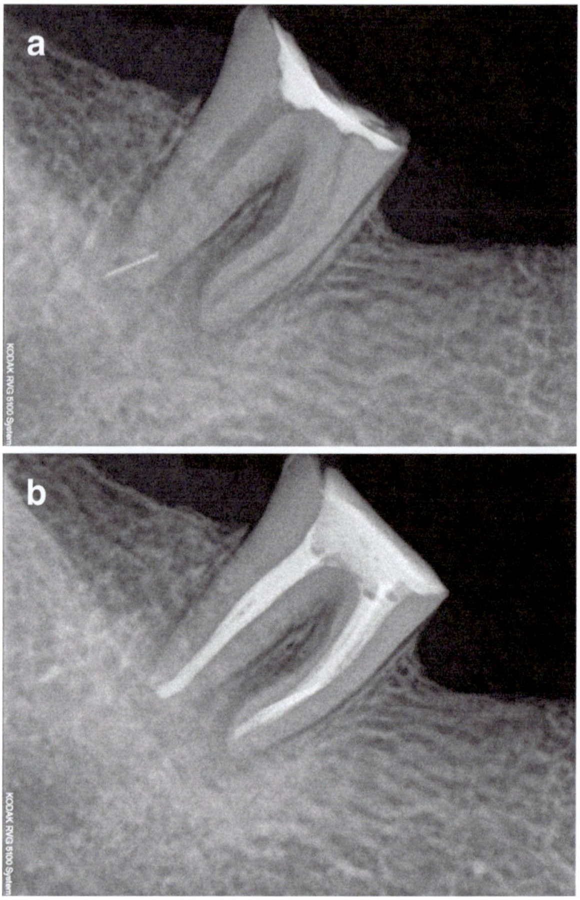

Fig. 4.74 (**a**) Fragment with one end protruding into the periapical tissues. (**b**) Immediate post-obturation radiograph after the retrieval of the fragment with a modification of the softened gutta-percha technique. The fragment was retrieved attached to the mass of the previously obtained unsatisfactory obturation of the distal canal (Courtesy of Dr. S. Giosis)

of the instrument (Fig. 4.74). Electrolytes used with the technique include normal saline, sodium hypochlorite in various concentrations, and saline with 0.1 N hydrochloric acid. Clinical and experimental in vitro and in vivo studies (Ito 1983; Saito et al. 1986; Ito et al. 1987; Okawauchi 1993) have demonstrated that this technique:

- Is more effective when the electrolyte contains hydrochloride acid.
- Is more effective on carbon steel than on SS instruments.
- Is more effective when the voltage is increased from 3 to 9 V.
- Is less effective when the fragment is lodged in the apical third.
- Is safe, as histologic examination did not reveal inflammation in periapical tissues. Deposits of Fe and Cr, mostly in the apical third, are found.
- Easily shows its degree of effectiveness. The electrolytic action and hence the effectiveness of the technique become directly visible when the color of the electrolyte changes because of the ions of the metal. Successfully used solutions become more brownish than the noneffective ones. Despite this, no tooth discoloration has been reported.

The major disadvantages of this technique are the need for special equipment, the use of acid in the electrolyte, and its limited effectiveness on SS instruments. Ormiga et al. (2010, 2011) expanded and used the concept of the electrolytic technique in a fluoride environment with NiTi instruments and concluded that they can be resolved but within a clinically unrealistic time frame of 6 h. In subsequent studies, the same group of researchers, by increasing fluoride concentration, achieved greater active dissolution of NiTi files and the partial dissolution of fractured NiTi files of different designs (Ormiga et al. 2015; Aboud et al. 2014) and of SS files (Amaral et al. 2015) in a simulated root canal during a 60-min period. The saturation of a fluoridated solution with sodium chloride led to an increase in electrical current and microscopic reductions in the length of the fragments within extracted human root canals that were subjected to electrochemical dissolution (Kowalczuck et al. 2016).

In this technique, regardless of the electrolyte used, contact between the fragment and the electrode used as the anode is absolutely essential (Ormiga et al. 2015).

4.3.26 Laser Irradiation (Laser-Assisted Removal of Fractured Instruments)

The neodymium-doped yttrium aluminum garnet lasers (Nd:YAG lasers) tested in laboratory studies have been claimed (Yu et al. 2000; Ebihara et al. 2003; Hagiwara et al. 2013; Cvikl et al. 2014; Tomov and Kissov 2014) to successfully manage instrument fragments in less than 5 min. This is done in four ways, all correlated to temperature effects:

1. The laser melts the dentin around the fragment, and then H-files are used to bypass and retrieve it.
2. The laser melts the fragment.
3. Laser energy melts the solder, connecting the fractured instrument with the brass tube charged with solder and placed at the exposed coronal end of the fragment.
4. The laser welds the file fragment positioned within the metal hollow tube (e.g., Endo-Eze® tip, Ultradent Products, Inc., USA) (Figs. 4.75, 4.76, and 4.77).

The claimed removal of a minimum amount of root dentin (Yu et al. 2000; Ebihara et al. 2003; Cvikl et al. 2014) can be attributed (Ebihara et al. 2003) to the capacity given to the user of Nd:YAG laser to distinguish (Ebihara et al. 2003) dentin from obstructions by the acoustic differences produced by the two materials.

4.4 Surgical Endodontics to Manage Fractured Instruments

Endodontic surgery has now evolved into endodontic microsurgery. This fundamental and radical change has broadened the range of therapeutic options. Utilization of the dental operating microscope for magnification and illumination and endoscopes in some cases combined with the application of microsurgical techniques that include accurate incisions, gentle flap reflections, small osteotomies, retro-cavity

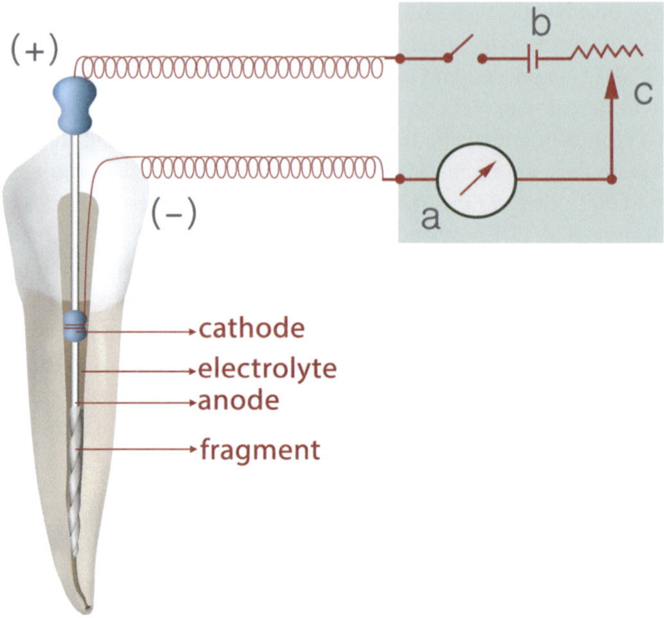

Fig. 4.75 Schematic illustration of the electrolytic technique. (**a**) Meter (mA). (**b**) Battery. (**c**) Voltage regulator

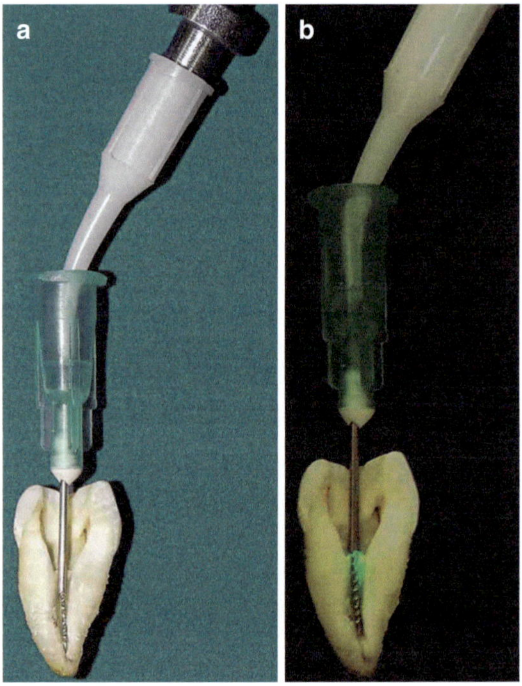

Fig. 4.76 Procedure of welding of a fractured K-file in an Endo-Eze® Tip (18ga) using Nd:YAG laser irradiation at 400 mJ/10 Hz (Courtesy of Prof. G. Tomov)

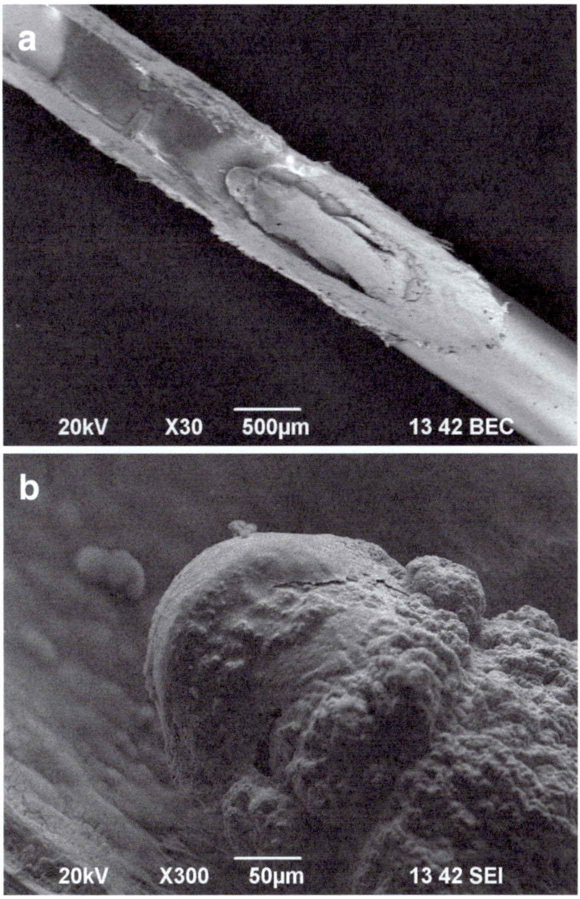

Fig. 4.77 SEM image of K-file after Nd:YAG laser irradiation at 400 mJ/10 Hz revealed the melted metal surface with an irregular granular structure after solidification (Courtesy of Prof. G Tomov)

preparation with sonic- or ultrasonic-driven micro-tips, primary closures using papilla preservation flaps, and precise flap approximations through micro-suturing, supported by the appropriate armamentarium, has benefited treatment procedures and resulted in less trauma to the patient and faster postsurgical healing. The many advances in the field of endodontic surgery and the routine use of microsurgical instrumentation, particularly ultrasonics, allowing for minimal root-end resection and beveling, thus preserving and conserving cortical bone (Kim and Kratchman 2006; Floratos and Kim 2017), coupled with magnification and biocompatible root-end filling materials, have significantly improved the outcome of therapies compared to traditional techniques (Tsesis et al. 2006; Setzer et al. 2012). The computer-aided surgical navigation system aided by an interocclusal splint for a stable, identically repeatable positioning of the mandible has also been used in a minimally invasive retrieval case of an instrument fragment with its one end extending beyond the apical foramen in a mandibular premolar (Sukegawa et al. 2017). This concept will possibly open a new era in the field of surgical endodontics by enabling the performance of more precise procedures.

Table 4.10 Factors to be carefully considered prior to endodontic surgery

Patient	Physical health (systemic disease)	
	Psychological status	
	General oral status (i.e., patient susceptibility to recurrent caries)	
	Patient's values and preferences after being fully informed of treatment options and rationales	
	Patient's expectations	
	Financial factors	
	Time factor	
Anatomic	Access to and visibility of surgical site	
	Bone quality	
	Inter-arch and intra-arch occlusal relationship	
	Relation/proximity to:	Maxillary sinus
		Nasal floor
		Greater palatine foramen and the associated neurovascular bundle
		Mandibular canal and its neurovascular bundle
		Mental foramen and its neurovascular bundle
Dental	Strategic (dental) value of the tooth in question	
	Root configurations	
	Restorability of the tooth	
	Supporting tissue	
	Bulk of the tooth structure to remain and its resistance to fracture	
	Quality of the coronal restoration	
Operator	Diagnostic and treatment planning skills	
	Surgical skills	
	Training in modern microsurgical techniques	
	Experience	
	Facilities (armamentarium) available	

It is imperative to justify when and which type of surgical intervention to choose. There are few absolute contraindications to endodontic surgery, but there are several factors that must be very carefully considered (Table 4.10) when surgical endodontic treatment is planned. Failure to consider all the factors may lead to questionable treatment plans which are not in the best interest of the patient. The majority of endodontic surgical procedures are better to be performed by trained endodontic specialists. General practitioners with extensive surgical training and experience can also perform them if they feel competent and provided that proper armamentarium is available. When administering care of a specialized nature, the standards applicable to specialists are to be maintained by the general practitioner who is doing the work of a specialist. When performing endodontic surgery, the current standard of practice requires the use of microscopy and ultrasonic tips for retro-cavity preparation for the subsequent retrofilling with a biocompatible material (Gluskin 2014). In every case of surgical endodontics, patients should be advised of any risks unique to their situation.

Timing and the type of surgical procedure are two parameters affecting the decision-making process in cases where surgical management is indicated. They are further influenced by a variety of factors as seen in Table 4.11.

Table 4.11 Issues to be decided in fractured instrument cases to be managed surgically

Timing	Prior to non-surgical management Immediately after non-surgical management At a later time upon future evaluation
Type of surgical procedure	Removal of the fragment with no resection of dental tissues Root-end resection (apicoectomy) Hemisection Root resection (root amputation) Intentional replantation

4.4.1 Timing of Surgical Management

Prior to non-surgical management. As a rule of thumb, surgical endodontics follows the non-surgical management of the mishap and is performed either immediately or postponed for a later time. There are some cases, though, where weighing of risks versus benefit changes this rule. When the failure of non-surgical orthograde management can be predicted and, additionally, there is an increased risk of creating another iatrogenic error, surgery is performed with no preceding non-surgical efforts.

A case scenario could be an instrument fragment in a root canal of a tooth which is part of an extensive satisfactory and relatively recent prosthetic restoration that the patient is not willing to replace. Additionally, the cast post and core present in this particular canal will inhibit any access through the prosthetic restoration. RCT through the prosthetics is a non-recommended procedure, which in this particular case cannot be applied at all due to the presence of the cast post and core. Breaking or disassembling the prosthetic restoration, removing the post, and retreating the canals would be more dramatic, more time-consuming, more expensive, and less predictable, with an increased risk of creating additional iatrogenic errors than a microsurgical approach (Fig. 4.78).

Immediate surgical endodontics, as the optimum management choice, upon completion of the non-surgical management efforts should be performed:

1. In cases of intense persistent clinical symptomatology (Figs. 4.79 and 4.80)
2. When a biopsy of periradicular tissue is required
3. If the patient, after being fully informed, insists for his own reasons on having the operation performed immediately (Figs. 4.81 and 4.82)

Surgical treatment at a later time upon future evaluation. Endodontic surgery should be the only answer to correct the problem by gaining access to it in failed non-surgical cases. In symptom-free cases though, the patient should be thoroughly informed of the relative benefits and risks, and the "wait-and-see approach" (monitoring) as a shared decision can also be followed. This occasionally leads to no surgery being required at all (Figs. 4.83, 4.84, and 4.85).

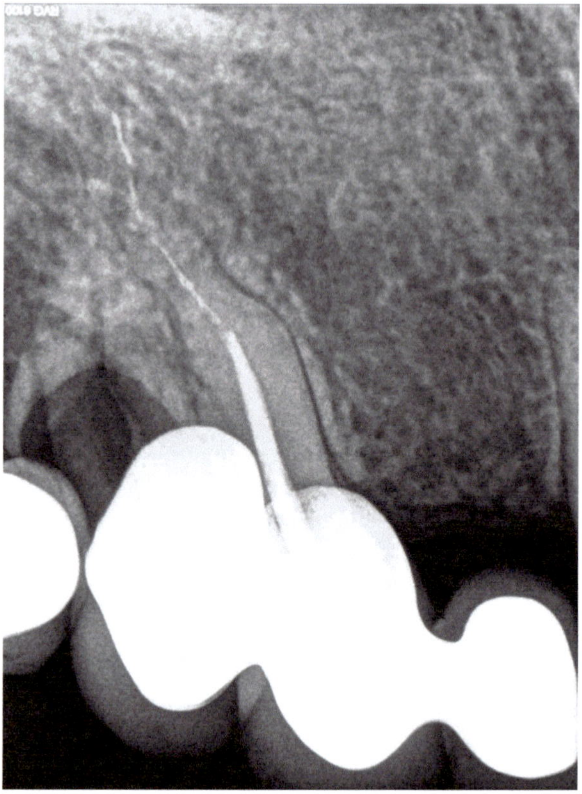

Fig. 4.78 An instrument fragment in a root canal of a maxillary canine with a cast post and core, part of an extensive, satisfactory, and relatively recent prosthetic restoration that the patient is not willing to replace. Surgical management will be the treatment of choice in the event of clinical and/or radiographic signs being present in the scheduled recall appointments

Surgical treatment at a later time upon future evaluation is performed when at the recall examination, the combined clinical and radiographic findings indicate symptoms and/or lesion development (Fig. 4.86) or increase in the size of the preexisting lesion.

The timing of the surgical intervention also depends on the kind of restoration that the tooth will undergo. Thus in cases where the fragment compromises the prognosis and an extensive prosthetic restoration is to follow, surgery should be performed immediately.

4.4.2 Type of Surgical Procedure

There is no predetermined surgical procedure that is appropriate for all clinical situations of instrument fragments. Several interdependent variable factors must be evaluated on an individual case-by-case basis and carefully considered prior to any surgical management attempt.

These include:

1. Anatomical factors:
   (a) The tooth location in the arch. This determines to a great extent the degree of accessibility to the area. This is also influenced by the degree of mouth opening. Obviously the access is the same regardless of whether traditional

or microsurgery is used. With the latter, vision is greatly enhanced by the highly focused illumination and the appropriate magnification.

(b) The tooth anatomy and especially the anatomy of the root and root canal with the fragment. This largely determines the type of surgical approach to be followed. For example, it is not possible to treat with hemisection a fragment in the proximal root of a mandibular molar when all its roots are fused, i.e., C-shaped tooth.

2. The location of the fragment in the root canal.

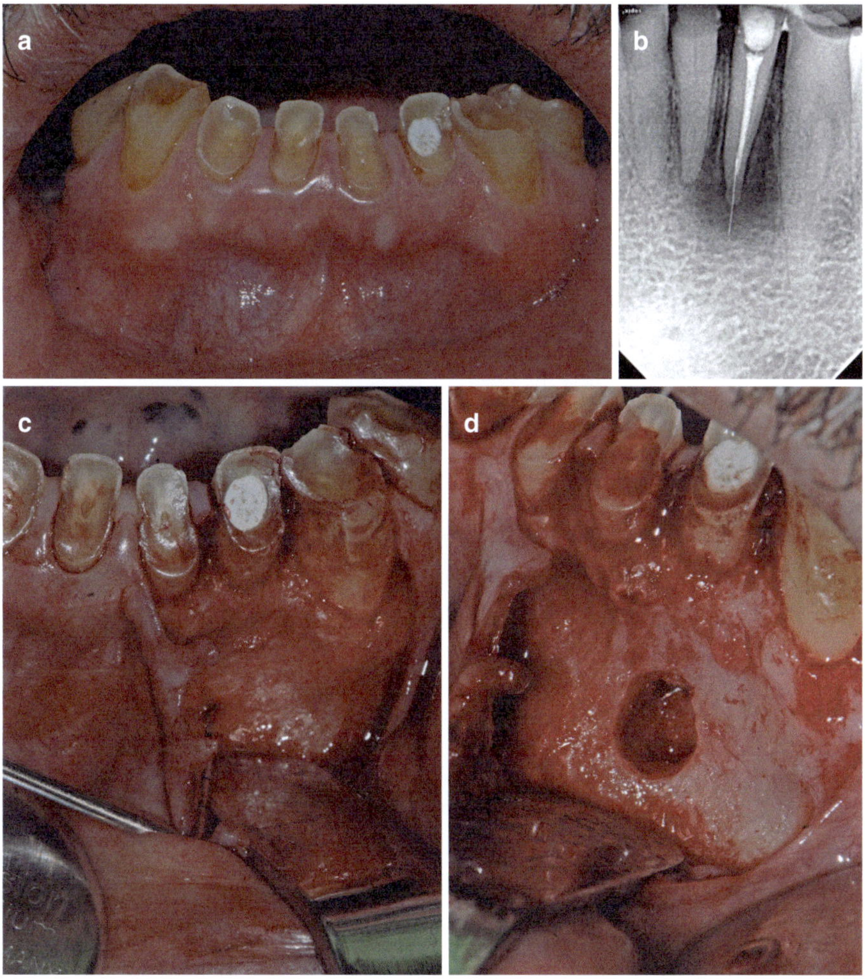

Fig. 4.79 (**a**, **b**) Clinical and radiographic appearance of a lower left lateral incisor with a fragment with its one end within the root canal and the other protruding into the periapical tissues. (**c**, **d**) Flap reflection and exposure of the fragment following instrumentation and obturation of the canal. (**e–g**) Removal of the fragment with forceps. (**h**) Apicoectomy and retrofilling with MTA. (**i**) One-year recall radiograph revealed good periradicular healing (From the Postgraduate Clinic of the Endodontic Department, Dental School, Aristotle University of Thessaloniki-Greece)

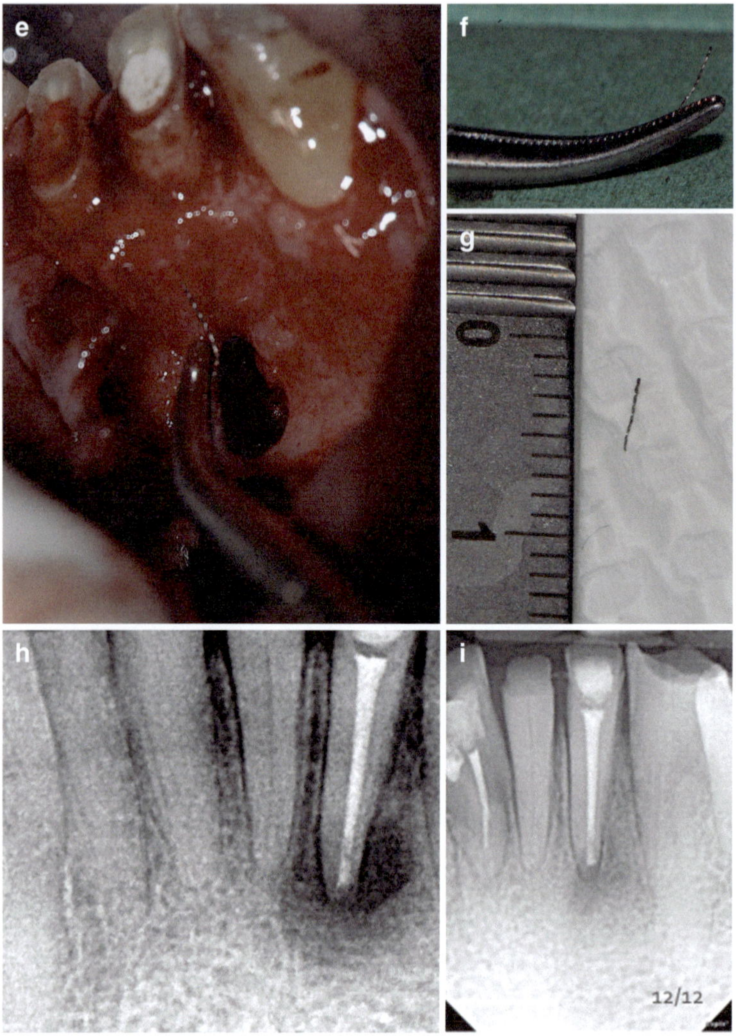

Fig. 4.79 (continued)

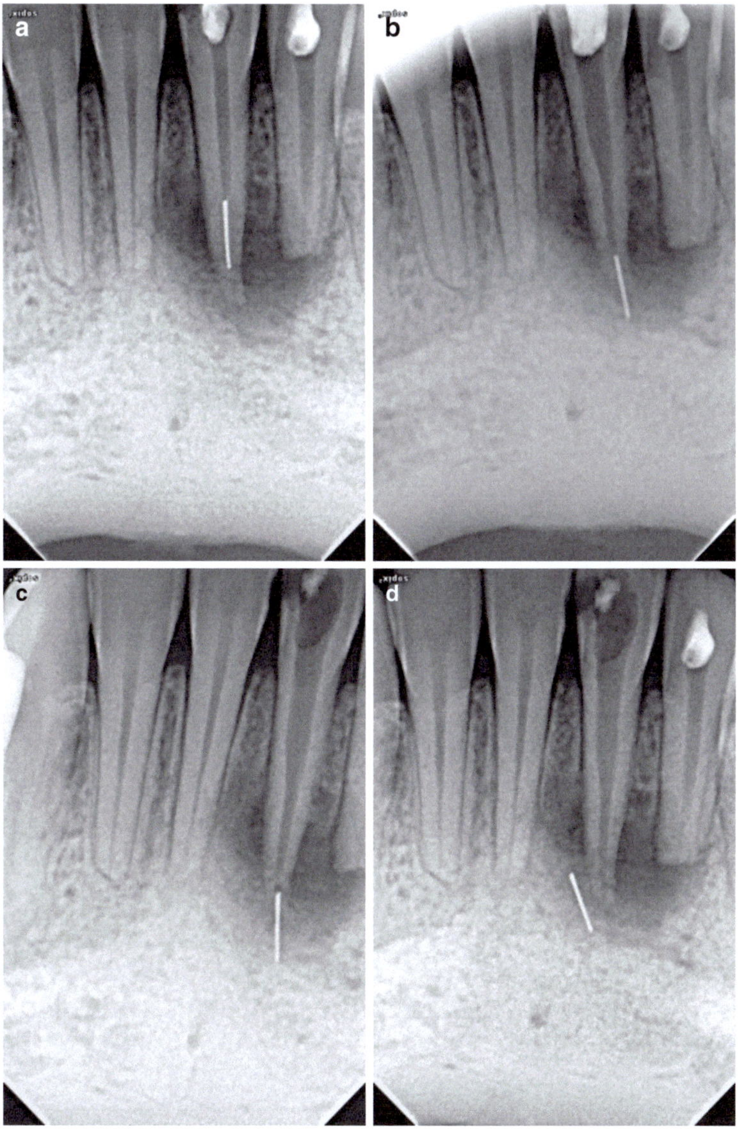

Fig. 4.80 (**a**) The lower left central incisor with a buccal fistula and an instrument fragment at the apical third of the root canal was referred for RCT. (**b–d**) Unsuccessful efforts to retrieve it with ultrasonics following exposure of its coronal segment and creation of a staging platform resulted in extrusion of the fragment to the periapical tissues. (**e**) The canal was instrumented to the desired working length, dressed with calcium hydroxide for 15 days, and eventually obturated with lateral compaction of gutta-percha and epoxy resin sealer (AH26, Dentsply DeTrey, GmbH, Konstanz, Germany), and the fragment was removed surgically. No resection of dental tissues was needed. (**f**) The scheduled recall clinical and radiographic follow-up at 1 year revealed uneventful healing (Courtesy of Dr. K. Kodonas)

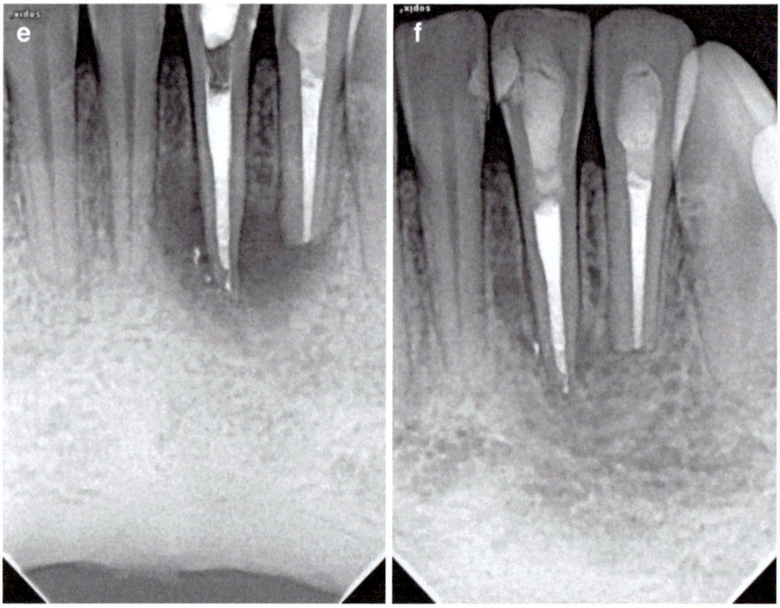

Fig. 4.80 (continued)

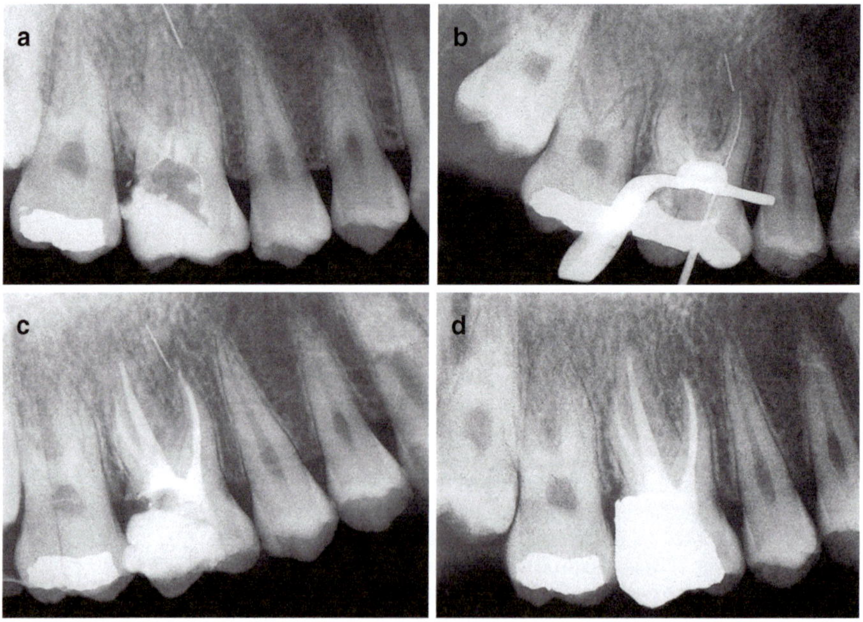

Fig. 4.81 (**a**) In the preoperative radiograph, it is not clear whether one end of the fragment is within the canal or the other protrudes in the periapical area. (**b**) In the working length radiograph, the fragment appears with both ends in the periapical area. (**c**) Immediate post-obturation radiograph. (**d**) Surgical removal of the fragment at the same appointment. No root-end resection was needed. (**e**) Three-month recall examination showed uneventful healing (with permission from Lambrianidis 2001)

Fig. 4.81 (continued)

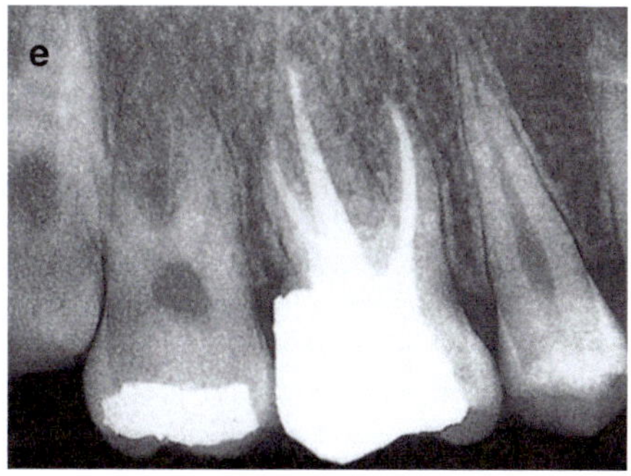

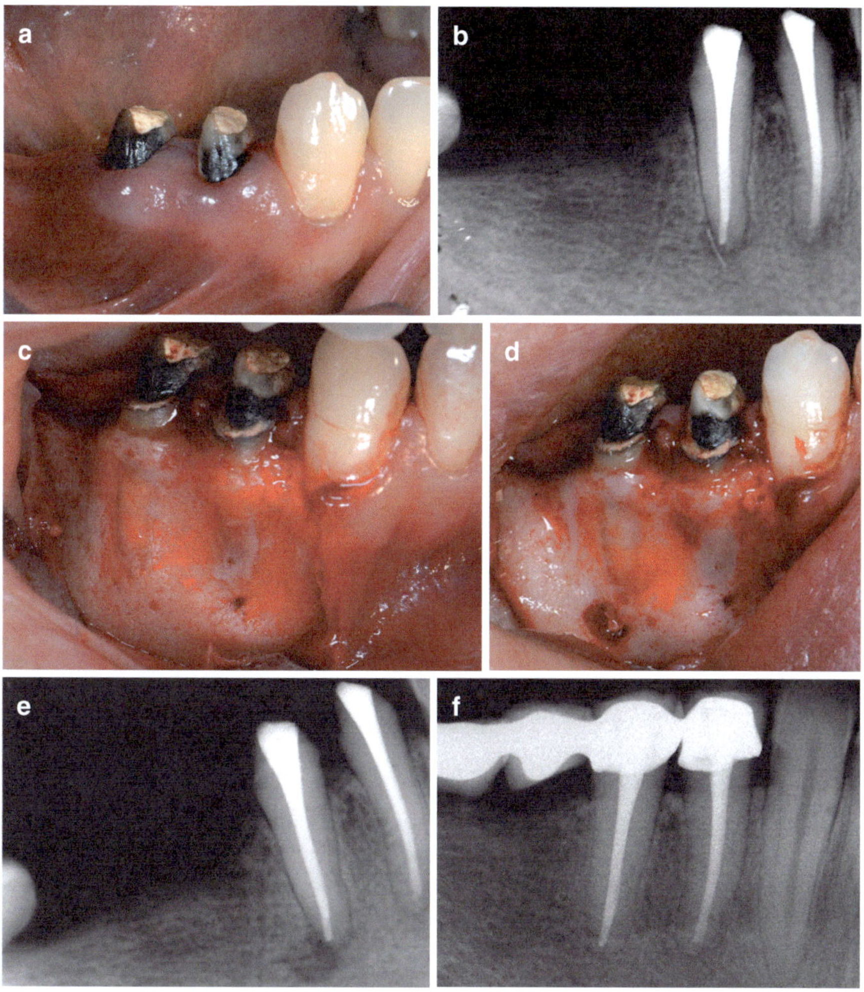

Fig. 4.82 (**a**, **b**) Preoperative clinical and radiographic image of a mandibular premolar with a fragment extruded in the periapical area. (**c**) Flap retraction and exposure of the buccal bone with the perforation of the area with the fragment. Retrieval of the fragment. No resection of dental tissues was needed. (**d**) Immediate postoperative radiograph. (**e**) Follow-up post-restoration radiograph (Courtesy of Dr. C. Boutsioukis and Prof. I. Lavrentiadis) (with permission from Lambrianidis et al. 2007)

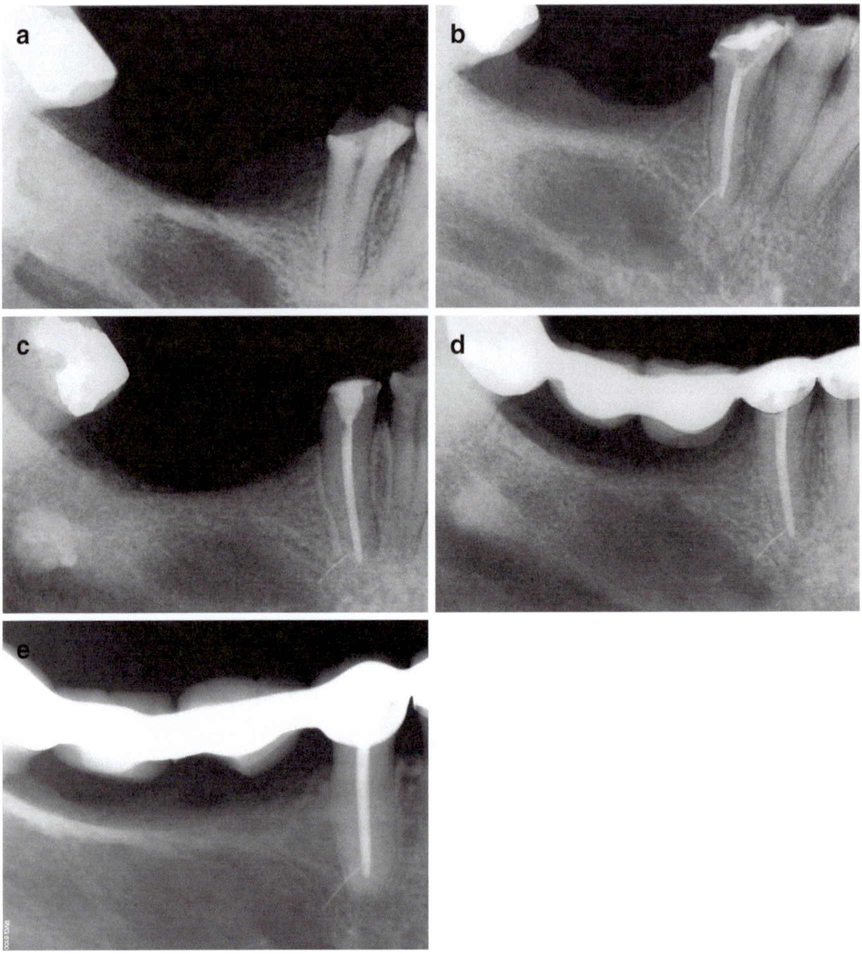

Fig. 4.83 (**a**) Preoperative radiograph of a mandibular premolar. (**b**) Immediate post-obturation radiograph where a fragment protruding into the periapical area can be seen. (**c**, **d**) Healthy periapical tissues can be seen at recall radiographs at 6 weeks and 3 and 19 years, respectively (Reprinted and modified with permission from Lambrianidis 2001)

3. The presence of periapical disease.
4. The condition of the periodontium.
5. The overall clinical evaluation. For example, the clinical picture of the crown and the patient's oral hygiene cannot be overlooked when deciding upon the type of surgical procedure.
6. The operator's skills and experience and the armamentarium available.

Careful consideration of all the factors cited in Table 4.10, based on case-specific criteria, will facilitate the selection of the most appropriate surgical procedure. There are some cases where one procedure only is indicated (Fig. 4.87) as opposed

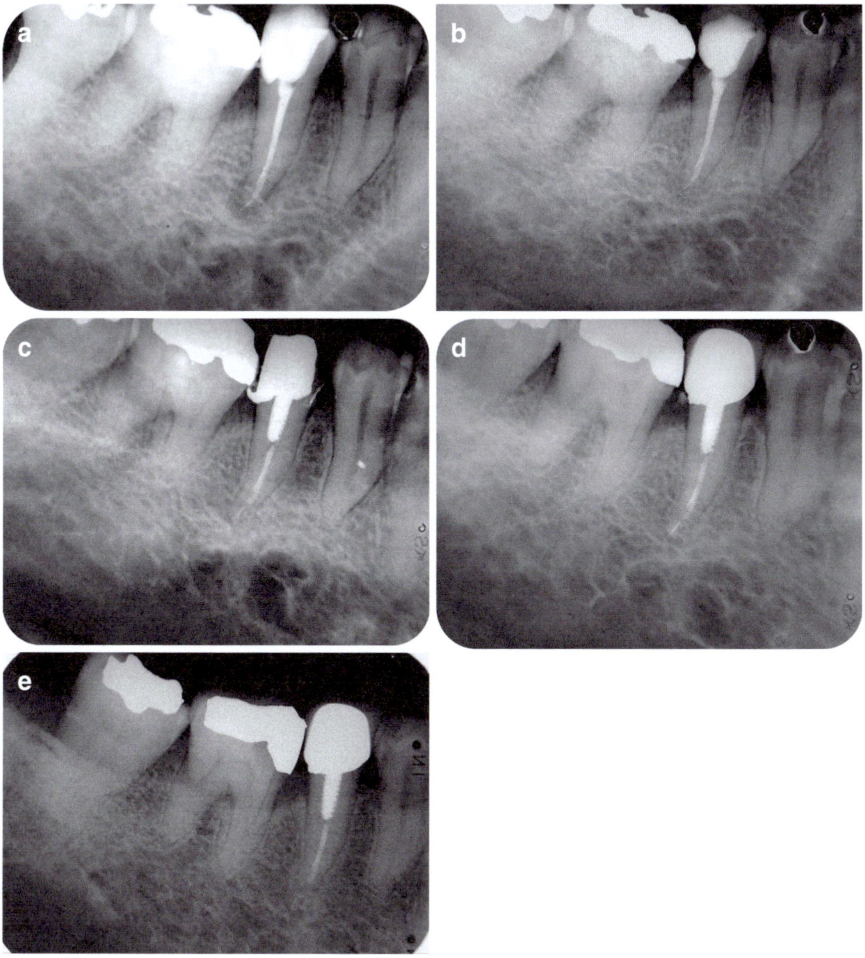

Fig. 4.84 (**a**) Mandibular right second premolar with two fragments, one at the apical third bypassed and incorporated into the mass of the obturating material and the other extruded to the periapical tissues. (**b–f**) Recall radiographs at 1, 4, 5, 18, and 32 years revealed gradual slow dissolution of the extruded fragment with healthy periapical tissues (reprinted and modified from Molyvdas et al. 1992)

to others where the decision has to be made among a variety of options. The surgical options include removal of the fragment with no resection of dental tissues (Figs. 4.80, 4.81, and 4.82), root-end resection (apicoectomy) (Figs. 4.79, 4.86, 4.87, and 4.88), hemisection (Fig. 4.89), root resection (amputation) (Figs. 4.90 and 4.91), and intentional replantation.

If apicoectomy is selected, the root canal is instrumented and obturated up to the fragment, and surgery follows. Special care is required in order to avoid "cutting" the fragment with the bur during apicoectomy. In cases where the tip of the fractured instrument protrudes into the periapical region and the fragment is quite long,

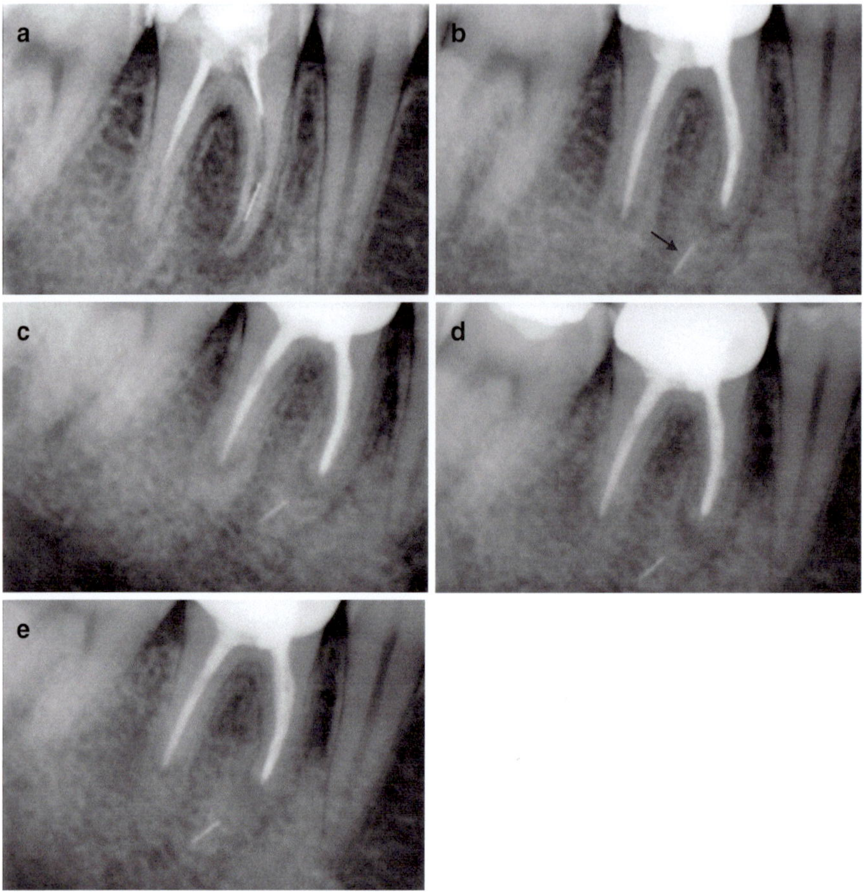

Fig. 4.85 (**a**) Mandibular right first molar with inadequate RCT and a fragment at the apical third of the mesiobuccal canal. (**b**) Immediate post-obturation radiograph. Note the inadvertent extrusion of the fragment to the periapical tissues (*arrow*) during retrieval efforts with the file bypass technique. (**c–e**) Recall radiographs at 4, 9, and 12 years revealed healthy periapical tissues (Courtesy of Prof. P. Beltes)

it is recommended that the root canal should not be obturated prior to the surgical procedure. Thus, after having surgically exposed the fragment that protrudes into the periapical tissues, ultrasonics can loosen the fragment from the apical direction and push it toward the crown and eventually remove it through the pulp chamber (Fig. 4.88). In retreatment cases and particularly when there is no access to the canal due to a post, the fragment is surgically exposed and removed from the apex, and the unprepared canal space is prepared with ultrasonic tips. Modern ultrasonic tips can facilitate the preparation of a 4 mm, 5 mm, 6 mm, or even 9 mm root-end cavity (Floratos and Kim 2017). The prepared space is retrofilled (Fig. 4.88).

If the iatrogenic error is to be corrected with hemisection (Fig. 4.89), the root canal in the root(s) to remain is instrumented and obturated, the access cavity is

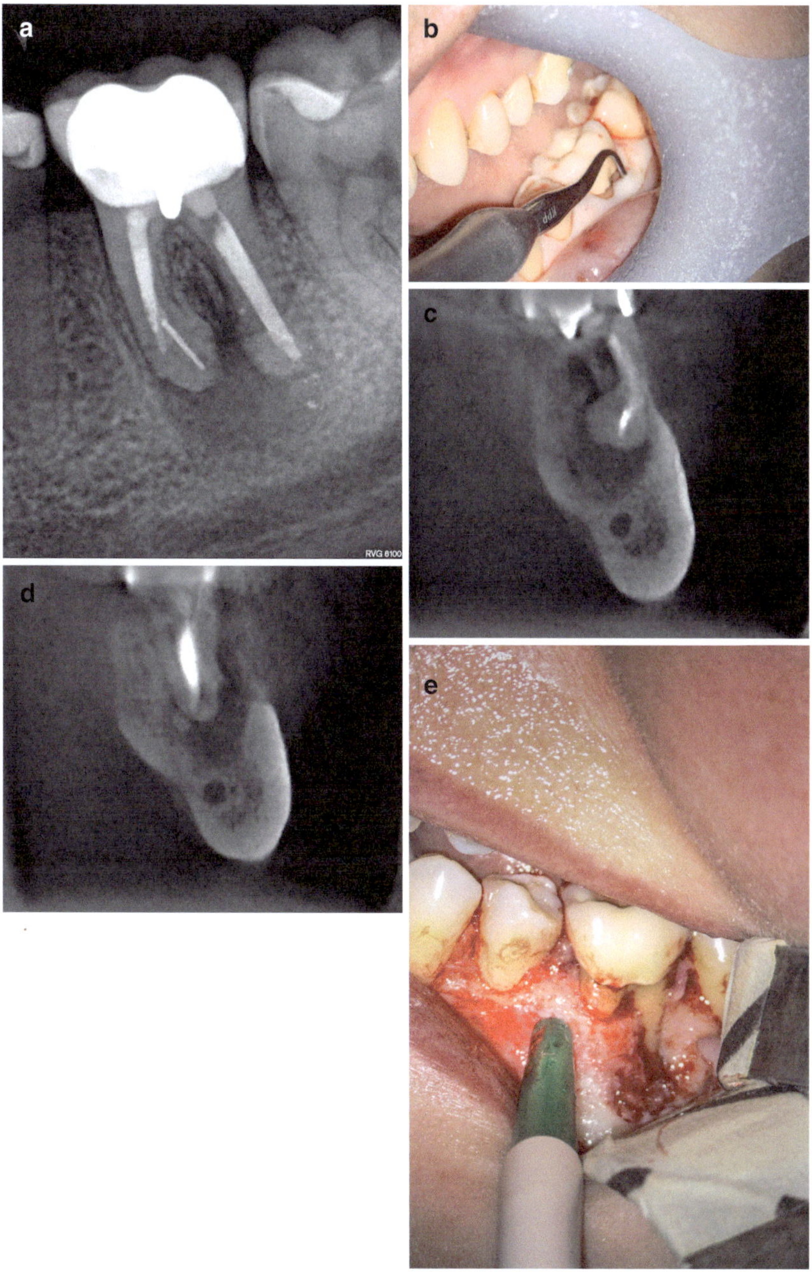

Fig. 4.86 (**a**) Preoperative radiograph of a mandibular first molar with a fragment at the apical third of the mesial root. The RCT was performed, according to the patient, 12 years earlier. (**b**) Periodontal involvement. (**c**, **d**) A CBCT image revealed the proximity of the periapical lesion to the mandibular canal. (**e**) Reflection of full mucoperiosteal flap. (**f–h**) Exposure of the fragment by use of an ultrasonic tip (JeTip 1B, B&L Biotech, USA). (**i**, **j**) Removal of the fragment. (**k**, **l**) Retrofilling with MTA. (**m**, **n**) Graft and membrane placement. (**o**) Immediate postoperative radiograph. (**p**) The 36-month recall radiograph revealed uneventful healing (Courtesy of Dr. S. Floratos)

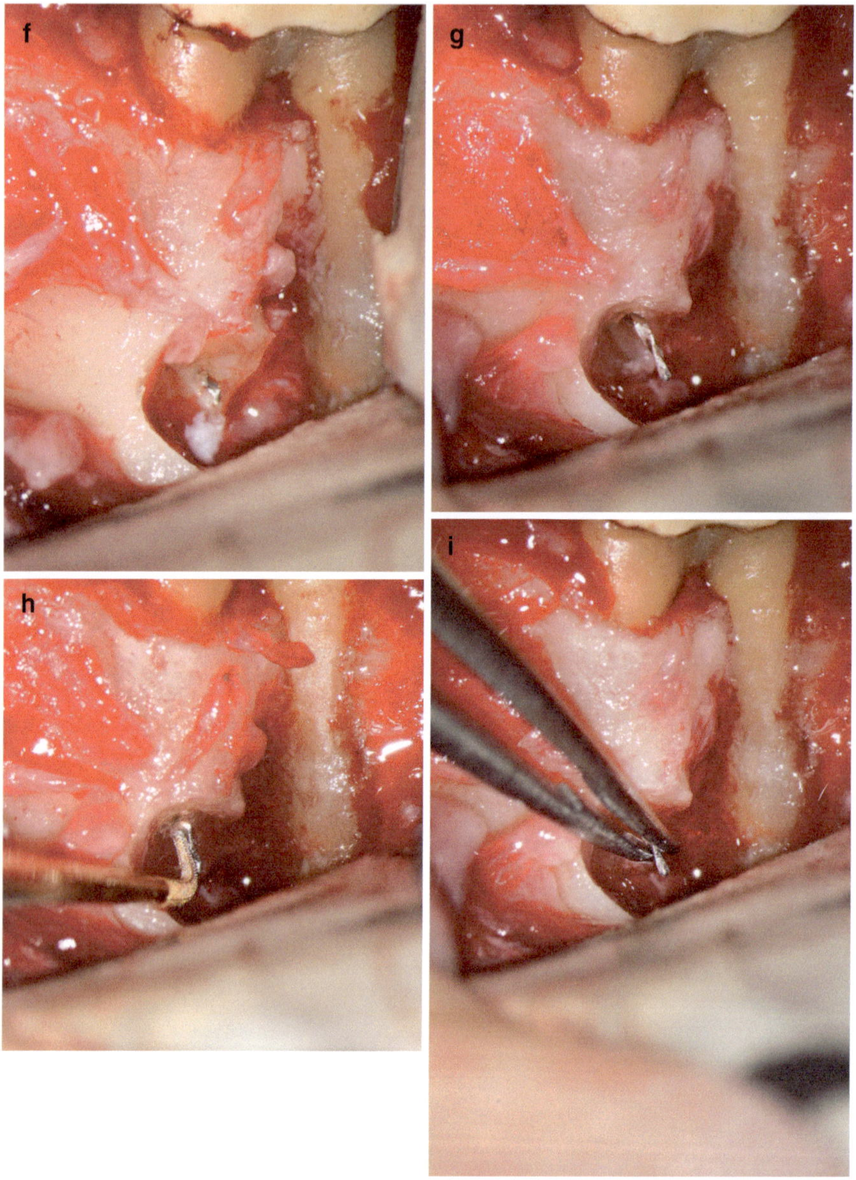

Fig. 4.86 (continued)

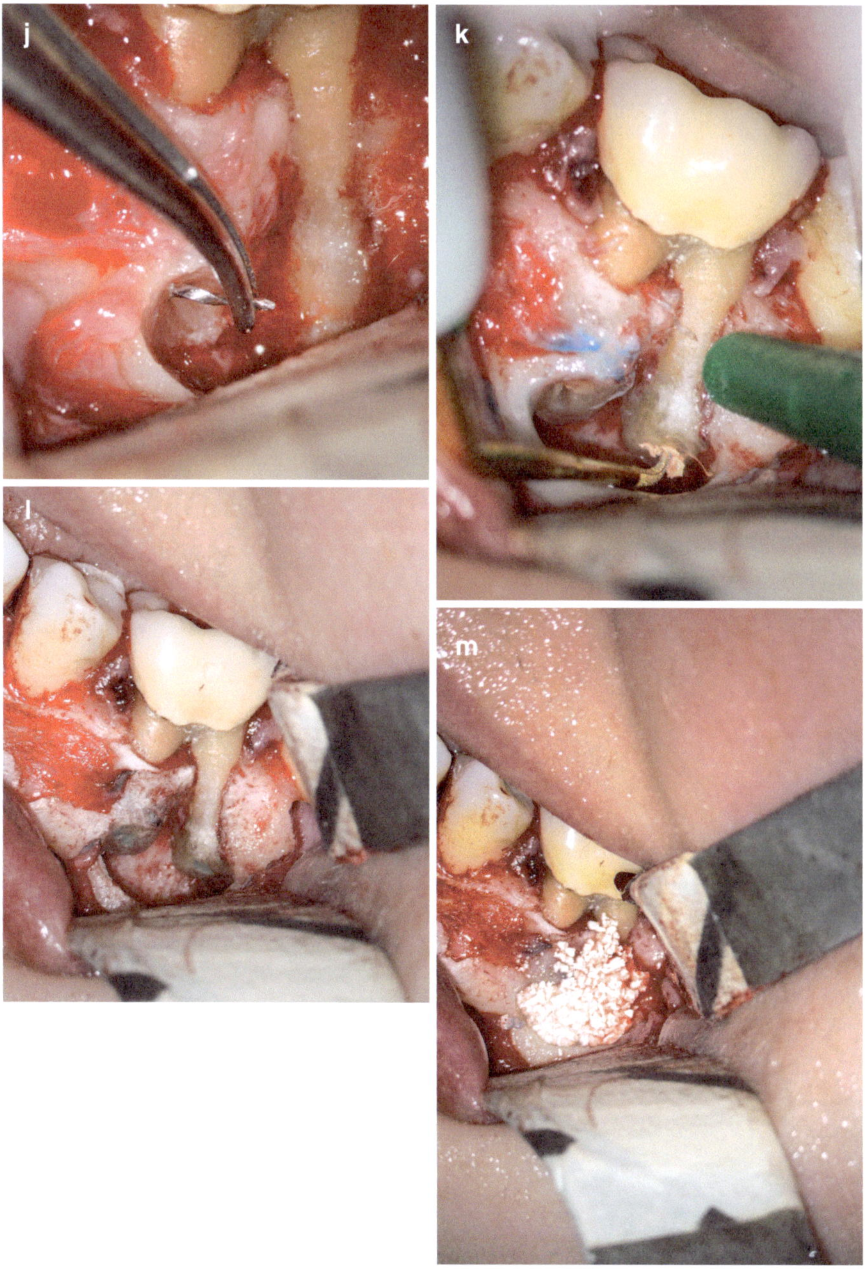

Fig. 4.86 (continued)

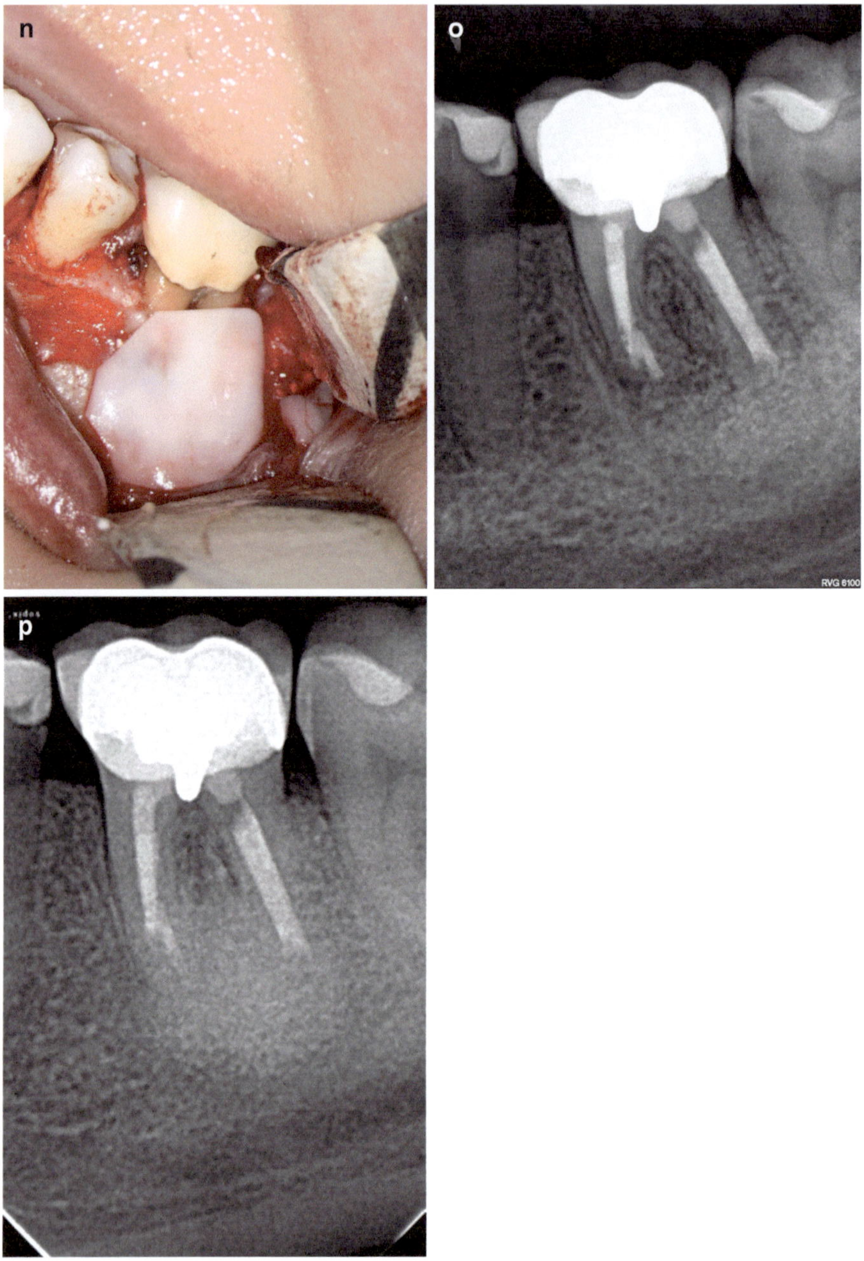

Fig. 4.86 (continued)

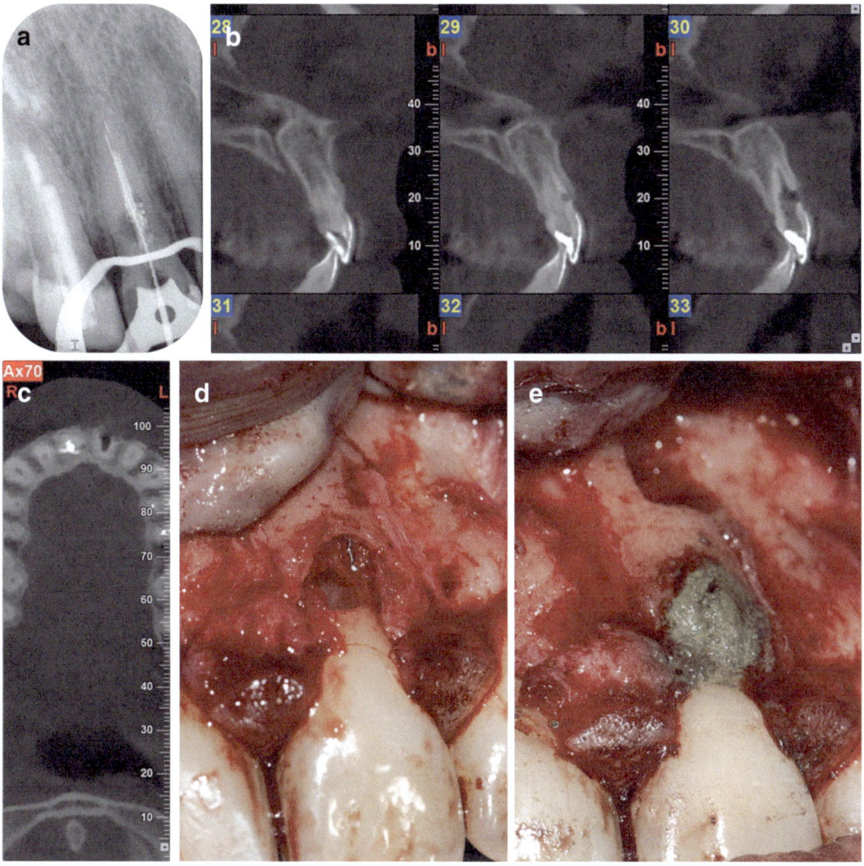

Fig. 4.87 (**a–g**) A case in which apicoectomy and obturation of the resorptive defect following surgical exposure were the only alternative to extraction. (**a**) Working length determination radiograph during retreatment and simultaneous efforts to bypass the fragment, which is located at the apical third. (**b**, **c**) Reconstructed cross-sectional and axial CBCT images revealed that the resorptive lesion had already perforated the buccal root wall—the lesion had also resorbed, but not perforated, the palatal aspect of the root. The buccal cortical plate has been destroyed as a result of chronic inflammation. (**d**) Following reflection of a flap, the resorption cavity can be seen. Complete absence of the buccal alveolar bone coronal to the resorption is evident. Note the presence of a second fragment in the periodontal ligament, opposite the resorptive defect, revealed upon reflection of the flap. This second fracture had probably happened during non-surgical retreatment efforts and was easily removed with forceps. (**e**) Root-end resection and retrofill with MTA and obturation of the resorption cavity with MTA. (**f**) Immediate postsurgical radiograph. (**g**) Six-week follow-up radiograph (From the Postgraduate Clinic of the Endodontic Department, Dental School, Aristotle University of Thessaloniki-Greece)

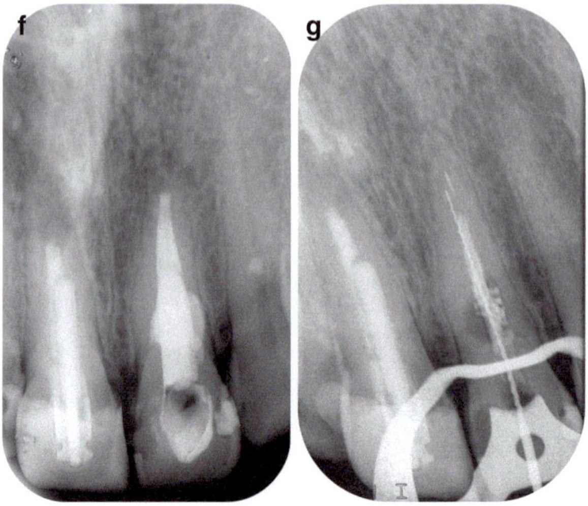

Fig. 4.87 (continued)

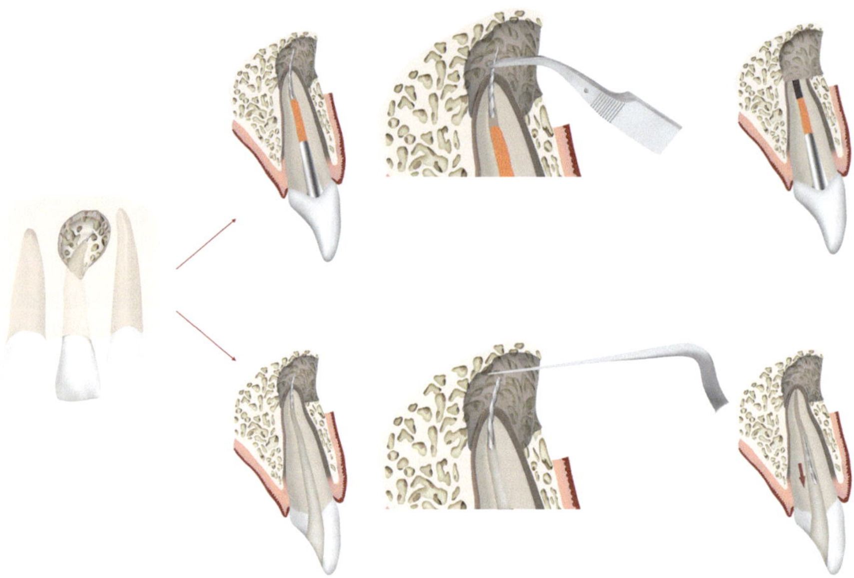

Fig. 4.88 Schematic illustration of the management of a long fragment extending into the periapical tissues. *Lower row* in cases of patent canals: surgical exposure of the fragment, loosening it ultrasonically and pushing the fragment in the canal to be retrieved in orthograde way. Root canal treatment is completed, and apical root-end resection and root-end filling are performed in one session. *Top row* in retreatment cases with no patent canal due to the presence of post and core: surgical removal of the fragment, retropreparation with ultrasonic tips, and retrofilling of the now prepared space up to the gutta-percha

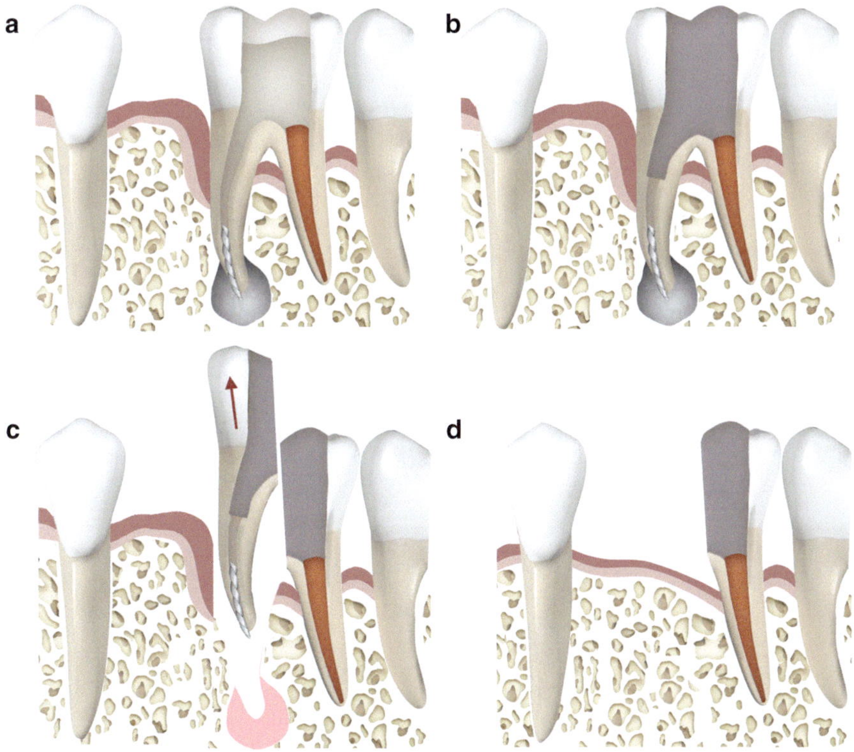

Fig. 4.89 (**a–d**) Schematic illustration of a case where hemisection is the only surgical option. (**a**) A mandibular molar with a severe bone loss limited to the mesial root with the fragment extending into the periapical tissues. (**b**) Instrumentation and obturation of the distal canal and of the access cavity with a permanent filling material. (**c**) Hemisection and extraction of the mesial root after the setting of the material. (**d**) Prosthetic restoration will follow after some weeks

sealed with a permanent filling material, and the surgery is scheduled after the setting of the material. Special care is required in cases of root resection (amputation) in order for the permanent filling materials used to seal the access cavity to be condensed 2–3 mm below the orifice within the root canal of the root to be removed.

Intentional replantation has been successfully used in few cases of teeth with instrument fragments (Filho et al. 2004, Shah et al. 2012, Shenoy et al. 2014, Soni et al. 2015). A case has also been published where, in a young healthy woman with restricted mouth opening, intentional replantation was performed in the mandibular second left molar mostly due to symptoms from furcal perforation and secondary for the management of instrument fragment in the mesial root of her poorly treated molar. She presented with symptoms of acute apical periodontitis in the area of the distal abutment of a four-unit fixed partial denture extending from the first right mandibular premolar to the second right mandibular molar (Fig. 4.92).

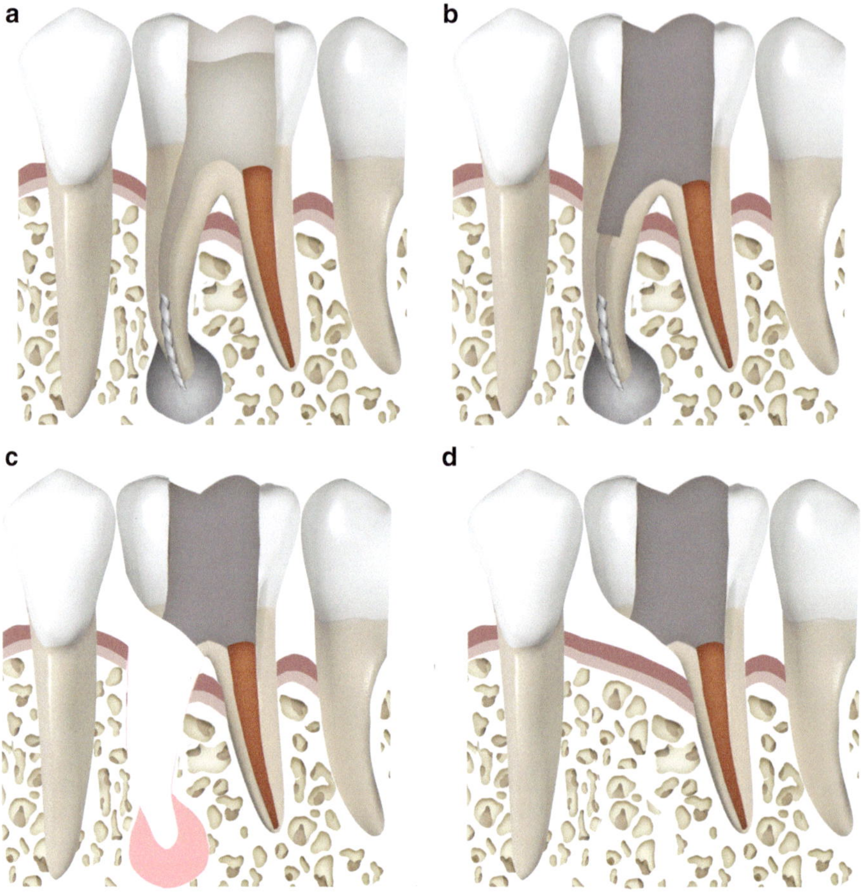

Fig. 4.90 (**a–d**) Schematic illustration of the management of an instrument fragment with root resection (amputation). (**a**) Radiographic confirmation of the presence of fragment and recognition of its location, size, and length and instrumentation and obturation of the root canal in the root(s) that will be preserved. (**b**) Enlargement with Gates Glidden bur of the coronal orifice of the root canal of the root to be sacrificed. Post-obturation restoration of the access cavity with a permanent material; care had to be taken in introducing the permanent filling material into be the space created with the Gates Glidden bur. (**c**) Surgical removal of the root with the fragment after the setting of the filling material. (**d**) Expected healing of the area

If intentional replantation is the treatment of choice, it must be performed preserving the integrity and vitality of the periodontal ligament because its condition is a key factor for the success of replantation (Andreasen 1981; Lambrianidis 1985; Zervas 1989; Andreasen et al. 1995). Extraction should be performed as atraumatically as possible with carefully pre-selected extraction forceps, taking care that the beak of the forceps should not go beyond the cementoenamel junction in order to prevent damage to the cementum and the periodontal ligament. Surgical elevators must not be used. Post-extraction socket must be carefully examined for fracture,

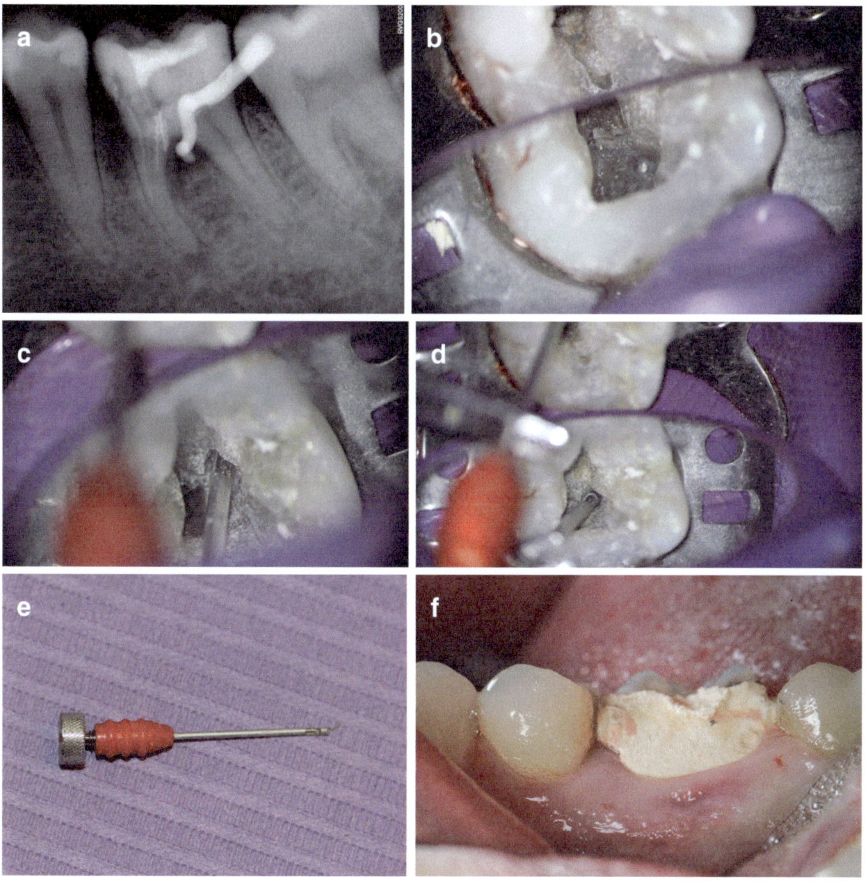

Fig. 4.91 (**a**) Preoperative radiograph of a mandibular first molar with inadequate RCT, three fragments, and chronic apical periodontics. The size #25 gutta-percha cone inserted into the sinus tract determines the furcal area as the source of the pathosis. (**b**) Exposure of one of the fragments. (**c–e**) Retrieval of the exposed fragment with the IRS (Dentsply Tulsa Dental, Tulsa, OK, USA). (**f**) Temporization with gutta-percha to achieve a healthy gingiva contouring. (**g**) Instrumentation and obturation of the distal canal. Note the presence of the two fragments. (**h**) Initiation of the restorative phase. Isolation with rubber dam. Removal of the existing OD restoration and modification of the proximal matrix to leave space for the splint fibers, taking care to preserve the full volume of the existing lingual enamel of the molar and eventual splinting with adjacent second premolar to equalize levering forces on the distal root of the molar. (**i**) Unilateral fibers, pre-embedded in resin (Evostick Post 900, GC Europe), used to splint and create a scaffold that supports the restoration. (**j**) Resin buildup around the scaffold. Dentin shade (IPS Empress, Ivoclar) and completion of the buildup with enamel-shade resin (IPS Empress, Ivoclar). (**k**, **l**) Clinical and radiographic appearance 1-week post-amputation (Courtesy of Dr. P. Kouros)

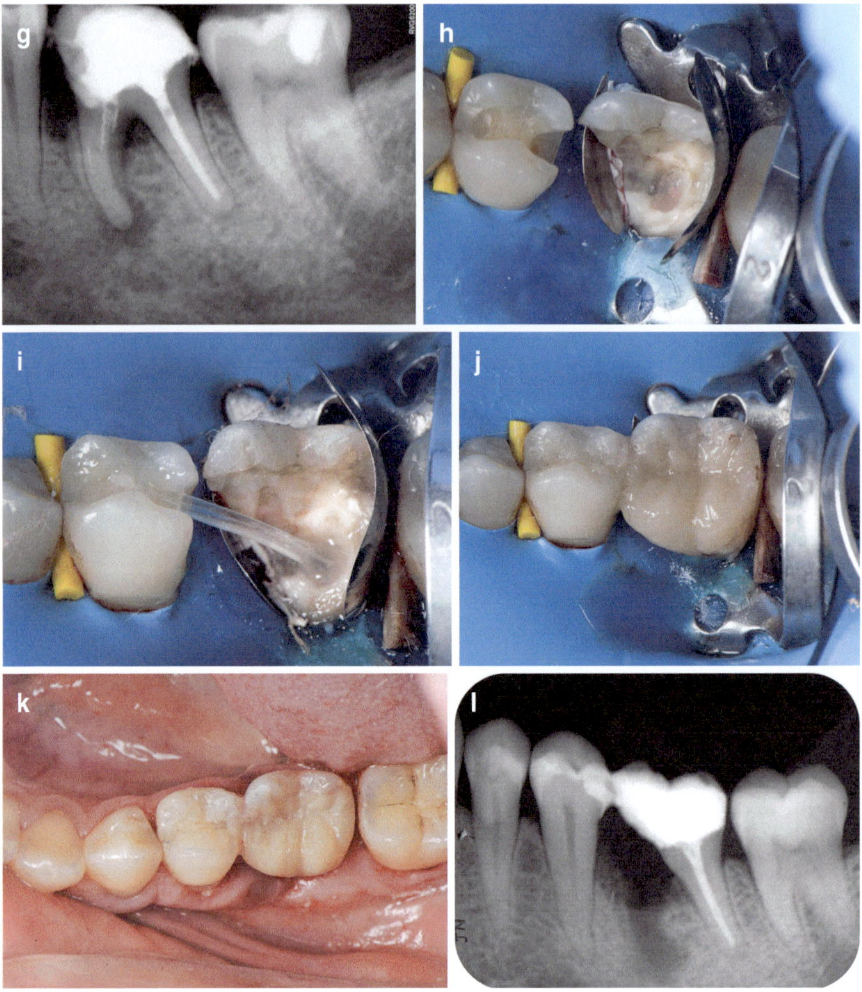

Fig. 4.91 (continued)

curated gently, and irrigated with normal saline. Extra-alveolar treatment should be the shortest possible. All extra-alveolar procedures must be performed by holding the tooth from its crown with sterile gauze soaked in saline. In order to minimize the extra-alveolar period, all patent canals in multi-rooted teeth should be instrumented and obturated prior to the extraction. Intentional replantation should be performed in cases where no other treatment can be applied and the situation comes down to the simple dilemma: extraction or replantation. Extraction in some cases is the treatment of choice (Fig. 4.93).

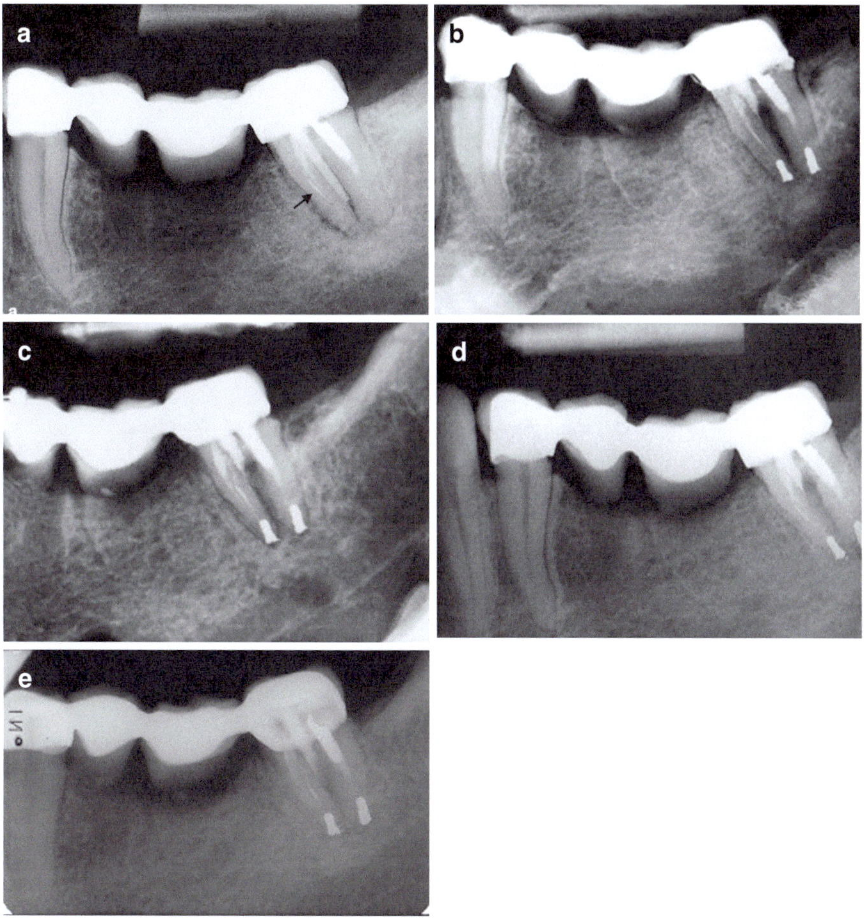

Fig. 4.92 (**a**) Preoperative radiograph of a poorly treated mandibular molar with an instrument fragment in the middle third of the mesial root (*arrow*) and a perforation of the furca by a post. Periapical radiolucent area involving the furca can be seen. (**b**) Removal of the fixed partial denture, tooth extraction, trimming of the post flash with the furca contour, apicectomy with amalgam retrofilling, tooth replantation, and re-cementation of the fixed partial denture. (**c–e**) 2, 4, and 8 years, respectively, recall examinations showed healing (Reprinted and modified with permission from Kafantaris and Lambrianidis 1999)

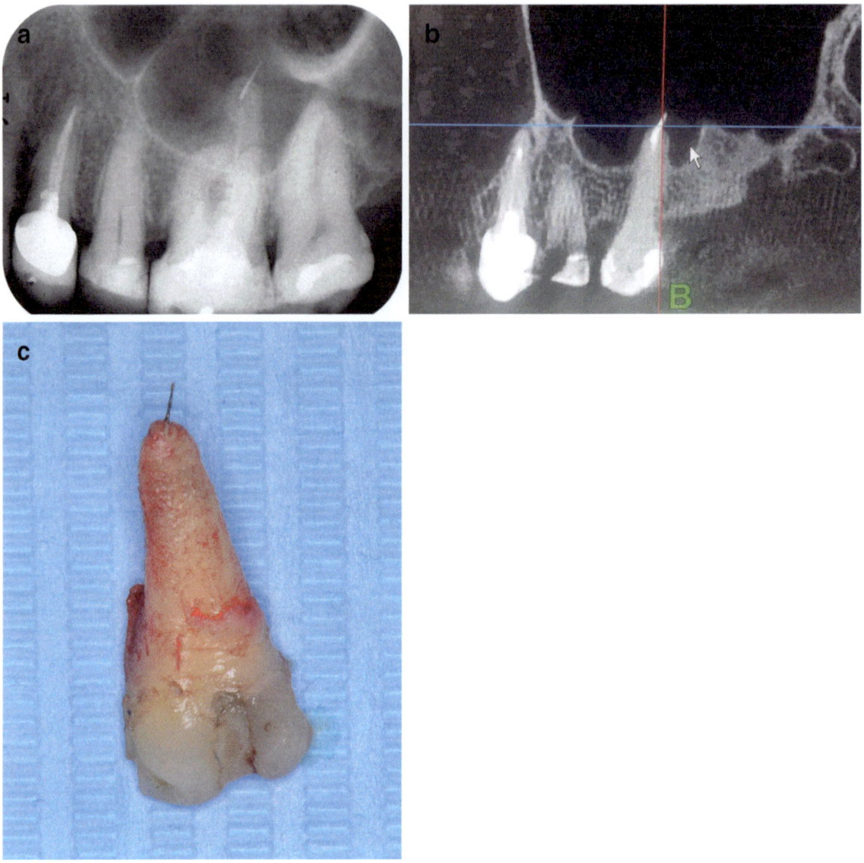

Fig. 4.93 (**a**) Preoperative radiograph of a maxillary left second molar with an inadequate root canal treatment and a fragment in the palatal root extruding beyond the foramen into the sinus in a 75-year-old patient with compromised general health. (**b**) CBCT image shows characteristic thickening of the inner lining (mucosa) of the sinus. (**c**) Palatal root of the extracted tooth

Conclusions

Patients should be informed if an instrument fractures during treatment or if a fractured file is discovered during a routine radiographic examination or retreatment. No management effort starts before completion of the patient briefing.

Localization of the fragment provides fundamental information for decision-making regarding the potential management of the fragment and the difficulty level of the case.

The prime therapeutic option for management of instrument fracture is non-surgical aiming in the retrieval of the fragment. If this attempt fails, bypassing is the option to follow and this also fails, instrumentation and obturation of the canal up to the fragment is performed. Surgical management is performed when the conservative approach fails or is considered from the outset to lead to failure.

A variety of methods have been proposed for the conservative and surgical management of fractured instruments. All require skilled use of the operating microscope and the appropriate armamentarium, training, experience, creativity, and patience and are generally considered within the remit of the endodontic specialist.

References

Aboud LR, Ormiga F, Gomes JACP. Electrochemical induced dissolution of fragments of a nickel–titanium endodontic files and their removal from simulated root canals. Int Endod J. 2014;37(2):155–62.

Amaral CC, Ormiga F, Gomes JA. Electrochemical-induced dissolution of stainless steel files. Int Endod J. 2015;48(2):137–44.

Andrabi SM, Kumar A, Iftekhar H, Alam S. Retrieval of a separated nickel-titanium instrument using a modified 18-guage needle and cyanoacrylate glue: a case report. Restor Dent Endod. 2013;38(2):93–7.

Andreasen JO. Traumatic injuries of the teeth. Copenhagen: Munksgaard; 1981.

Andreasen JO, Borum MK, Jacobsen HL, Andreasen FM. Replantation of avulsed permanent incisors. 4. Factors related to periodontal ligament healing. Endod Dent Traumatol. 1995;11(2):76–89.

Berbert A, Filho MT, Ueno AH, Bramante CM, Ishikiriama A. The influence of ultrasound in removing intraradicular posts. Int Endod J. 1995;28(2):100–2.

Brito-Junior M, Normanha JA, Camilo CC, Faria-e-Silva AL, Saquy PC, Ferraz MA, et al. Alternative techniques to remove fractured instrument fragments from the apical third of root canals: report of two cases. Braz Dent J. 2015;26(1):79–85.

Brown DW. Paper point revisited: risk of cellulose fibres shedding during canal length confirmation. Int Endod J. 2016; doi:10.1111/iej.12663. [Epub ahead of print].

Charara K, Friedman S, Sherman A, Kishen A, Malkhassian G, Khakpour M, et al. Assessment of apical extrusion during root canal irrigation with the novel gentlewave system in a simulated apical environment. J Endod. 2016;42(1):135–9.

Chauhan R, Chandra A, Singh S. Retrieval of a separated instrument from the root canal followed by non-surgical healing of a large periapical lesion in maxillary incisors – a case report. Endodontology. 2013;25:68–73.

Cohen S, Schwartz S. Endodontic complications and the law. J Endod. 1987;13(4):191–7.

Cohen S, Gary D, Glassman G, Mounce R. Rips, strips and broken tips: handling the endodontic mishap Part II: the separated instrument. In: Oral Health; 2005. p. 10–20.

Cuje J, Bargholz C, Hülsmann M. The outcome of retained instrument removal in a specialist practice. Int Endod J. 2010;43(7):545–54.

Cvikl B, Klimscha J, Holly M, Zeitlinger M, Gruber R, Moritz A. Removal of fractured endodontic instruments using an Nd:YAG laser. Quintessence Int. 2014;45(7):569–75.

D'Arcangelo C, Varvara G, De Fazio P. Broken instrument removal–two cases. J Endod. 2000;26(6):368–70.

Davies GM, Worthington HV, Clarkson JE, Thomas P, Davies RM. The use of fibre-optic transillumination in general dental practice. Br Dent J. 2001;191(3):145–7.

Ebihara A, Takashina M, Anjo T, Takeda A, Suda H. Removal of root canal obstructions using pulsed Nd:YAG laser. Int Congr Ser. 2003;1248:257–9.

Feldman G, Solomon C, Notaro P, Moskowitz E. Retrieving broken endodontic instruments. J Am Dent Assoc. 1974;88(3):588–91.

Filho T, Krebs R, Berlinck T, Galindo R. Retrieval of a broken endodontic instrument using cyanoacrylate adhesive. Case report. Braz Dent J. 1998;9(1):57–60.

Filho F, Vanni J, Limongi S, Fariniuk L, Travassos R, Albuauerance D. Intentional replantation: case report of an alternative treatment for endodontic therapy failure. IRSBO. 2004;1:36–40.

Floratos S, Kim S. Modern endodontic microsurgery concepts: a clinical update. Dent Clin N Am. 2017;61(1):81–91.
Fors UG, Berg JO. A method for the removal of broken endodontic instruments from root canals. J Endod. 1983;9(4):156–9.
Fu M, Zhang Z, Hou B. Removal of broken files from root canals by using ultrasonic techniques combined with dental microscope: a retrospective analysis of treatment outcome. J Endod. 2011;37(5):619–22.
Gettleman BH, Spriggs KA, ElDeeb ME, Messer HH. Removal of canal obstructions with the Endo Extractor. J Endod. 1991;17(12):608–11.
Gluskin A. Standard of practice in contemporary endodontics. In: Endodontics: Colleagues for Excellence newsletter; 2014.
Grossman LI. Endodontic case reports. Dent Clin N Am. 1974;18(2):509–27.
Haapasalo M, Wang Z, Shen Y, Curtis A, Patel P, Khakpour M. Tissue dissolution by a novel multisonic ultracleaning system and sodium hypochlorite. J Endod. 2014;40(8):1178–81.
Haapasalo M, Shen Y, Wang Z, Park E, Curtis A, Patel P, Vandrangi P. Apical pressure created during irrigation with the GentleWave™ system compared to conventional syringe irrigation. Clin Oral Investig. 2016;20(7):1525–34.
Hagiwara R, Suehara M, Fujii R, Kato H, Nakagawa K, Oda Y. Laser welding method for removal of instruments debris from root canals. Bull Tokyo Dent Coll. 2013;54(2):81–8.
Hülsmann M. Removal of silver cones and fractured instruments using the Canal Finder System. J Endod. 1990a;16(12):596–600.
Hülsmann M. [Removal of fractured root canal instruments using the Canal Finder System]. Dtsch Zahnarztl Z. 1990b;45(4):229–32.
Hülsmann M. Methods for removing metal obstructions from the root canal. Endod Dent Traumatol. 1993;9(6):223–37.
Hülsmann M, Schinkel I. Influence of several factors on the success or failure of removal of fractured instruments from the root canal. Endod Dent Traumatol. 1999;15(6):252–8.
Iqbal MK, Rafailov H, Kratchman SI, Karabucak B. A comparison of three methods for preparing centered platforms around separated instruments in curved canals. J Endod. 2006;32(1):48–51.
ISO 9626:1991/Amd.1:2001(en) Stainless steel needle tubing for the manufacture of medical devices Amendment 1.
Ito K. The effect of voltage and electrolyte on the dissolubility of separated root canal instrument by electrolytic method. Jpn J Conserv Dent. 1983;26:178.
Ito K, Mototsugu O, Nishihara H, Shiono M, Hattori N, Asano M, Yamashita Y, Takahashi T, Saito T. A study on broken instrument removal from root canal. Influence of voltage on the dissolubility, current and temperature change. Jpn J Conserv Dent. 1987;30:172.
Jeng HW, ElDeeb ME. Removal of hard paste fillings from the root canal by ultrasonic instrumentation. J Endod. 1987;13(6):295–8.
Johnson WB, Beatty RG. Clinical technique for the removal of root canal obstructions. J Am Dent Assoc. 1988;117(3):473–6.
Kafantaris N, Lambrianidis T. Intentional replantation. Report of two cases. Stoma. 1999;27:205–10.
Kim S, Kratchman S. Modern endodontic surgery concepts and practice: a review. J Endod. 2006;32(7):601–23.
Koppang HS, Koppang R, Solheim T, Aarnes H, Stolen SO. Cellulose fibers from endodontic paper points as an etiological factor in postendodontic periapical granulomas and cysts. J Endod. 1989;15(8):369–72.
Kowalczuck A, Silva Neto UX, Fariniuk LF, Westphalen VP, Laurindo CA, Carneiro E. Electrochemical dissolution of fractured nickel-titanium instruments on human extracted teeth. Int Endod J. 2016; doi:10.1111/iej.12654. [Epub ahead of print].
Krell KV, Neo J. The use of ultrasonic endodontic instrumentation in the re-treatment of a paste-filled endodontic tooth. Oral Surg Oral Med Oral Pathol. 1985;60(1):100–2.
Krell KV, Fuller MW, Scott GL. The conservative retrieval of silver cones in difficult cases. J Endod. 1984;10(6):269–73.

Lambrianidis T. Tooth reimplantation. Monograph; 1985 (in Greek).
Lambrianidis T. Risk management in root canal treatment. Thessaloniki: University Studio Press; 2001. p. 199–247.
Lambrianidis T, Molyvdas J, Mazinis E. Roentgenology in endodontics. Athens: Odontiatriko Vima; 2007, p. 229–53 (in Greek).
Liewehr FR. An inexpensive device for transillumination. J Endod. 2001;27(2):130–1.
Lubisich EB, Hilton TJ, Ferracane J, Northwest P. Cracked teeth: a review of the literature. J Esthet Restor Dent. 2010;22(3):158–67.
Ma J, Shen Y, Yang Y, Gao Y, Wan P, Gan Y, Patel P, Curtis A, Khakpour M, Haapasalo M. In vitro study of calcium hydroxide removal from mandibular molar root canals. J Endod. 2015;41(4):553–8.
Madarati AA, Watts DC, Qualtrough AJ. Opinions and attitudes of endodontists and general dental practitioners in the UK towards the intra-canal fracture of endodontic instruments. Part 2. Int Endod J. 2008;41(12):1079–87.
Masserann J. [The extraction of posts broken deeply in the roots]. Actual Odontostomatol (Paris). 1966;75:329–42 (in French).
Masserann J. "Entfernen metallischer Fragmente aus Wurzelkanalen" (Removal of metal fragments from the root canal). J Br Endod Soc. 1971;5(3):55–9.
Meidinger DL, Kabes BJ. Foreign object removal utilizing the Cavi-Endo ultrasonic instrument. J Endod. 1985;11(7):301–4.
Mitropoulos CM. The use of fibre-optic transillumination in the diagnosis of posterior approximal caries in clinical trials. Caries Res. 1985;19(4):379–84.
Molina B, Glickman G, Vandrangi P, Khakpour M. Evaluation of Root Canal debridement of human molars using the GentleWave system. J Endod. 2015;41(10):1701–5.
Molyvdas I, Lambrianidis T, Zervas P,Veis A. Clinical study on the prognosis of endodontic treatment of teeth with broken endodontic instruments. Stoma. 1992;20:63–72 (in Greek).
Monteiro JC, Kuga MC, Dantas AA, Jordao-Basso KC, Keine KC, Ruchaya PJ, Faria G, Leonardo Rde T. A method for retrieving endodontic or atypical nonendodontic separated instruments from the root canal: a report of two cases. J Contemp Dent Pract. 2014;15(6):770–4.
Nagai O, Tani N, Kayaba Y, Kodama S, Osada T. Ultrasonic removal of broken instruments in root canals. Int Endod J. 1986;19(6):298–304.
Nair PN. On the causes of persistent apical periodontitis: a review. Int Endod J. 2006;39(4):249–81.
Nair PN, Sjogren U, Krey G, Sundqvist G. Therapy-resistant foreign body giant cell granuloma at the periapex of a root-filled human tooth. J Endod. 1990;16(12):589–95.
Nair M, Levin M, Nair U. In: Hargreaves KM, Berman LH, editors. Cohen's pathways of the pulp. 11th ed. St. Louis: Elsevier Health Sciences; 2016. p. 63–5.
Nehme W. A new approach for the retrieval of broken instruments. J Endod. 1999;25(9):633–5.
Nevares G, Cunha RS, Zuolo ML, Bueno CE. Success rates for removing or bypassing fractured instruments: a prospective clinical study. J Endod. 2012;38(4):442–4.
Okawauchi T. Removal of separated instruments from the root canal. The change of Fe, Cr, Ca, and P on the root canal by electrolytic method. Jpn J Conserv Dent. 1993;36:562.
Okiji T. Modified usage of the Masserann kit for removing intracanal broken instruments. J Endod. 2003;29(7):466–7.
Ormiga F, da Cunha Ponciano Gomes JA, de Araujo MC. Dissolution of nickel-titanium endodontic files via an electrochemical process: a new concept for future retrieval of fractured files in root canals. J Endod. 2010;36(4):717–20.
Ormiga F, da Cunha Ponciano Gomes JA, de Araujo MC, Barbosa AO. An initial investigation of the electrochemical dissolution of fragments of nickel-titanium endodontic files. J Endod. 2011;37(4):526–30.
Ormiga F, Aboud LR, Gomes JA. Electrochemical-induced dissolution of nickel-titanium endodontic instruments with different designs. Int Endod J. 2015;48(4):342–50.
Patel J, Morawala A, Talathi R, Shirol D. Retrieval of a broken instrument from root canal in primary anterior teeth. Univ Res J Dent. 2015;5:203–6.

Pessoa de Andrade L, Chacon de Oliveira Conde N, Sponchiado Junior EC, Franco Marques AA, Pereira JV, Garcia LF. Contamination of absorbent paper points in clinical practice: a critical approach. Gen Dent. 2014;62(4):e38–40.
Pitt Ford TR, Rhodes JS, Pitt Ford HE. Endodontics problem-solving in clinical practice. London: Martin Dunitz; 2002. p. 142.
Pk M, Sc K, As S. Broken instrument retrieval with indirect ultrasonics in a primary molar. Eur Arch Paediatr Dent. 2016;17(1):71–4.
Plotino G, Pameijer CH, Grande NM, Somma F. Ultrasonics in endodontics: a review of the literature. J Endod. 2007;33(2):81–95.
Rahimi M, Parashos P. A novel technique for the removal of fractured instruments in the apical third of curved root canals. Int Endod J. 2009;42(3):264–70.
Ramos Brito AC, Verner FS, Junqueira RB, Yamasaki MC, Queiroz PM, Freitas DQ, Oliveira-Santos C. Detection of fractured endodontic instruments in root canals: comparison between different digital radiography systems and cone-beam computed tomography. J Endod. 2017;43(4):544–9.
Roig-Greene JL. The retrieval of foreign objects from root canals: a simple aid. J Endod. 1983;9(9):394–7.
Rosen E, Azizi H, Friedlander C, Taschieri S, Tsesis I. Radiographic identification of separated instruments retained in the apical third of root canal-filled teeth. J Endod. 2014;40(10):1549–52.
Rosen E, Venezia NB, Azizi H, Kamburoglu K, Meirowitz A, Ziv-Baran T, Tsesis I. A comparison of cone-beam computed tomography with periapical radiography in the detection of separated instruments retained in the apical third of root canal-filled teeth. J Endod. 2016;42(7):1035–9.
Ruddle C. Nonsurgical endodontic retreatment. J Endod. 2004;30(12):827–45.
Saito T, Yamaguchi M, Tamura K, Tanabe K, Nagai S, Ito K. A clinical study of removing the separated root canal instrument by electrolytic method. Jpn J Conserv Dent. 1986;29:81–95.
Schafer E. Irrigation of the root canal. Endod Pract Today. 2007;1:11–27.
Schindler WG, Walker WA III. Transillumination of the beveled root surface: an aid to periradicular surgery. J Endod. 1994;20(8):408–10.
Schneiderman A, Elbaum M, Shultz T, Keem S, Greenebaum M, Driller J. Assessment of dental caries with Digital Imaging Fiber-Optic TransIllumination (DIFOTI): in vitro study. Caries Res. 1997;31(2):103–10.
Sedgley CM, Messer H. Long-term retention of a paper point in the periapical tissues: a case report. Endod Dent Traumatol. 1993;9(3):120–3.
Setzer FC, Kohli MR, Shah SB, Karabucak B, Kim S. Outcome of endodontic surgery: a meta-analysis of the literature–Part 2: comparison of endodontic microsurgical techniques with and without the use of higher magnification. J Endod. 2012;38(1):1–10.
Shah N, Logani A, Kumar A. Intentional replantation: A viable treatment option for specific endodontic conditions. Roots 2012;1:10–2.
Shenoy A, Mandava P, Bolla N, Vemuri S. A novel technique for removal of broken instrument from root canal in mandibular second molar. Indian J Dent Res. 2014;25(1):107–10.
Shiyakov KK, Vasileva RI. Success for removing or bypassing instruments fractured beyond the root canal curve-45 clinical cases. J IMAB Annu Proc. 2014;20(3):567–71.
Sigurdsson A, Le KT, Woo SM, Rassoulian SA, McLachlan K, Abbassi F, Garland RW. Six-month healing success rates after endodontic treatment using the novel GentleWave System: the pure prospective multi-center clinical study. J Clin Exp Dent. 2016;8(3):e290–8.
Soni D, Raisingani D, Mehta P, Swarnkar P, Meel R, Beniwal A. Intentional replantation: a case report. Int J Res Dent. 2015;5(6):12–22.
Souyave LC, Inglis AT, Alcalay M. Removal of fractured endodontic instruments using ultrasonics. Br Dent J. 1985;159(8):251–3.
Spriggs K, Gettleman B, Messer HH. Evaluation of a new method for silver point removal. J Endod. 1990;16(7):335–8.
Stamos DG, Haasch GC, Chenail B, Gerstein H. Endosonics: clinical impressions. J Endod. 1985;11(4):181–7.
Stasinopoulos E. Dental pathology and therapeutics. Athens: Parisianos; 1978. p. 2. (in Greek).
Stock CJ. Current status of the use of ultrasound in endodontics. Int Dent J. 1991;41(3):175–82.

Sukegawa S, Kanno T, Shibata A, Matsumoto K, Sukegawa-Takahashi Y, Sakaida K, Furuki Y. Use of an intraoperative navigation system for retrieving a broken dental instrument in the mandible: a case report. J Med Case Rep. 2017;11:14.

Suter B. A new method for retrieving silver points and separated instruments from root canals. J Endod. 1998;24(6):446–8.

Terauchi Y. Separated file removal. Dent Today. 2012;31(5):108, 110–3

Terauchi Y, O'Leary L, Suda H. Removal of separated files from root canals with a new file-removal system: case reports. J Endod. 2006;32(8):789–97.

Terauchi Y, O'Leary L, Kikuchi I, Asanagi M, Yoshioka T, Kobayashi C, et al. Evaluation of the efficiency of a new file removal system in comparison with two conventional systems. J Endod. 2007;33(5):585–8.

Terauchi Y, O'Leary L, Yoshioka T, Suda H. Comparison of the time required to create secondary fracture of separated file fragments by using ultrasonic vibration under various canal conditions. J Endod. 2013;39(10):1300–5.

Tomov G, Kissov H. Laser-assisted endodontic retreatment. Evidences and critique. On-line J Bulgarian Dent Assoc. 2014 (in Bulgarian).

Tsesis I, Rosen E, Schwartz-Arad D, Fuss Z. Retrospective evaluation of surgical endodontic treatment: traditional versus modern technique. J Endod. 2006;32(5):412–6.

Tzanetakis GN, Kontakiotis EG, Maurikou DV, Marzelou MP. Prevalence and management of instrument fracture in the postgraduate endodontic program at the Dental School of Athens: a five-year retrospective clinical study. J Endod. 2008;34(6):675–8.

Walton RE, Tamse A. Diagnosis of vertical root fractures. In: Tamse A, Tsesis I, Rosen E, editors. Vertical root fractures in dentistry. 2015. p. 60, Walton.

Wefelmeier M, Eveslage M, Burklein S, Ott K, Kaup M. Removing fractured endodontic instruments with a modified tube technique using a light-curing composite. J Endod. 2015;41(5):733–6.

Wohlgemuth P, Cuocolo D, Vandrangi P, Sigurdsson A. Effectiveness of the GentleWave System in removing separated instruments. J Endod. 2015;41(11):1895–8.

Yang Q, Shen Y, Huang D, Zhou X, Gao Y, Haapasalo M. Evaluation of two trephine techniques for removal of fractured rotary nickel-titanium instruments from root canals. J Endod. 2017;43(1):116–20.

Yu DG, Kimura Y, Tomita Y, Nakamura Y, Watanabe H, Matsumoto K. Study on removal effects of filling materials and broken files from root canals using pulsed Nd:YAG laser. J Clin Laser Med Surg. 2000;18(1):23–8.

Zeigler P, Serene T. Failures in therapy. CV Mobsy: St. Louis; 1984.

Zervas P. Evaluation of the effects of citric acid application on the outcome of replanted teeth. Clinical and histologic investigation in dogs. PhD Thesis, University of Thessaloniki; 1989 (in Greek).

Parameters Influencing the Removal of Fractured Instruments

5

Theodor Lambrianidis and Emmanuel Mazinis

The likelihood of successfully management of fractured instruments ranges greatly (see Tables 6.1–6.9 in Chap. 6). It has been reported that the longer the time needed to manage a fractured instrument, the greater the chance/possibility for complications and the lower the success rate (Ward et al. 2003; Suter et al. 2005). The wide variation in the reported results and time needed to manage a fractured instrument can be attributed to the variety of factors influencing the possibility of their retrieval. These factors can be grouped into:

- Tooth factors
- Localization of the fragment
- Fractured instrument factors
- Operator factors
- The technique chosen
- Patient factors

5.1 Tooth Factors

The type of tooth, the root canal morphology and particularly its cross-sectional shape and diameter, the thickness of the dentin, the depth of the external root concavities, the presence of root canal curvature, and the radius and degree of the root

T. Lambrianidis, D.D.S., Ph.D. (✉)
Department of Endodontology, Dental School, Aristotle University of Thessaloniki, Thessaloniki, Greece
e-mail: thlampri@dent.auth.gr

E. Mazinis, D.D.S., Ph.D.
Private Practice, Veria, Greece

T. Lambrianidis (ed.), *Management of Fractured Endodontic Instruments*,
DOI 10.1007/978-3-319-60651-4_5

canal curvature are among the decision-making and influencing factors in the management of fractured instruments. *As a generalized finding, the success rate of retrieving instrument fragments is higher in straight and wide canals than in curved and narrow canals* (Hülsmann and Schinkel 1999; Shen et al. 2004; Cuje et al. 2010; McGuigan et al. 2013). In canals with severe curvature, the retrieval success rate was found considerably low as opposed to the success rate in canals with moderate or slight curvature (Hülsmann and Schinkel 1999; Shen et al. 2004; Cuje et al. 2010; McGuigan et al. 2013). To our knowledge, there is only one study that found no statistically significant difference in the success rate with respect to the location (tooth/root type) of the fractured instrument (Suter et al. 2005). A statistical model for predicting the retrieval rate of fragments in relation to root canal curvature and the depth and length of fragments has been established (Chen et al. 2015). Data on the tooth position, root canal curvature, and the depth and length of fragments were collected from 210 clinical cases with fragments in the lower segments of curved root canal. The correlations of these factors and the retrieval rate were analyzed. It was concluded that root canal curvature and the depth of the fractured instrument were significantly correlated with the retrieval rate. With the increase of curvature and depth, the retrieval rate decreased significantly (Chen et al. t2015). Depth in this study was defined as the straight-line length on the radiograph film from the root canal orifice to the coronal end of the fragment.

In all cases of management of instrument fragments, it should be born in mind that:

- Curved canals often curve in more than one plane.
- Even if the canal appears straight, a curve in the plane of the radiographic beam might be present.
- Establishment of straight-line access to the fragment, particularly if it is located in the apical third, necessitates sacrificing a significant amount of root dentin, which eventually weakens the tooth.

Instrument fracture among molars is reported as occurring particularly in the mesial roots of mandibular molars (Molyvdas et al. 1992; Hülsmann and Schinkel 1999; Ward et al. 2003; Skyttner 2007). The presence of isthmus, the narrow, ribbon-shaped communication between the mesiobuccal and mesiolingual canals, in the mandibular molars which is present in more than half of mandibular molars (de Pablo et al. 2010; Estrela et al. 2015), can be of great assistance when dealing with a fragment in one of these canals. It is easier and safer to remove dentin at the isthmus between the two canals in order to free the fragment (Fig. 5.1). The presence of isthmus detected also in maxillary molars and maxillary premolars (de Pablo et al. 2010; Estrela et al. 2015; Pecora et al. 2013) can be particularly useful for the management of instrument fragments in these teeth as well. Therefore, a thorough knowledge of tooth and root morphology and meticulous interpretation of available radiographs of the tooth under treatment are essential. The use of CBCT could contribute to the detection, location, and estimation of the extent of isthmi and the

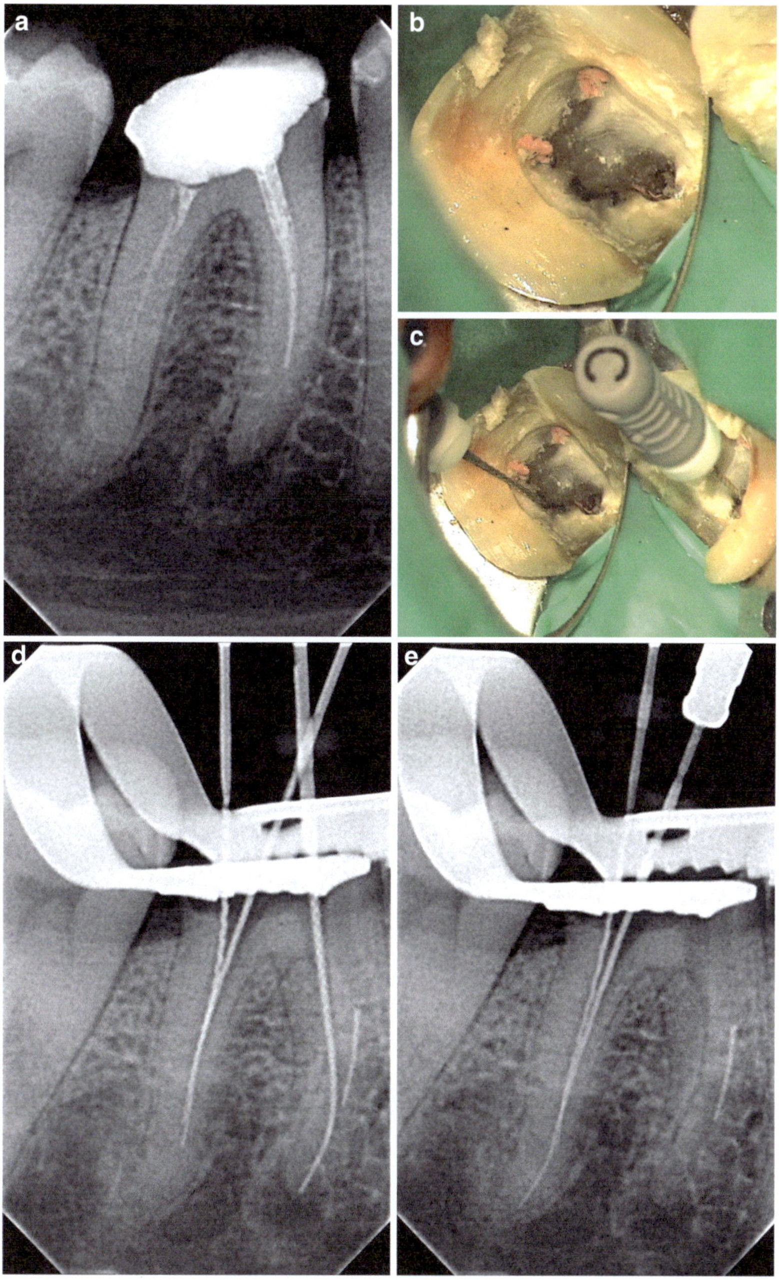

Fig. 5.1 (**a**) Preoperative radiograph of a mandibular right first molar with a fragment in the middle third of the mesial root. (**b**, **c**) Operative microscope photographs of the pulp chamber floor. (**d**, **e**) Working length radiographs with different angulations to aid in the localization the fragment. (**f**, **g**) CBCT images of the fragment present in the isthmus. (**h**) Operative microscope photograph after exposure of the coronal part of the fragment. (**i**) Master cone radiograph. (**j**) Immediate post-operative radiograph. (**k**) Two-year follow-up radiograph (Courtesy Dr. K. Kalogeropoulos)

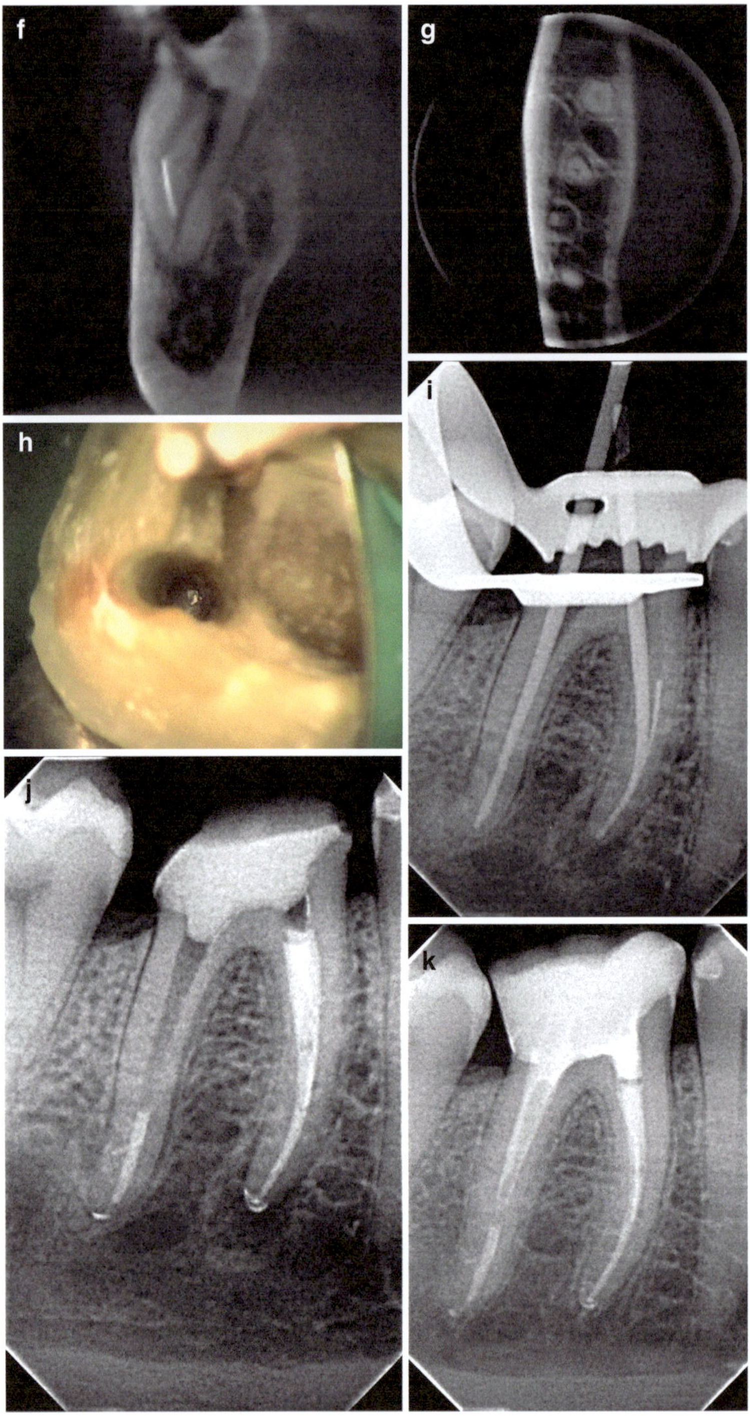

Fig. 5.1 (continued)

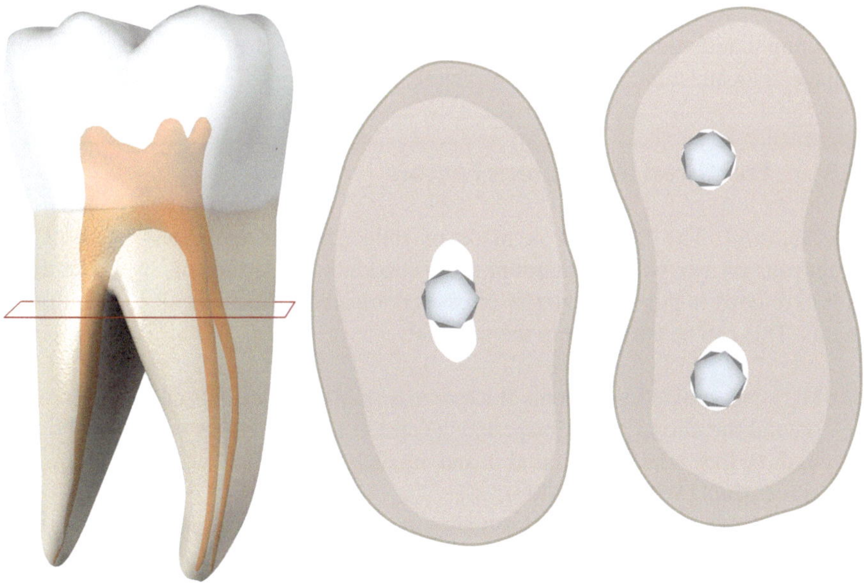

Fig. 5.2 Cross section of the distal and mesial root of a lower first molar. The cross-sectional shape of the root canal determines to a great extend the available space between the fragment and the canal walls. The space around a fragment in an oval root canal provides access for manipulations as opposed to the available space in case of fragments in narrow canals with round cross section

identification of oval or round cross-sectional shape of the root canal which determines to a great extend the available space between the fragment and the canal wall (Fig. 5.2).

5.2 Localization of the Fragment

It is widely recognized that the location of the fragment in relation to the curvature of the root canal is the main determinant, rather than the method used to retrieve it. Fragments in the coronal third that is, more or less, the straight visible portion of the root canal are managed more easily and with a higher success rate compared to the corresponding rates for fragments in the middle or apical third (Souter and Messer 2005; Madarati et al. 2008; Tzanetakis et al. 2008; Cuje et al. 2010). As a rule of thumb, *what cannot be seen cannot be properly managed.* When a fractured instrument lies partially around the canal curvature, and particularly when it lies totally beyond the curvature, safe nonsurgical management usually cannot be accomplished unless a straight-line access can be established to their most coronal portion (Ruddle 2002). This straight-line access might be possible in cases of fragments lying partially around curvatures (Ruddle 2002). There are several success rates reported in in vivo and ex vivo studies using a variety of techniques in different modifications for the removal of fractured instruments located partly or totally beyond the curvature (see Tables 6.1–6.9 in Chap. 6).

In conclusion, tooth factors and fragment location factors favorable for retrieval are straight and wide canals, localization in the coronal or mesial third of the root canal and localization prior to the curvature.

5.3 Fractured Instrument Factors

The material. The fragment is made of influences the likelihood of retrieval. Fragments of rotary nickel-titanium (NiTi) endodontic instruments are more difficult to remove in the vast majority of cases compared to stainless steel (SS) instruments. This can be attributed to the fact that:

(a) NiTi endodontic instruments fracture at a smaller length, further apically, at or around the curves of narrow canals (Ward et al. 2003). Due to their rotational motion, they tend to be wound in and impacted in the canal walls, occluding the entire canal (Ward et al. 2003).
(b) SS fragments absorb the ultrasonic energy bodily during retrieval efforts and thus move early on in contrast to NiTi fragments which absorb the energy at and/or near the point of contact with the tip (Cohen et al. 2005).
(c) NiTi instruments have also a greater tendency to fracture repeatedly, becoming smaller and smaller when ultrasonic energy is applied to them, whereas SS instruments are more robust (Ruddle 2002; Cohen et al. 2005; Suter et al. 2005; Madarati et al. 2008). The presence or absence of supporting dentinal wall as a contributing factor affecting the tendency of a file fragment to undergo secondary fracture has been investigated (Terauchi et al. 2013). It was concluded that whenever the coronal portion of NiTi fragments lacked dentin wall opposite to the area where the ultrasonic tip was applied, it tended to break significantly faster than those with dentinal wall support (Terauchi et al. 2013). It is possible that ultrasonic energy applied to the fragments was transmitted to the dentin, dissipating some of the stress that would have contributed to file breakage. Therefore, this secondary fracture of fragments can be reduced by applying the ultrasonic tip to the inner curvature of the canal (Terauchi et al. 2013).
(d) The increasing taper of NiTi compared with SS instruments (Fig. 5.3) makes access and trephining around the coronal aspect of the NiTi fragments more difficult and thus harder to retrieve (McGuigan et al. 2013).

The type of the instrument. This is another largely unaddressed issue in the literature, and the available information is inconclusive. It has been found that the instrument type does not affect the removal success rate (Shen et al. 2004; Suter et al. 2005) and that it also influences removal efficacy (Hülsmann and Schinkel 1999). Thus, Lentulo spirals, for example, have been found to be easier to remove than reamers or Hedstroem files, with which the lowest success rate was recorded (Hülsmann and Schinkel 1999). In the case of Lentulo spiral fillers, this could be attributed to their ability to be bypassed via their empty centers (Hülsmann and Schinkel 1999) and, of course, to the fact that these instruments are used in

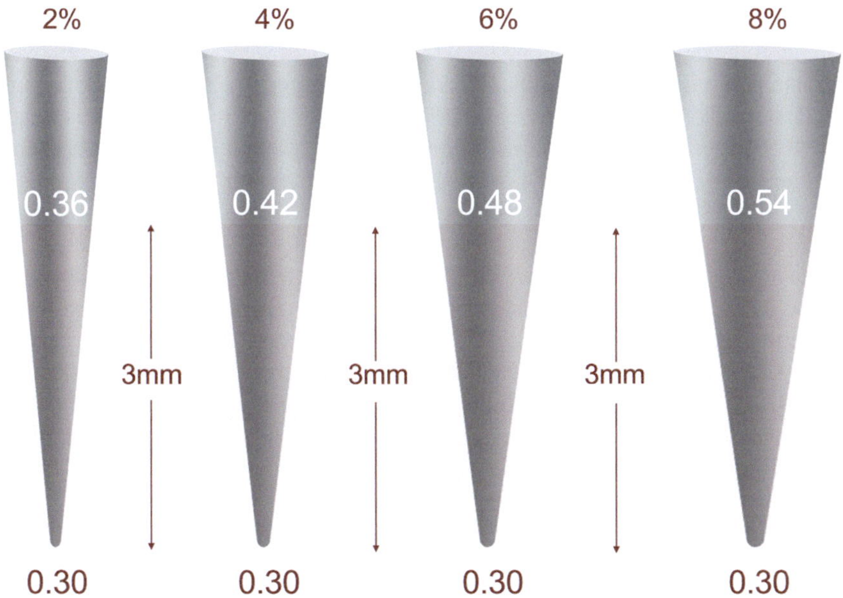

Fig. 5.3 Diameter differences 3 mm from the tip of instruments with various tapers

completely instrumented and thus wider canals where easier manipulations are allowed.

Theoretically, a segment of a LightSpeed LSX (LSX, LightSpeed Technology) can quite easily be retrieved as, due to its flat spade-shaped, non-cutting blade and the lack of traditional flutes, it does not screw and bind into dentin. In addition, the space provided due to its flat spade-shaped blade explains the reported bypassing in clinical practice of irretrievable segments in 75% (9/12) of cases (Hansen et al. 2013).

The length of the fragment. The influence of fragment length as a variable on the success or failure of removal attempts has not been investigated extensively. Additionally, there are contradictory views among the few studies that have been carried out. A correlation between fragment length and success of removal (Hülsmann and Schinkel 1999) and no such finding (Suter et al. 2005; Cuje et al. 2010) has been reported. An increased successful retrieval of longer fragments was reported but the difference was not statistically significant (Shen et al. 2004). Therefore, at present, there is insufficient evidence-based data on the topic. Anecdotal findings, however, suggest that long fragments are easier to remove than short ones. This can be attributed to the fact that probably only the tip of the fragment is engaged into the root dentin, leaving at the coronal segment enough space for its loosening and removal. Additionally, it is more or less possible that the coronal part of long fragments lies in the visible and thus easier to be handled portion of the root canal. The length of the fragment as a factor influencing the outcome of management attempts, which has also been highlighted by (Hülsmann and Schinkel

1999), is particularly accentuated in the study of Skyttner (2007) where 19 out of 20 lengthy fragments stretched along the whole root length were successfully removed. Similar findings with fragments extending over the complete length of the root canal were also reported (Suter et al. 2005). The important role of fragment length probably triggered (Bahcall et al. 2005) the design of the controlled fracture endodontic rotary NiTi files with a predetermined fracture point. The concept was to incorporate a small hub with a smaller diameter placed near the shaft of the file that would allow the file to fracture at the hub rather than the tip and make the fragment long and easier to manage. To our knowledge these instruments have never appeared on the market. To our knowledge also, only LightSpeed LSX (LSX, LightSpeed Technology) instruments are designed to twist up, pull out of the handle, or separate at the shaft-handle junction when subjected to excessive twisting forces (Hansen et al. 2013). This separation resembles the one that occurs with Gates Glidden burs as they are designed to separate to their weakest point, which is near the hub of the drill. In both instruments, this type of separation allows easier retrieval.

5.4 Operator Factors

The knowledge, skill, experience, creativity, and patience of the operator are crucial in the management of fractured instruments (Hülsmann and Schinkel 1999; Lambrianidis 2001; Madarati et al. 2013). All retrieval/bypassing techniques are technically challenging procedures, depending solely on the tactile sensitivity and sheer perseverance of the clinician. Thus, for instrument fragment management, an experienced operator knows the most appropriate techniques and applies the particular one with which he/she is most familiar with and has most experience. In all cases, manipulations should be very meticulous to avoid unnecessary sacrifice of tooth structure.

5.5 The Technique Chosen

The technique chosen can be a key factor in the successful removal of an instrument fragment from a root canal. It has been suggested, though, that it may not be as important as anatomical factors (Shen et al. 2004; Madarati et al. 2013). Obviously, the application of any technique is closely related to the operator factors. The comparative evaluation of the techniques applied shows differences in the success rates (see Chap. 6).

5.6 Patient Factors

The extent of mouth opening and difficulties in accessing the canal with the fragment are the two main anatomical factors to be carefully evaluated before commencing any attempt as they greatly influence management efficiency and eventually decision-making.

The patient's anxiety and agony level as well as his/her attitude toward dentistry and in particular toward retention of the tooth in question might also influence the operator's manipulations and efforts.

References

Bahcall JK, Carp S, Miner M, Skidmore L. The causes, prevention, and clinical management of broken endodontic rotary files. Dent Today. 2005;24(11):74, 76, 78–80, quiz 80.

Chen L, Li X, Yang-xi C, Yuan L, Xiao-lin C, Yao L, et al. A statistical model for predicting the retrieval rate of separated instruments and clinical decision-making. J Dent Sci. 2015;10(4):423–30.

Cohen S, Gary D, Glassman G, Mounce R. Rips, strips and broken tips: handling the endodontic mishap Part II: the separated instrument. Oral Health; 2005, p. 10–20.

Cuje J, Bargholz C, Hülsmann M. The outcome of retained instrument removal in a specialist practice. Int Endod J. 2010;43(7):545–54.

de Pablo OV, Estevez R, Peix Sanchez M, Heilborn C, Cohenca N. Root anatomy and canal configuration of the permanent mandibular first molar: a systematic review. J Endod. 2010;36(12):1919–31.

Estrela C, Rabelo LE, de Souza JB, Alencar AH, Estrela CR, Sousa Neto MD, et al. Frequency of root canal isthmi in human permanent teeth determined by cone-beam computed tomography. J Endod. 2015;41(9):1535–9.

Hansen JR, Beeson TJ, Ibarrola JL. Case series: tooth retention 5 years after irretrievable separation of LightSpeedLSX instruments. J Endod. 2013;39(11):1467–70.

Hülsmann M, Schinkel I. Influence of several factors on the success or failure of removal of fractured instruments from the root canal. Endod Dent Traumatol. 1999;15(6):252–8.

Lambrianidis T. Risk management in root canal treatment. Thessaloniki: University Studio Press; 2001. p. 199–247.

Madarati AA, Watts DC, Qualtrough AJ. Opinions and attitudes of endodontists and general dental practitioners in the UK towards the intra-canal fracture of endodontic instruments. Part 2. Int Endod J. 2008;41(12):1079–87.

Madarati AA, Hunter MJ, Dummer PM. Management of intracanal separated instruments. J Endod. 2013;39(5):569–81.

McGuigan MB, Louca C, Duncan HF. Endodontic instrument fracture: causes and prevention. Br Dent J. 2013;214(7):341–8.

Molyvdas I, Lambrianidis T, Zervas P, Veis A. Clinical study on the prognosis of endodontic treatment of teeth with broken endodontic instruments. Stoma. 1992;20:63–72. (in Greek).

Pecora JD, Estrela C, Bueno MR, Porto OC, Alencar AH, Sousa-Neto MD, et al. Detection of root canal isthmuses in molars by map-reading dynamic using CBCT images. Braz Dent J. 2013;24(6):569–74.

Ruddle C. Broken instrument removal: the endodontic challenge. 2002 [cited 2016]. Available from: www.dentistrytoday.com/endodontics/997--sp-2132305201. Accessed 15 Dec 2016.

Shen Y, Peng B, Cheung GS. Factors associated with the removal of fractured NiTi instruments from root canal systems. Oral Surg Oral Med Oral Pathol Oral Radiol Endod. 2004;98(5):605–10.

Skyttner B. Endodontic instrument separations. Evaluation of a patient cases series with separated endodontic instruments and factors related to the treatment regarding separated instruments. Master of Medical Science in Odontology, Karolinska Institute for Odontology; 2007. p. 1–34.

Souter NJ, Messer HH. Complications associated with fractured file removal using an ultrasonic technique. J Endod. 2005;31(6):450–2.

Suter B, Lussi A, Sequeira P. Probability of removing fractured instruments from root canals. Int Endod J. 2005;38(2):112–23.

Terauchi Y, O'Leary L, Yoshioka T, Suda H. Comparison of the time required to create secondary fracture of separated file fragments by using ultrasonic vibration under various canal conditions. J Endod. 2013;39(10):1300–5.

Tzanetakis GN, Kontakiotis EG, Maurikou DV, Marzelou MP. Prevalence and management of instrument fracture in the postgraduate endodontic program at the Dental School of Athens: a five-year retrospective clinical study. J Endod. 2008;34(6):675–8.

Ward JR, Parashos P, Messer HH. Evaluation of an ultrasonic technique to remove fractured rotary nickel-titanium endodontic instruments from root canals: clinical cases. J Endod. 2003;29(11):764–7.

Comparative Evaluation of Techniques and Devices for the Removal of Fractured Instruments

6

Michael Hülsmann and Theodor Lambrianidis

In most cases fractured instruments do not present diagnostic problems, with the exception of retreatment cases where the fragment in some instances might be "hidden," obscured by root filling material and not very clearly visible. The recognition of remaining fragments is important for treatment planning. This involves the need to choose between various acceptable nonsurgical orthograde and surgical options. Evaluating, analyzing, and comparing the performance of the techniques proposed for the management of intracanal fractured endodontic instruments are important prerequisites for the selection of the most appropriate strategy and for the prediction of the outcome. For the best modality of treatment, good clinical judgment and experience in assessing objective findings are absolutely essential.

6.1 Comparative Evaluation of Nonsurgical Removal Techniques

Although a variety of techniques and devices have been described and used, no standardized procedure for the safe, successful, and consistent retrieval of instrument fragments in the root canal exists. The decisive factor for a successful intervention in the vast majority of proposed techniques is the preparation of a straight-line access to the fragment. Surgical operating microscopes and powerful piezoelectric ultrasonic units along with refined ultrasonic instruments are among the technological advances that have considerably increased the potential for

M. Hülsmann, D.D.S., Ph.D.
Department of Preventive Dentistry, Periodontology and Cariology, University Medicine Göttingen, Göttingen, Germany

T. Lambrianidis, D.D.S., Ph.D. (✉)
Department of Endodontology, Dental School, Aristotle University of Thessaloniki, Thessaloniki, Greece
e-mail: thlampri@dent.auth.gr

T. Lambrianidis (ed.), *Management of Fractured Endodontic Instruments*,
DOI 10.1007/978-3-319-60651-4_6

retrieval of instrument fragments. Some of the techniques proposed for the management of fractured instruments have been examined in clinical and/or experimental studies, and a variety of success rates have been reported, ranging from 33 to 100%. Nevertheless, it should be emphasized that the results from experimental studies should be carefully interpreted as they are of limited clinical relevance because the experimental setup cannot replicate the clinical situation for five main reasons:

(a) The instruments in experimental studies are intentionally fractured with the obvious consequence of a more or less different kind and degree of binding to the root dentin. Usually instruments are fractured intentionally following notching the instruments at a predetermined position. Therefore, the friction of the fractured tip of an endodontic file may not reflect the friction of an inadvertently fractured instrument inside a root canal.
(b) As two types of instrument fracture—ductile and torsional fracture and, of course, a combination of both—can occur inside a root canal; widely differing degrees of friction can be expected under clinical conditions. So far, no study has been published investigating differences in the removal of instruments fractured as a result of ductile or torsional failure. The time required for removal, the ease of bypassing, and the equipment and techniques for removal may differ between both groups, as well as the success rates and the incidence of perforations or other mishaps.
(c) There is more favorable access to the pulp cavity in experimental studies, in contrast to many clinical cases with restricted access. Most of the studies have been performed on extracted teeth not mounted in a mannequin head, thus allowing unlimited movement of the tooth and allowing unrestricted access to the cavity which is not limited by an opposite jaw or limited mouth opening.
(d) The responsibility to preserve dental tissues and avoid additional iatrogenic errors in clinical practice may result in less aggressive manipulations as compared to those in extracted teeth.
(e) The patients themselves, as their anxiety level and attitude toward dentistry and in particular toward retention of the tooth in question, might influence the operator's manipulations and efforts.

6.1.1 Ultrasonics

The ultrasonic removal technique is the most popular technique among both general dental practitioners and endodontic specialists (Madarati et al. 2008). This is probably due to the high overall success rate reported with this technique when used in conjunction with a dental operating microscope, providing the clinician with increased illumination and direct vision inside the root canal. Concerns, though, have been raised regarding the effect of ultrasonic vibration during removal efforts on the external root temperature, the loss of tooth structure, and the creation of ledges (See Chap. 7). The ultrasonic technique is considered superior to the Masserann technique (Friedman et al. 1990; Gencoglu and Helvacioglu 2009).

Although associated with some inherent risks, such as ledge formation, straightening, perforation, or excessive loss of tooth substance, this technique shows a high success rate (Table 6.1).

Table 6.1 Success rates as reported from in vivo and ex vivo studies using ultrasonics in different modifications for the removal of fractured instruments

Author(s)	Study design and sample size	Methods, devices, instruments, techniques, and protocol used	Microscope	Definition of success	Success rate
Shiyakov and Vasileva (2014)	In vivo ($n = 26$)	Ultrasonics	Yes	Removal	84.6% (22/26)
Shahabinejad et al. (2013)	In vitro ($n = 35$)	Ultrasonics preceded by 5 min efforts to bypass the fragment using #8 and #10K-files	Yes	Removal	Overall: 80% (28/35) Middle third 100% (8/8) Apical third 74% (20/27)
Nevares et al. (2012)	Prospective clinical study ($n = 112$)	Ultrasonics alone or associated with bypassing the fragment with hand files	Yes	Removal or bypassing	Overall: 70.5% (79/112) Visible fragment: 85.3% (58/66) Invisible fragment: 47.7% (21/44)
Fu et al. (2011)	In vivo retrospective study ($n = 66$)	Ultrasonics	Yes	Removal	88% (58/66)
Cuje et al. (2010)	In vivo retrospective study ($n = 170$)	Ultrasonics	Yes	Removal	Overall: 95% (162/170)
Gencoglu and Helvacioglu (2009)	Ex vivo ($n = 90$)	– K-files in straight and curved canals	Yes	Removal or bypassing	K-files overall 75% (27/36 In curved canals 66.6% (10/15) In straight canals 80.9% (17/21)
		– Ultrasonics in straight and curved canals K-files			Ultrasonics overall 94% (34/36) In curved canals 93.3%(14/15) In straight canals 95.2% (20/21)
Alomairy (2009)	Ex vivo ($n = 15$)	Ultrasonics	Yes	Removal	Ultrasonics: 80% (12/15)

(continued)

Table 6.1 (continued)

Author(s)	Study design and sample size	Methods, devices, instruments, techniques, and protocol used	Microscope	Definition of success	Success rate
Tzanetakis et al. (2008)	In vivo retrospective study (*n* = 134)	Ultrasonics	Yes	Removal or bypassing	Coronal third 100% Middle third 45.4% Apical third 37.5%
Skyttner (2007)	In vivo (*n* = 142)	Ultrasonics File bypass technique (braiding) Micro-forceps Tube technique with glue	Yes	NA	15 cases no treatment 20 cases extraction 64/107 removed 20/107 bypassed 4/107 retro endo 19/107 root filling, fragment retained
Terauchi et al. (2007)	Ex vivo (*n* = 98)	Ultrasonics (*n* = 35)	Yes		86% (30/35)
Souter and Messer (2005)	Ex vivo (*n* = 45) In vivo (*n* = 60)	Ultrasonics with staging platform	Yes	Removal	Ex vivo 91% (41/45) Coronal third 100% (14/14) Middle third 100% (16/16) Apical third 73% (11/15) In vivo overall: 70% (42/60) Coronal third 100% (11/11) Middle third 100% (22/22) Apical third 33% (9/27)
Souter and Messer (2005)	In vivo prospective study (*n* = 97)	Ultrasonics	Yes	Removal	80% (66/78)
Shen et al. (2004)	In vivo retrospective study (*n* = 72)	Ultrasonics	Yes	Removal or bypassing	Overall: 75% (34/47)

Table 6.1 (continued)

Author(s)	Study design and sample size	Methods, devices, instruments, techniques, and protocol used	Microscope	Definition of success	Success rate
Wei et al. (2004)	In vivo retrospective study (*n* = 47)	Ultrasonics	Yes	Removal	Extracted mandibular first molars 86.6% (26/30)
Ward et al. (2003b)	In vivo clinical cases (*n* = 24)	Ultrasonics	Yes	Removal	Overall: 67% (16/24)
Ward et al. (2003a)	(A) In vitro simulated canals (*n* = 60)	Bypassing the fragment with hand files and then removing it using ultrasonic vibration of a modified spreader	Yes	Removal	Overall: 67% (16/24)
	(B) Ex vivo (extracted mandibular teeth) (*n* = 30)				Overall: 91% (20/22)
Nehme (1999)	In vivo (*n* = 22)	Bypassing the fragment by hand files and then removing it by ultrasonic vibration of a modified spreader	Not available at the time	Removal	Overall: 91% (20/22)
Nagai et al. (1986)	Ex vivo-1 (*n* = 39)	Ultrasonic vibration of K-files	Not available at the time	Removal	In vivo: 67% (26/39)
	Ex vivo-1 (*n* = 42)	Ultrasonic vibration of K-files (visible fragment)			Ex vivo-1: 79% (33/42)
	Ex vivo (*n* = 57)	Ultrasonic vibration of K-files (not visible fragment)			Ex vivo: 68% (39/57)

One of the first studies on the use of ultrasonics for fragment removal by Nagai et al. (1986) reported a success rate of 68% (39 out of 57 fragments) in extracted teeth. In vivo 33 out of 42 fragments (79%) were removed. In another in vitro study by Alomairy (2009) on 30 extracted teeth, fairly balanced allocated to two groups of 15 teeth each, the application of ultrasonics was successful in 80% of the cases, whereas the Instrument Removal System (IRS) was able to remove only 60% of the fragments. Ward et al. (2003a) in an in vitro study investigated the so-called Ruddle technique, including preparation of a staging platform and use of ultrasonic tips, and reported success rates of 75% (resin blocks) and 86.8% (extracted teeth). In 24 clinical cases, this technique performed successfully in 66.7% (16 out of 24) of the cases (Ward et al. 2003b). Nevares et al. (2012) in 112 clinical cases achieved a success rate of 70.5%. For fragments visible under the microscope, the success rate was 85.3%, while that for fragments not visible was only 47.7%. In each of both subgroups, one perforation occurred. Gencoglu and Helvacioglu (2009) in an experimental study using the Ruddle technique were able to remove 95.2% (20 out of 21) of intentionally fractured instruments from straight root canals and 93.3% (14 out of 15) from curved root canals. The comparative values for a so-called conventional technique, also using a dental operating microscope, were 80.9% and 66.6%, respectively. The Masserann technique was successful only in 47.6% in straight canals. Souter and Messer (2005) in an experimental study on 45 extracted mandibular molars with intentionally fractured instruments, using a modified Ruddle technique, successfully removed 41 fragments (91%). Four cases failed with three perforations, all of these in the apical third of the roots. In 60 clinical cases 42 fragments were removed (70%), while 18 attempts failed. Suter et al. (2005) in 97 consecutive clinical cases removed 87% (84 out of 97) of the fragments. In 78 cases ultrasonics was successful, while in 12 cases this technique failed. Cuje et al. (2010) reported on a 95% (162 out of 170) success rate for the removal of fractured instruments in a dental office limited to endodontics. The authors used a strictly standardized procedure based on the Ruddle technique. The highest success rates were achieved for fragments in the coronal third (100%, 16 out of 16), in the coronal and middle third (100%, 19 out of 19), and straight root canal (100%, 14 out of 14). Six fragments could not be removed, one was only bypassed, and one perforation occurred.

There are no studies demonstrating the superiority of any available ultrasonic device or tip.

6.1.2 Tube Technique

After nearly more than half a century since its introduction, the Masserann system, the first tube technique described in the literature, is still in use (Okiji 2003; Suter et al. 2005; Pai et al. 2006; Terauchi et al. 2007; Gencoglu and Helvacioglu 2009) and is considered effective in selected cases, especially in those where the instrument fragment is located in a readily accessible position. The Masserann system and a variety of other tube techniques in different modifications have been investigated in in vivo and ex vivo studies (Table 6.2). The Masserann system has limited application in posterior teeth, particularly in patients with limited mouth opening and in teeth with thin and curved roots. More or less the same restrictions apply for the Mounce extractor, which can be used eventually only when fragments are located in the most accessible coronal portion of the root canal due to its relatively

Table 6.2 Success rates as reported from in vivo and ex vivo studies using the Masserann kit or any other tube technique in different modifications for the removal of fractured instruments

Author(s)	Study design and sample size	Methods, devices, instruments, techniques, and protocol used	Microscope	Definition of success	Success rate
Gencoglu and Helvacioglu (2009)	Ex vivo ($n = 90$)	Masserann only in straight canal	Yes	Removal or bypassing	Masserann: 47.6% (10/21)
Alomairy (2009)	Ex vivo ($n = 15$)	Instrument Removal System	Yes	Removal	Instrument Removal System: 60% (9/15)
Suter et al. (2005)	In vivo ($n = 12$)	Tube and Hedstrom file method		Removal	91% (11/12)
Hassan (2012)	In vitro ($n = 112$)	Ultrasonics ($N = 57$) EndoRescue ($N = 55$)	Yes	Removal	Ultrasonics: 81.8% (45/55) EndoRescue: 54.4% (31/57)
Terauchi et al. (2007)	Ex vivo ($n = 98$)	Masserann kit ($N = 33$) File Removal System ($N = 30$)	Yes	Removal	Masserann kit ($N = 33$) 91% (30/33) File Removal System ($N = 30$) 100% (30/30)
Sano et al. (1974)	In vivo ($n = 100$)	Masserann kit	Not Available		Removal: 55% (55/100) Bypassing: 45% (45/100)

large ball tip. Yoldas et al. (2004) found Masserann drills to increase the risk of perforations in curved canals. There are great variations in the sizes of the instruments used in the various holding techniques; for example, the trephine burs in the Endo Rescue Kit are considerably smaller than those in the Masserann kit. Nevertheless, all holding techniques such as the Masserann technique, the Feldman et al. (1974) technique, the Meitrac Endo Safety System (Hager and Meisinger, Neuss, Germany), the Instrument Removal System (IRS) (Dentsply, Ballaigues, Switzerland), and the Endo Rescue Kit (Komet/Brasseler, Savannah, GA) are able to gain a strong mechanical grip on a fragment. However, the bulk and rigidity of their armamentarium does not allow their use in narrow and curved root canals, and actually the external diameter of some of them limits their application only to the coronal segment of larger root canals. For example, the approximately 1.50 mm external diameter of the smallest Meitrac I (Hager and Meisinger, Neuss, Germany) trephine and extractor obviously permits its use only in the coronal part of root canals with a very large diameter.

In an early study by Sano et al. (1974), a success rate of 55% was reported, but no data are available on the location of the fragments inside the root canal. Removal in anterior teeth was more successful (73%, 8 out of 11) than in posterior teeth (44%, 4 out of 9). Gencoglu and Helvacioglu (2009) removed 47.6% of intentionally fractured instruments from straight root canal in an in vitro study with the Masserann technique, which was significantly less than with the ultrasonic technique (95.2%). Further tube retrieving techniques such as the Instrument Removal System (Dentsply, Ballaigues, Switzerland), Meitrac (Hager and Meisinger, Neuss, Germany), Endo Extractor (Brasseler, Savannah, USA), Cancellier Extractor Kit (Sybron Endo, Orange, CA), Endo Rescue Kit (Komet, Lemgo, Germany), and the hypodermic surgical needle techniques, along with the holding techniques and the technique described by Fors and Berg (1983) that utilize a modified needle holder used in microsurgery by ophthalmologists, frequently require over-enlargement of the root canal down to the fragment. Thus, excessive removal of hard dental tissue eventually structurally weakens the root and predisposes creation of ledges, perforations, or root fractures. When cyanoacrylate is used as an adhesive for bonding the fragment to the tube, it should be remembered that it is not "designed" to bridge a gap of >0.1 mm (Wefelmeier et al. 2015) and also care should be exercised to use only a few drops as excessive adhesive when set could inadvertently block the root canal. The same care should be exercised when using auto-polymerizing resins or Core Paste XP (DenMat Company, CA, USA), instead of cyanoacrylate adhesive. The Core Paste XP is radiopaque, and thus any excess left in the canal can be seen in the radiograph. In an in vitro study on the tube technique in which cyanoacrylate, dual-curing (Rebilda DC; Voco, Cuxhaven, Germany), or light-curing (Surefil SDR, Dentsply, York, PA) composite resin were utilized as adhesives, the amount of force required to break the connection between the microtube and the instrument was investigated (Wefelmeier et al. 2015). The results revealed that significantly higher values in pullout tests were achieved with both tested composites than with cyanoacrylate, and the best results were achieved with light-cured composite used for fixation (Wefelmeier et al. 2015). Polymerization of the light-cured composite through an optical fiber inserted into the microtube and pushed forward until the fiber came into contact with the endodontic instrument resulted in leaving the excess material outside the tube not polymerized and thus easily removable (Wefelmeier et al. 2015).

For the Endo Extractor, comparable to the Masserann kit but using a trephine bur, a hollow tube, and an adhesive to fix the fragment inside the hollow tube (Brasseler, Savannah, USA), only a case series comprising four successful clinical cases (two posts, one fractured instrument, and one silver point) has been published (Gettleman et al. 1991). The fractured instrument extended from near the orifice to the apical part of the root canal in a maxillary incisor, thus being easy to grasp even with a large tube. Suter et al. (2005) applied the tube-and-Hedstrom file technique in 12 clinical cases and were successful in 11 cases (91%), with one failure. It should be noted that this technique was applied only in 11% of 97 cases with fractured instruments.

In a study on 30 extracted teeth (Alomairy 2009), the Instrument Removal System (IRS) performed successfully in 60% of 15 teeth while ultrasonics in 80%.

The Endo Rescue Kit (Komet, Lemgo, Germany) represents a modified tube technique: following preparation of an access cavity and cutting around the top of the fragment, a center drill, named Pointer, excavates the last few millimeters of the canal coronal to the fragment, providing access to the broken instrument. A drill exposes the fragment's surface, and an extremely fine trephine bur is placed onto it, holding it in place using residual dentin shavings. The broken file is removed from the canal in a counterclockwise rotational motion of the trephine bur. In a comparative experimental study on 112 extracted teeth with intentionally fractured instruments, the total success rate was 67.9%, with a success rate of 81.8% for ultrasonics and only 54.4% for the Endo Rescue Kit. The difference was statistically significant. In curved canals the ratio was 78% (Ultrasonics) to 21% (Endo Rescue). In cases of successful removal, the working time was not significantly different for both systems (Hassan 2012).

6.1.3 Loop Techniques

Although the wire loop technique has been essentially replaced by more practical or successful techniques (Ruddle 2004), it remains a technique which utilizes equipment available in almost all dental offices and it is still in use (Terauchi 2012). Four successful cases have been demonstrated with the use of the Terauchi technique by the inventor of the device himself (Terauchi et al. 2006). The technique starts with the preparation of a staging platform, followed by ultrasonically troughing the fragment and finally grasping and removal using a wire loop. A similar device has just recently been developed and has not been investigated so far: the Frag Remover (HanCha-Dental, Zwenkau, Germany).

6.1.4 Canal Finder System

The Canal Finder is a rotary preparation system with a relatively flexible working mode variably combining rotary and vertical movement of the inserted instrument. The removal of fractured instruments is based on forced attempts to bypass fragments and then trying to remove the fragments in a pulling motion. The system has been used for instrument removal, but has been investigated for that purpose only in three studies (Table 6.3) reporting acceptable success rates (Hülsmann 1990a, b; Hülsmann and Schinkel 1999). Operating microscopes were not available at that time.

6.1.5 Laser Technique

To our knowledge, there are no clinical studies in peer review journals on the clinical management of instrument fragments with laser irradiation. There are three ex vivo studies only (Table 6.4). The harmful effects of temperature on root

Table 6.3 Success rates as reported from in vivo and ex vivo studies using the Canal Finder System for the removal of fractured instruments

Author(s)	Study design and sample size	Methods, devices, instruments, techniques, and protocol used	Microscope	Definition of success	Success rate
Hülsmann and Schinkel (1999)	In vivo retrospective (*n* = 113)	A combination of two or more of the following: Canal Finder System, ultrasonics, file bypass technique	Not available	Removal or bypassing	Overall: 68% (77/113) Removal: 49% (55/113) Bypassing: 19% (22/113)
Hülsmann (1990a, b)	Ex vivo (*n* = 22)	Canal Finder System Removal or bypassing	Not available	Removal or bypassing	Overall: 60% (13/22) Removal: 32% (7/22) Bypassing: 27% (6/22)
Hülsmann (1990a, b)	In vivo (*n* = 62)	Canal Finder System and ultrasonics	Not available	Removal or bypassing	Overall: 58% (36/62) Removal: 37% (23/62) Bypassing: 21% (13/62)

dentin, i.e., carbonization and melting, and on periodontal tissues as a result of temperature rise on the internal and external root surface, as well as the probability of root perforation in curved root canal or thin roots, remain ongoing concerns when this energy is used within the root canal (Yu et al. 2000; Hagiwara et al. 2013).

6.1.6 Electrochemical Dissolution Techniques

The electrochemical dissolution of stainless steel (SS) or Ni-Ti endodontic instruments has not been clinically attempted yet, as this technique could be dangerous if the electrical current is conducted by the soft tissues. Therefore, our knowledge is based mostly on ex vivo studies (Table 6.5). Additionally, there is missing evidence regarding the cytotoxic effect onto the periapical tissues. Studies on the effects of the dissolution products on periodontal ligament fibroblasts have revealed that they are cytotoxic (Mitchell et al. 2013). Concern has also been raised regarding the heat generated during the dissolution process, the optimal current needed in clinical practice, and the possible discoloration effect of the precipitate produced (Mitchell et al. 2013), and thus further investigation is needed.

Table 6.4 Success rates as reported from ex vivo studies using laser irradiation for the removal of fractured instruments

Author(s)	Study design and sample size	Methods, devices, instruments, techniques, and protocol used	Definition of success	Success rate
Cvikl et al. (2014)	Ex vivo ($n = 33$)	Nd:YAG laser was used to melt the solder, connecting the fragment with the brass tube placed at the coronal end of the fragment. The assembly was removed altogether	Removal	77.3% (17/22) when more than 1.5 mm of fragment was tangible 27.3% (3/11) if less than 1.5 mm of fragment was tangible
Ebihara et al. (2003)	Ex vivo ($n = 8$)	Nd:YAG laser	Removal	Overall: 63% (5/8)
Yu et al. (2000)	Ex vivo ($n = 18$)	Nd:YAG laser to melt the fragment completely or to bypass it and then to remove it with a Hedstrom file	Removal	Overall: 56% (10/18)

Table 6.5 Results from ex vivo studies using electrochemical dissolution techniques for the management of fractured instruments

Author(s)	Study design and sample size	Methods, devices instruments, techniques, and protocol used	Results
Amaral et al. (2015)	Experimental $n = 12$ #20 $n = 12$ #30 SS hand K-files	Evaluation of dissolution process of 6-mm-long portion of the experimental files exposed to the solution	Time-related progressive consumption of the files Files with the larger diameters exhibited greater weight loss and longer times of dissolution and generated a greater electrical charge
Ormiga et al. (2010)	Experimental $n = 20$ Ni-Ti K3 files #25/.04	Evaluation of the dissolution process in three time periods	Progressive consumption of the files with increasing polarization time
Ormiga et al. (2015)	Experimental $n = 20$ K3 files, #20/.06 $n = 20$, F1 ProTaper $n = 20$ Mtwo files #20/.06	Evaluation of the dissolution process in four time periods	Progressive consumption according to the file investigated. K3 and ProTaper instruments had significantly greater weight loss than Mtwo instruments after 30 min of polarization. K3 instruments had the highest values of total electrical charge and Mtwo instruments the lowest
Aboud et al. (2014)	Experimental K3 Ni-Ti file #20/.06	Evaluation of the dissolution process in four NaF solutions with different concentrations	Increasing fluoride concentration resulted in higher active dissolution of Ni-Ti files

6.1.7 Chemicals

The use of chemical means, mostly iodine compounds (Stasinopoulos 1978; Hülsmann 1993), for the removal or bypassing of fragments within the root canal is not an actual technique. It is a preparatory stage to decalcify the dentinal wall around the fragment and/or corrode it and thus facilitate its loosening with mechanical means. Their ineffectiveness combined with the fact that any chemical used in the root canal may be harmful to the periapical tissues if inadvertently extruded through the foramen or leaking into the gingiva resulted in a significant reduction in the frequency of their use. No studies are available on the efficacy of this technique.

6.1.8 Magnets

The magnet has been proposed for removal of instrument fragments (Grossman 1974) in the expectation that it might "attract" the fragment, but it has had very limited success in retrieving fragments and is not used anymore. No studies are available on the efficacy of this technique.

6.1.9 Multisonic Ultracleaning System

The Multisonic Ultracleaning System (Gentle Wave System, Sonendo, Laguna Hills, CA) seems promising, but the currently available data (Table 6.6) are too limited to allow a reliable evaluation of its effectiveness. Among the promising aspects of this method are: (1) preservation of dental tissue as minimal instrumentation is required and (2) time required for the successful management, which is minimal as compared to the time required in all the other techniques reviewed. No studies are available on the efficacy of this device.

Table 6.6 Results from an ex vivo study on the effectiveness of the Multisonic Ultracleaning System

Author(s)	Study design and sample size	Methods, devices, instruments, techniques, and protocol used	Microscope	Definition of success	Success rate
Wohlgemuth et al. (2015)	Ex vivo ($n = 36$)	Multisonic Ultracleaning System (Gentle Wave)	No	Removal	Middle third 83.3% (15/18) Apical third 61.1% (11/18)

6.1.10 Softened Gutta-Percha

The softened gutta-percha point technique as published in a case report (Rahimi and Parashos 2009) or its modification which is the obturation of the root canal with the remaining fragment with laterally or vertically compacted gutta-percha and the subsequent immediate removal of the filling might be successful in the cases of loosely bound fragments. It is a simple technique that does not require any special sophisticated armamentarium nor any additional removal of hard dental tissue, and thus it can be tried in selected cases when the fragment is partly bypassed and loosened. However, care should be exercised to avoid the extrusion of softened gutta-percha to the periapical tissues. No studies are available on the efficacy of this device.

6.1.11 File Removal System

Terauchi et al. (2006, 2007) reported that the File Removal System could successfully retrieve instrument fragments from the root canal in a relatively short time with minimal removal of root dentin. The extremely elongated ultrasonic tips made of ductile stainless steel are mostly helpful. To our knowledge, since then, no similar report nor clinical or experimental studies or even further case reports have been published in peer-reviewed dental journals. However, anecdotal opinions among endodontists rank it among the most efficient ways of managing intracanal fractured instruments.

6.1.12 Bypassing

It should be seriously considered that not only the removal but also the bypassing of a fractured instrument can and should be regarded as a success as it may allow proper cleaning and disinfection of the space apical to the retained fragment and eventually complete and tight obturation of the most apical part of the root canal.

Several techniques have been described for this purpose of bypassing, among them hand files and the Canal-Finder-System. This technique has been evaluated in several studies either as the sole technique used or in comparison with other techniques (Table 6.7).

6.1.13 Dental Operating Microscope

Although the microscope itself cannot remove a fractured endodontic instrument from the root canal, a comparison of respective studies (Tables 6.8 and 6.9) demonstrates that the use of a microscope results in clearly increased success rates.

Training, patience, and creativity still seem to be the most important prerequisites for the successful removal of instrument fragments from root canal. The combined use of improved armamentaria and management techniques by an experienced trained clinician starting in the vast majority of cases with the file bypass technique

Table 6.7 Success rates as reported from in vivo and ex vivo studies using hand file bypassing and the Canal Finder System

Author(s)	Study design and sample size	Methods, devices, instruments, techniques, and protocol used	Microscope	Definition of success	Success rate
Shiyakov and Vasileva (2014)	In vivo ($n = 19$)	File bypass technique	Yes	Bypassing	36.84(7/19)
Hülsmann and Schinkel (1999)	In vivo retrospective ($n = 113$)	A combination of two or more of the following: Canal Finder System, ultrasonic, file bypass technique	Not available at the time	Removal or bypassing	Overall: 68% (77/113) Removal: 49% (55/113) Bypassing: 19% (22/113)
Nehme (1999)	In vivo ($n = 22$)	Bypassing the fragment by hand files and then removing it by ultrasonic vibration of a modified spreader	Not available at the time	Removal	Overall: 91% (20/22)
Molyvdas et al. (1992)	In vivo retrospective study ($n = 70$)	File bypass technique	Not available at the time	Removal bypassing	Overall: 54% Removal:8.5% (6/70) Bypassing:44.2% (31/70)
Hülsmann (1990a, b)	Ex vivo ($n = 22$)	Canal Finder System	Not available at the time	Removal or bypassing	Overall: 60% (13/22) Removal: 32% (7/22) Bypassing: 27% (6/22)
Hülsmann (1990a, b)	In vivo ($n = 62$)	Canal Finder System and ultrasonics	Not available at the time	Removal or bypassing	Overall: 58% (36/62) Removal: 37% (23/62) Bypassing: 21% (13/62)
Gencoglu and Helvacioglu (2009)	Ex vivo ($n = 90$)	K-files in straight and curved canals	Yes	Removal or bypassing	Overall 75% (27/36) In straight canals 80.9% (17/21) In curved canals 66.6% (10/15)

Table 6.7 (continued)

Author(s)	Study design and sample size	Methods, devices, instruments, techniques, and protocol used	Microscope	Definition of success	Success rate
Al-Fouzan (2003)	In vivo Prospective study ($n = 21$)	Bypassing the fragment by using hand k-files	Not mentioned	Bypassing	Overall 33.33% (7/21) Apical third 21.42% (3/14) Middle third 57.14% (4/7)

Table 6.8 Success rates as reported from in vivo and ex vivo studies using a variety of techniques without use of a dental operating microscope

Author(s)	Method	Type of study	Success rate (%)
Sano et al. (1974)	Masserann	In vivo	55.0
Ketterl (1975)	Masserann	In vivo	37.7
Nagai et al. (1986)	Ultrasonics	Ex vivo (visible fragment)	79
		Ex vivo (fragment not visible)	68
		In vivo	67
Hülsmann (1990a, b)	Canal Finder	In vitro	59
		In vivo	48
Hülsmann and Schinkel (1999)	Different techniques	In vivo	68
Molyvdas et al. (1992)	File bypass technique	Clinical study	54

Table 6.9 Success rates as reported from in vivo and ex vivo studies using a variety of techniques with the use of a dental operating microscope

Author(s)	Method	Type of study	Success rate
Ward et al. (2003b)	Ultrasonics	Clinical study	66.7% (16/24)
Ward et al. (2003a)	Ultrasonics	In vitro resin blocks	75.0% (45/60)
		Ex vivo	86.6% (26/30)
Shen et al. (2004)	Hand files Ultrasonics	Clinical study	53% (3872)
Cuje et al. (2010)		Clinical study	95% (162/170)
Gencoglu and Helvacioglu (2009)	Ultrasonics Hand files Masserann	Ex vivo	82.2%
Nevares et al. (2012)	Ultrasonics alone or associated with bypassing with hand files	Clinical study	70.5% (79/112)
Fu et al. (2011)	Ultrasonics	Clinical study	88% (58/66)
Suter et al. (2005)	Ultrasonics Tube and Hedstrom files method Masserann Pliers	Clinical study	87% (84/97)

and always bearing in mind that saving hard tissue and avoiding perforations is most important for the long-term survival of the tooth involved (see respective chapter) is very important. The fact that *no retrieval technique is successful in all cases* should be constantly kept in mind when dealing with an intracanal fractured instrument. Interestingly, Suter et al. (2005), Hülsmann and Schinkel (1999), Shen et al. (2004), and Cuje et al. (2010), in their retrospective studies on the success rates of retrieval attempts, mentioned the use of different techniques, i.e., ultrasonics, tube techniques, loop techniques, Hedstrom file techniques, and more.

This once again highlights the importance of familiarization with as many techniques as possible.

6.2 Comparative Evaluation of Surgical Techniques

If the removal of a fragment is indicated and nonsurgical attempts have remained without success in terms of removal or bypassing, a surgical approach can be considered. In surgical endodontics, knowledge and understanding of the prognostic predictors of any type of surgical intervention are important in the process of decision-making.

Comparative evaluation among the variety of surgical techniques that can be applied is difficult and probably impossible to be assessed. In cases with a variety of options considering the cost benefit for tooth preservation and durability the selection of the surgical procedure with minimal removal of tooth structure and surrounding tissues is recommended. *In each single case it has to be considered first of all, whether removal of the fragment is necessary at all!*

References

Aboud LR, Ormiga F, Gomes JA. Electrochemical induced dissolution of fragments of nickel-titanium endodontic files and their removal from simulated root canals. Int Endod J. 2014;47(2):155–62.

Al-Fouzan KS. Incidence of rotary ProFile instrument fracture and the potential for bypassing in vivo. Int Endod J. 2003;36(12):864–7.

Alomairy KH. Evaluating two techniques on removal of fractured rotary nickel-titanium endodontic instruments from root canals: an in vitro study. J Endod. 2009;35(4):559–62.

Amaral CC, Ormiga F, Gomes JA. Electrochemical-induced dissolution of stainless steel files. Int Endod J. 2015;48(2):137–44.

Cuje J, Bargholz C, Hülsmann M. The outcome of retained instrument removal in a specialist practice. Int Endod J. 2010;43(7):545–54.

Cvikl B, Klimscha J, Holly M, Zeitlinger M, Gruber R, Moritz A. Removal of fractured endodontic instruments using an Nd:YAG laser. Quintessence Int. 2014;45:569–75.

Ebihara A, Takashina M, Anjo T, Takeda A, Suda H. Removal of root canal obstructions using pulsed Nd:YAG laser. Int Cong Ser. 2003;1248:257–9.

Feldman G, Solomon C, Notaro P, Moskowitz E. Retrieving broken endodontic instruments. J Am Dent Assoc. 1974;88(3):588–91.

Fors UG, Berg JO. A method for the removal of broken endodontic instruments from root canals. J Endod. 1983;9(4):156–9.

Friedman S, Stabholz A, Tamse A. Endodontic retreatment–case selection and technique. 3. Retreatment techniques. J Endod. 1990;16(11):543–9.

Fu M, Zhang Z, Hou B. Removal of broken files from root canals by using ultrasonic techniques combined with dental microscope: a retrospective analysis of treatment outcome. J Endod. 2011;37(5):619–22.

Gencoglu N, Helvacioglu D. Comparison of the different techniques to remove fractured endodontic instruments from root canal systems. Eur J Dent. 2009;3(2):90–5.

Gettleman BH, Spriggs KA, ElDeeb ME, Messer HH. Removal of canal obstructions with the Endo Extractor. J Endod. 1991;17(12):608–11.

Grossman LI. Endodontic case reports. Dent Clin N Am. 1974;18(2):509–27.

Hagiwara R, Suehara M, Fujii R, Kato H, Nakagawa K, Oda Y. Laser welding method for removal of instruments debris from root canals. Bull Tokyo Dent Coll. 2013;54:81–8.

Hassan M. Success rates in removal of fractured instruments using ultrasonics or the EndoRescue-Kit: an in vitro study on extracted teeth. Master Thesis, Düsseldorf Dental Academy (DDA); 2012.

Hülsmann M. Removal of silver cones and fractured instruments using the Canal Finder System. J Endod. 1990a;16(12):596–600.

Hülsmann M. [Removal of fractured root canal instruments using the Canal Finder System]. Dtsch Zahnarztl Z. 1990b;45(4):229–32.

Hülsmann M. Methods for removing metal obstructions from the root canal. Endod Dent Traumatol. 1993;9(6):223–37.

Hülsmann M, Schinkel I. Influence of several factors on the success or failure of removal of fractured instruments from the root canal. Endod Dent Traumatol. 1999;15(6):252–8.

Ketterl W. Instrumentenfraktur im Wurzelkanal. Munich: Hanser; 1975.

Madarati AA, Watts DC, Qualtrough AJ. Opinions and attitudes of endodontists and general dental practitioners in the UK towards the intra-canal fracture of endodontic instruments. Part 2. Int Endod J. 2008;41(12):1079–87.

Mitchell Q, Jeansonne BG, Stoute D, Lallier TE. Electrochemical dissolution of nickel-titanium endodontic files induces periodontal ligament cell death. J Endod. 2013;39(5):679–84.

Molyvdas I, Lambrianidis T, Zervas P, Veis A. Clinical study on the prognosis of endodontic treatment of teeth with broken endodontic instruments. Stoma. 1992;20:63–72. (in Greek).

Nagai O, Tani N, Kayaba Y, Kodama S, Osada T. Ultrasonic removal of broken instruments in root canals. Int Endod J. 1986;19(6):298–304.

Nehme W. A new approach for the retrieval of broken instruments. J Endod. 1999;25(9):633–5.

Nevares G, Cunha RS, Zuolo ML, Bueno CE. Success rates for removing or bypassing fractured instruments: a prospective clinical study. J Endod. 2012;38(4):442–4.

Okiji T. Modified usage of the Masserann kit for removing intracanal broken instruments. J Endod. 2003;29(7):466–7.

Ormiga F, da Cunha Ponciano Gomes JA, de Araujo MC. Dissolution of nickel-titanium endodontic files via an electrochemical process: a new concept for future retrieval of fractured files in root canals. J Endod. 2010;36(4):717–20.

Ormiga F, Aboud LR, Gomes JA. Electrochemical-induced dissolution of nickel-titanium endodontic instruments with different designs. Int Endod J. 2015;48(4):342–50.

Pai AR, Kamath MP, Basnet P. Retrieval of a separated file using Masserann technique: a case report. Kathmandu Univ Med J. 2006;4(2):238–42.

Rahimi M, Parashos P. A novel technique for the removal of fractured instruments in the apical third of curved root canals. Int Endod J. 2009;42(3):264–70.

Ruddle CJ. Nonsurgical retreatment. J Endod. 2004;30(12):827–45.

Sano S, Miyake K, Osada T. A clinical study on the removal of the broken instrument in the root canal using Masserann Kit. Kanagawashigaku. 1974;9(1):50–7.

Shahabinejad H, Ghassemi A, Pishbin L, Shahravan A. Success of ultrasonic technique in removing fractured rotary nickel-titanium endodontic instruments from root canals and its effect on the required force for root fracture. J Endod. 2013;39(6):824–8.

Shen Y, Peng B, Cheung GS. Factors associated with the removal of fractured NiTi instruments from root canal systems. Oral Surg Oral Med Oral Pathol Oral Radiol Endod. 2004;98(5):605–10.
Shiyakov K, Vasileva R. Success for removing or bypassing instruments fractured beyond the root canal curve-45 clinical cases. In: Journal of IMAB – Annual Proceeding; 2014.
Skyttner B. Endodontic instrument separations. Evaluation of a patient cases series with separated endodontic instruments and factors related to the treatment regarding separated instruments. Master of Medical Science in Odontology, Karolinska Institute for Odontology; 2007. p. 1–34.
Souter NJ, Messer HH. Complications associated with fractured file removal using an ultrasonic technique. J Endod. 2005;31(6):450–2.
Stasinopoulos E. Dental pathology and therapeutics, Vol. II: Therapeutics. Athens: Parisianos; 1978. p. 212–5. (in Greek).
Suter B, Lussi A, Sequeira P. Probability of removing fractured instruments from root canals. Int Endod J. 2005;38(2):112–23.
Terauchi Y. Separated file removal. Dent Today. 2012;31(5):108, 110–3.
Terauchi Y, O'Leary L, Suda H. Removal of separated files from root canals with a new file-removal system: case reports. J Endod. 2006;32(8):789–97.
Terauchi Y, O'Leary L, Kikuchi I, Asanagi M, Yoshioka T, Kobayashi C, et al. Evaluation of the efficiency of a new file removal system in comparison with two conventional systems. J Endod. 2007;33(5):585–8.
Tzanetakis GN, Kontakiotis EG, Maurikou DV, Marzelou MP. Prevalence and management of instrument fracture in the postgraduate endodontic program at the Dental School of Athens: a five-year retrospective clinical study. J Endod. 2008;34(6):675–8.
Ward JR, Parashos P, Messer HH. Evaluation of an ultrasonic technique to remove fractured rotary nickel-titanium endodontic instruments from root canals: an experimental study. J Endod. 2003a;29(11):756–63.
Ward JR, Parashos P, Messer HH. Evaluation of an ultrasonic technique to remove fractured rotary nickel-titanium endodontic instruments from root canals: clinical cases. J Endod. 2003b;29(11):764–7.
Wefelmeier M, Eveslage M, Burklein S, Ott K, Kaup M. Removing fractured endodontic instruments with a modified tube technique using a light-curing composite. J Endod. 2015;41(5):733–6.
Wei X, Ling JQ, Gao Y, Huang XY, Li XX. [Management of intracanal separated instruments with the microsonic technique and its clinical outcome]. Zhonghua Kou Qiang Yi Xue Za Zhi. 2004;39(5):379–81.
Wohlgemuth P, Cuocolo D, Vandrangi P, Sigurdsson A. Effectiveness of the GentleWave System in Removing Separated Instruments. J Endod. 2015;41(11):1895–8.
Yoldas O, Oztunc H, Tinaz C, Alparslan N. Perforation risks associated with the use of Masserann endodontic kit drills in mandibular molars. Oral Surg Oral Med Oral Pathol Oral Radiol Endod. 2004;97(4):513–7.
Yu DG, Kimura Y, Tomita Y, Nakamura Y, Watanabe H, Matsumoto K. Study on removal effects of filling materials and broken files from root canals using pulsed Nd:YAG laser. J Clin Med Surg. 2000;18:23–8.r

Complications During Attempts of Retrieval or Bypassing of Fractured Instruments

7

Theodor Lambrianidis and Michael Hülsmann

The delicate manipulations necessary for the management of a fractured instrument using an orthograde and/or a surgical approach include the risk of creating additional complications that might jeopardize the treatment outcome. These include:

1. Complications during and following orthograde attempts
2. Complications during and following surgical attempts

7.1 Complications During and Following Orthograde Attempts of Removing or Bypassing Fractured Instruments

Even with the most sophisticated equipment and techniques, and regardless of the outcome, several complications may occur during orthograde attempts to remove or bypass fragments of endodontic instruments (Lambrianidis 2001; Ward et al. 2003a, b; Souter and Messer 2005; Suter et al. 2005; Hülsmann and Scafer 2009). This is particularly true in cases of narrow and curved root canal when a fragment is locked apically of the curvature. Thus, prior to commencing any attempt to retrieve or bypass fragments, the chances of success in every case should be balanced against the potential complications. The complications that may arise include:

T. Lambrianidis, D.D.S., Ph.D. (✉)
Department of Endodontology, Dental School, Aristotle University of Thessaloniki, Thessaloniki, Greece
e-mail: thlampri@dent.auth.gr

M. Hülsmann, D.D.S., Ph.D.
Department of Preventive Dentistry, Periodontology and Cariology, University Medicine Göttingen, Göttingen, Germany

T. Lambrianidis (ed.), *Management of Fractured Endodontic Instruments*,
DOI 10.1007/978-3-319-60651-4_7

- Root perforation
- Excessive removal of tooth structure
- Fracture of another file
- Inadvertent fracture, repeatedly sometimes, of the original fragment
- Ledge formation
- Transportation of the root canal
- Thermal injury of dental and periodontal tissues
- Transportation of the instrument fragment deeper into the root canal
- Extrusion of the fragment beyond the apex
- Dislodgement of the fragment into another root canal
- Predisposition of the root to a vertical root fracture

Most of these complications have still not been thoroughly investigated; thus, no conclusions on the frequency and impact of complications on treatment outcome, nor on strategies for prevention, are justified.

7.1.1 Incidence of Complications

As an overall figure, 61.8% of respondents to a questionnaire addressed to general practitioners and endodontists practicing in the UK concerning their opinions and attitudes toward the intra-canal failure of endodontic instruments reported that they experienced complications while managing fractured instruments; more precisely, a significantly higher proportion of endodontists (71.6%) compared with general dental practitioners (55.6%) reported so (Madarati et al. 2008a).

As the chances of successful removal decrease with time of treatment (Suter et al. 2005), an increase in the possibility of complications can be expected. Some studies suggest a working time of approximately 45 min for the majority of successful cases. To avoid time-related complications, it seems necessary to have a defined cutoff point, ensuring an acceptable relation between successful treatment and the risk of complications. This time frame and cutoff point have to be defined individually for each dentist with regard to his/her experience and equipment (and be modified—if necessary—for each single case).

- Root perforation

  Perforation of the root wall constitutes one of the major risks during management of instrument fragments (Nagai et al. 1986; Hülsmann 1990; Hülsmann and Schinkel 1999; Yoldas et al. 2004; Souter and Messer 2005; Suter et al. 2005; Fu et al. 2011; Nevares et al. 2012). Using ultrasonics under the dental operating microscope, an overall incidence ranging from 1.8 (Nevares et al. 2012) to 7.2% (Suter et al. 2005) has been reported. Thus, this catastrophic violation of the integrity of the root canal wall might adversely affect tooth prognosis. The closer the fragment is located to the apex, the greater is the risk of perforation (Souter and Messer 2005). Perforation can occur with all proposed techniques, i.e., during preparation of the staging platform, when size 3 or 4 modified Gates Glidden drills are used, and during efforts to bypass the fragment with small-sized endodontic instruments with the file bypass technique (Figs. 7.1, 7.2, 7.3, and 7.4). Radiographic evaluation of the residual dentine thickness in the course of preparation of the staging platform can be misleading due to the inaccuracy of radiographic interpretation. Radiographic follow-up of the route of the bypassing file with the file bypass technique might reveal its misdirection toward causing root perforation (Fig. 7.2b).

Perforation can occur at the inner side of the curve, similar to a strip perforation, as well as on the outer side of the curve. In the latter case bypassing initially results in ledging, which can then eventually perforate the root canal wall.

Prevention

Good illumination of the cavity, magnification, and a dry working field deep inside the root canal are the most important prerequisites to avoid perforations. It should be born in mind that moisture around a fractured instrument can reflect light from a loup or a dental operating microscope, thereby providing the dentist with false information on the location of the fragment.

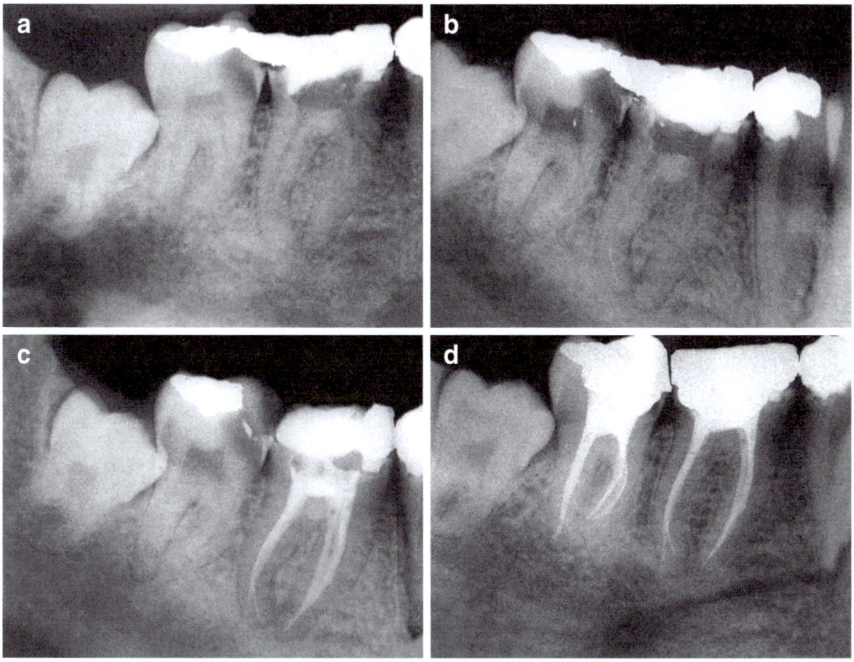

Fig. 7.1 (**a**) Preoperative radiograph. (**b**) Fractured instrument in the apical third of the curved distal root of a first mandibular molar. (**c**) Root perforation and creation of "iatrogenic" canal during unsuccessful efforts to retrieve or bypass the fragment with the file bypass technique. Immediate post-obturation radiograph. Note gutta-percha in the artificially created canal and separated instrument still in place. (**d**) Three-year recall radiograph showing complete healing (with permission from Lambrianidis 2001)

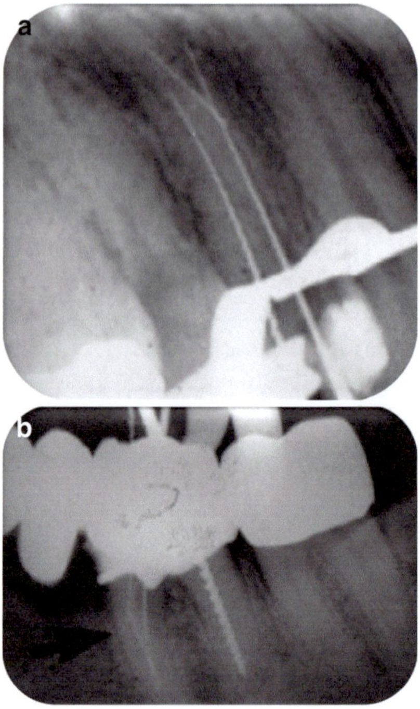

Fig. 7.2 (**a**) The attempt to bypass the fragment with a Hedstrom file, used in rotary motion, resulted in root perforation. (**b**) Etiology of a perforation during attempted bypassing of a fragment: the file is “directed” outward by the top of the fragment. Early radiographic control in some cases can help to avoid a perforation

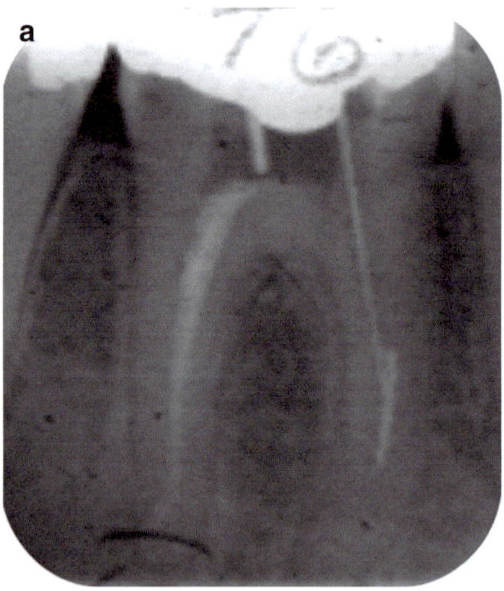

Fig. 7.3 (**a**) Fractured instrument in the apical part of the root canal. (**b**) Successful removal of the fragment. (**c**) The post-obturation control reveals substantial loss of dentine in the coronal and middle third of the root canal and a perforation at the furcational inner side of the curvature

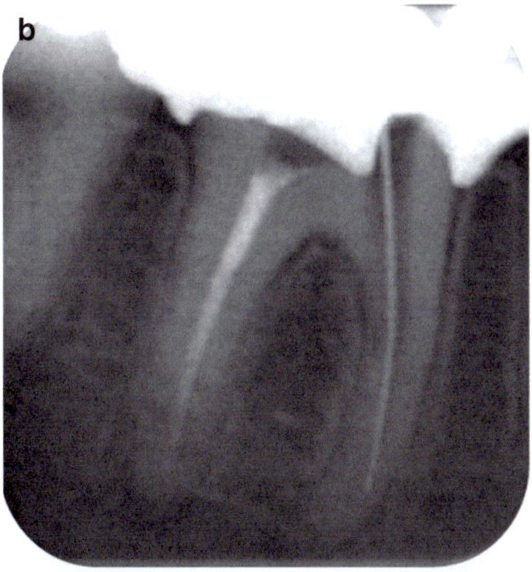

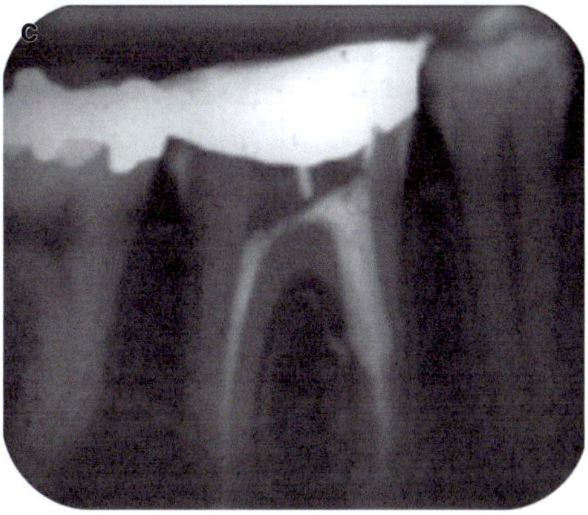

Fig. 7.3 (continued)

To prevent perforation of the root, it is important to keep any preparation centered around the fragment. This requires proper pre- and intraoperative treatment planning. After location of the fragment, a decision has to be made with respect to the root anatomy on which side of the fragment safe bypassing can be attempted. This should consider root canal curvature as well as the estimated residual dentine thickness and concavities of the root. Excessive screwing of instruments into the dentine should be avoided. Radiographic control of the direction of the inserted instrument may be necessary in some cases (Fig. 7.2b).

- Excessive removal of tooth structure
  The most common complication reported in many studies (Lertchirakarn et al. 2003; Souter and Messer 2005; Madarati et al. 2008a, b) is the excessive removal of tooth structure (Figs. 7.5 and 7.6). Removal or bypassing of a fragment without removing of dentine is virtually impossible. The more dentine is cut away around the fragment, the greater the chances of complete bypassing, loosening,

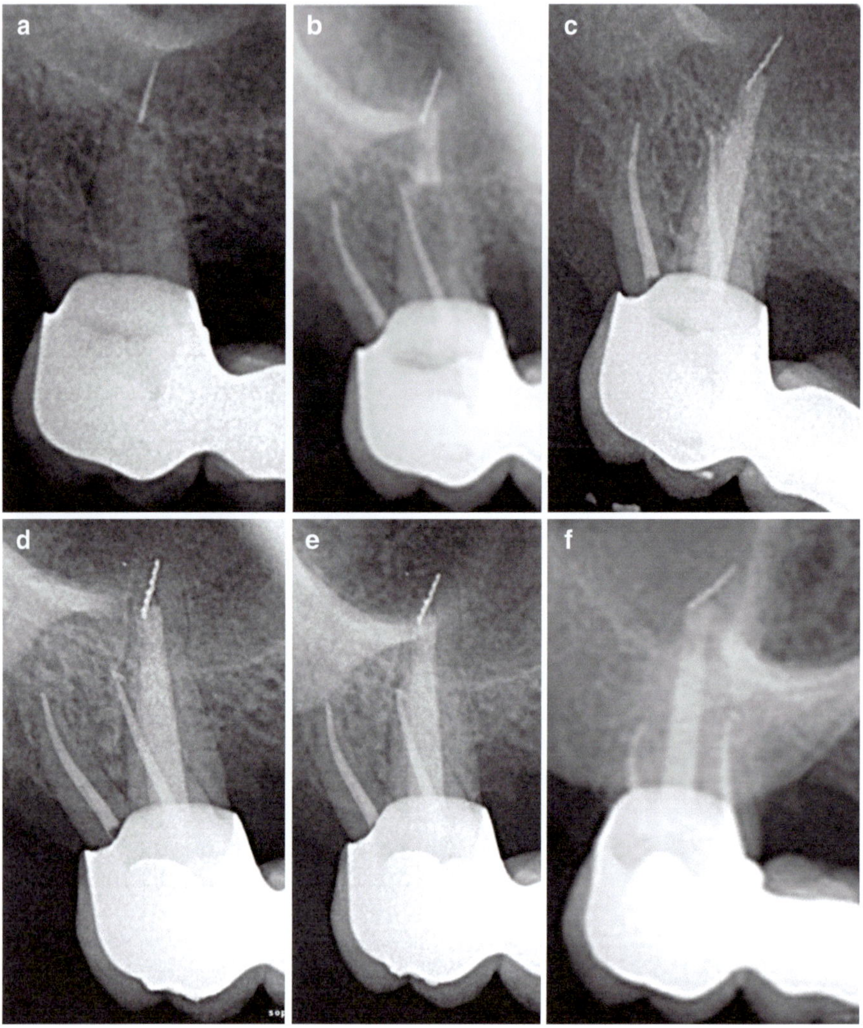

Fig. 7.4 (**a**) A maxillary second molar with a small fragment of a #30 Hedstrom file referred for endodontic treatment. (**b**) Lateral perforation was created at the apical third of the palatal root during efforts to remove the fragment, and thus 4 mm of the apical third including the perforation site were sealed with MTA. (**c**) The remaining palatal canal was obturated with injection of thermoplasticized gutta-percha and the buccal root canal with lateral compaction of gutta-percha and epoxy-resin sealer. (**d–f**) The scheduled clinical and radiographic recall examinations at 6 months, a year, and 2 years, respectively, revealed uneventful healing (Courtesy Dr. K. Kodonas)

and removal of the fragment. The greatest loss of root dentine occurs when fragments are retrieved from the apical third of the root canal and the least when fragments are located at the coronal third (Madarati et al. 2009b). This loss of tooth structure from the apical or middle third significantly affects the integrity of the tooth. It is interesting to note that the removal procedure decreased root

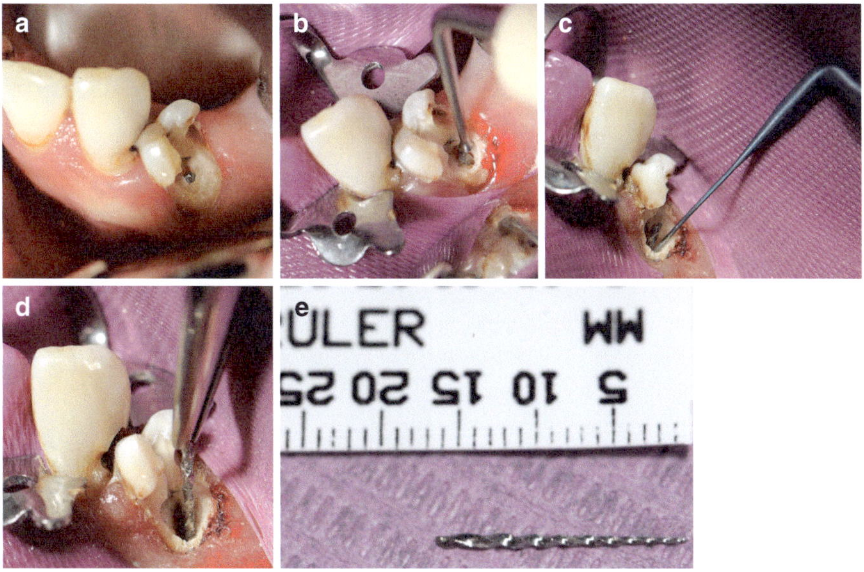

Fig. 7.5 (**a**) Clinical appearance of a mandibular canine with a fragment. (**b–d**) Excessive removal of tooth structure during fragment removal with ultrasonics. (**e**) Removed fragment

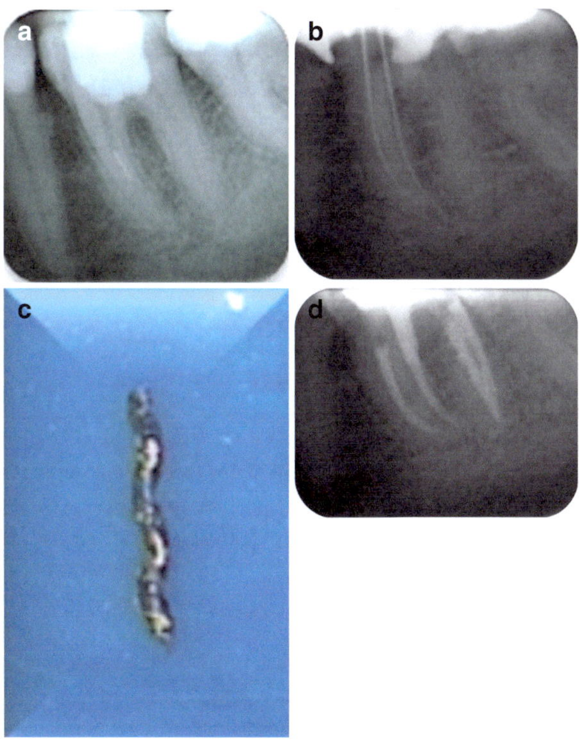

Fig. 7.6 (**a**) Fractured instrument in the mesiolingual root canal. (**b**, **c**) Control radiograph following removal of the fragment. (**d**) The radiographic control reveals massive loss of dental hard tissue in the coronal part of the root canal

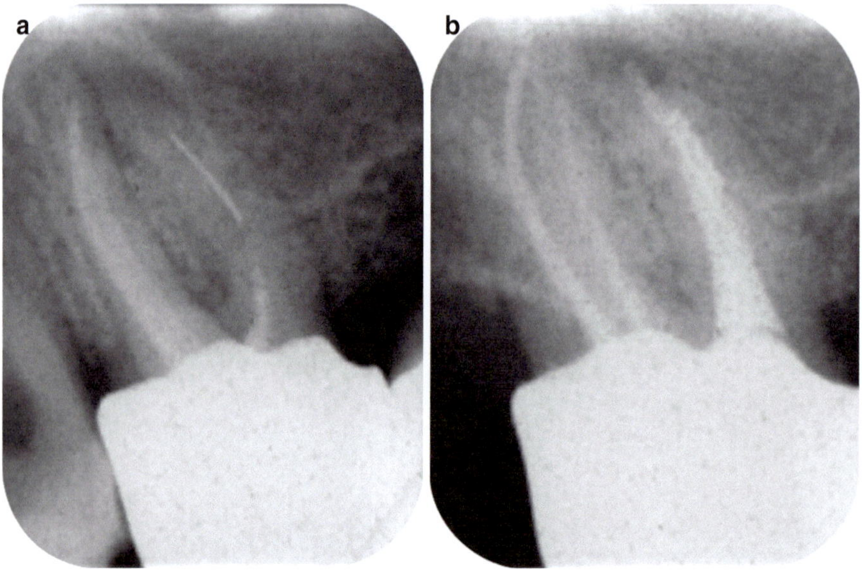

Fig. 7.7 (**a**) Preoperative radiograph showing a fractured instrument in the mesiobuccal root canal of a maxillary molar. (**b**) During successful removal of the fragment, a second instrument (Hedstrom file) fractured. Despite this second fracture, the root canal could be prepared and obturated to its apical terminus

strength by 30% and 40%, when the file was located in the middle and apical third, respectively, compared with controls (Souter and Messer 2005). This decrease in root strength may predispose to vertical root fractures (Lertchirakarn et al. 2003; Souter and Messer 2005). The force required to fracture roots vertically after the removal of instrument fragments using ultrasonic tips has been investigated in some studies (Souter and Messer 2005; Madarati et al. 2010; Shahabinejad et al. 2013) with controversial findings. In some studies, a significant difference was found between the force required for root fracture in the control and experimental groups (Souter and Messer 2005); in others, no significant difference was noted (Shahabinejad et al. 2013). The influence of the location of the fragment on fracture resistance was also highlighted in a study by Madarati et al. (2010). Removal of fractured instruments from the coronal one-third of the root canal had no impact on fracture resistance, as opposed to the removal of fragments from deeper locations within the root canal, which eventually jeopardized root resistance to vertical fracture. In a comparative study, it was found that the force required to cause vertical root fractures was similar regardless of the technique (ultrasonics or Masserann system) utilized for fragment retrieval although the Masserann system due to its rigid components seems to be a more aggressive instrument (Gerek et al. 2012). This inconsistency might be attributed to tooth-related factors (sample type, morphology of canals evaluated), mode of preparation, dimensions of the staging platform, and method of force application. It is interesting to note that leaving instruments that had broken in the apical one-third of the root canal did not affect the force required to fracture the root (Madarati et al. 2010).

- Therefore, any removal attempts should be undertaken in a dentine-saving, minimally invasive approach. This holds true especially in cases in which removal of a fragment is not absolutely necessary.
  Prevention

The use of high magnification and good illumination once more are the best prerequisites to avoid this complication. Preferably small instruments should be used, such as small ultrasonic tips and orifice openers. Dry work will allow better placement of instruments and better control of dentine removal.

- Fracture of a second instrument
  During the attempt to bypass a fragment completely or partially with a second instrument, the latter can be severely engaged between the fragment and the dentine, resulting in a strain exceeding the file's fracture limit and provoking an additional fracture inside this root canal (Fig. 7.7).
  Prevention

The best way to prevent a fracture of a second instrument is its use with controlled power. Especially rotary Ni-Ti instruments are not suited at all for attempts of bypassing a fractured instrument.

- Inadvertent second fracture of the original fragment
  When working with high energy (ultrasonics) or mechanical power (tube or wire techniques, use of a forceps), separation of just the coronal part of a fragment

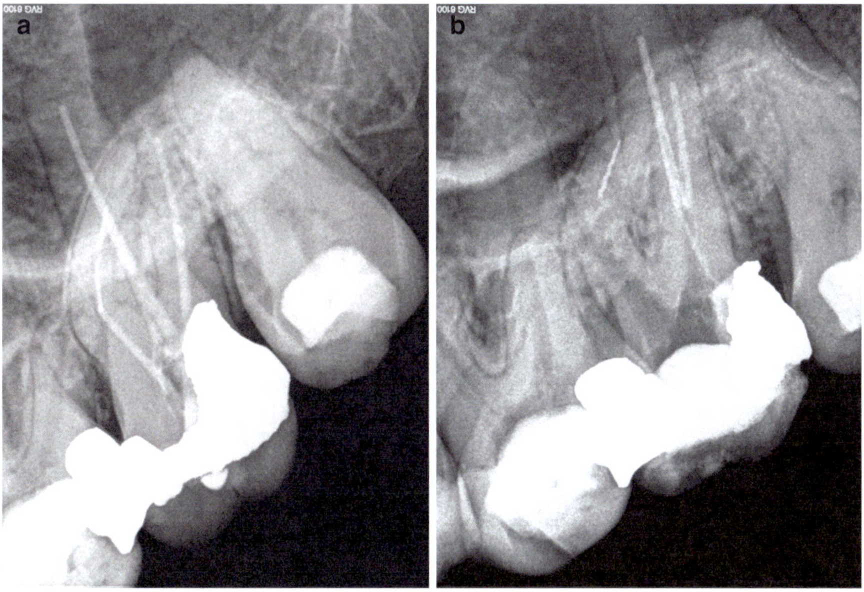

Fig. 7.8 (**a**) Preoperative radiograph of a maxillary second left molar with inadequate root canal treatment and an instrument fragment approximately 5 mm long at the mesiobucall root canal. (**b**) Second fracture of the original fragment during efforts to retrieve it with ultrasonics under the dental operating microscope. Note the preparation of the canal up to the original site of the fragment

may occur (Fig. 7.8). The risk depends on the type of fragment, e.g., that Ni-Ti fragments are more susceptible to secondary fracture than stainless steel instruments. Anyway, this complication cannot be avoided completely.

Prevention

In cases of fractured Ni-Ti instruments, ultrasonic tips should be used only with low power. Consideration should be given to whether tube or wire loop techniques can be used with a lower risk of secondary fracture.

- Ledge formation

  File removal with the vast majority of proposed mechanical techniques typically results in ledge formation (Figs. 7.9, 7.10 and 7.11) and therefore creates a possible point of stress concentration, which is considered to be a crucial factor in the generation of vertical root fractures (Lertchirakarn et al. 2003). Additionally, for effective management of fractured instruments, regardless of the technique or devices used, sufficient enlargement of the root canal coronal to the fragment is required. The deeper the broken file, the more tooth structure is removed, jeopardizing root resistance to vertical root fracture. Thus, only fracture removal attempts from the coronal one-third can be considered safe, as opposed to

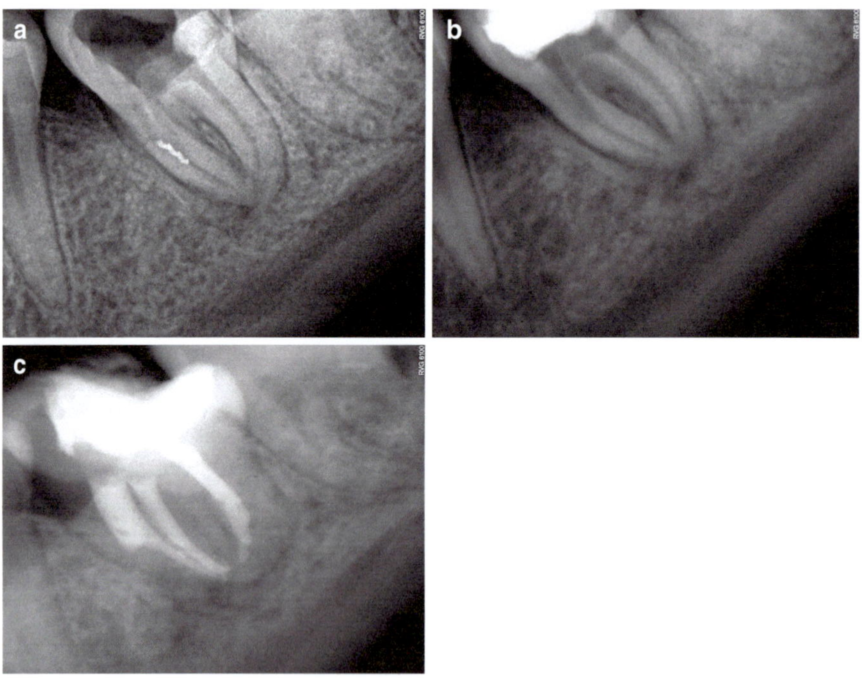

Fig. 7.9 (**a**) Preoperative radiograph with a 2.5 mm fragment of Hedstrom file #30 in the mesial third of the mesiobuccal root canal of a mandibular second molar. (**b**) Preparation of a staging platform with a #2 Gates Glidden bur and removal of the fragment with an ultrasonic technique under the dental operating microscope. (**c**) Immediate post-obturation radiograph. Note the characteristic appearance of the ledge at the outer side of the curvature

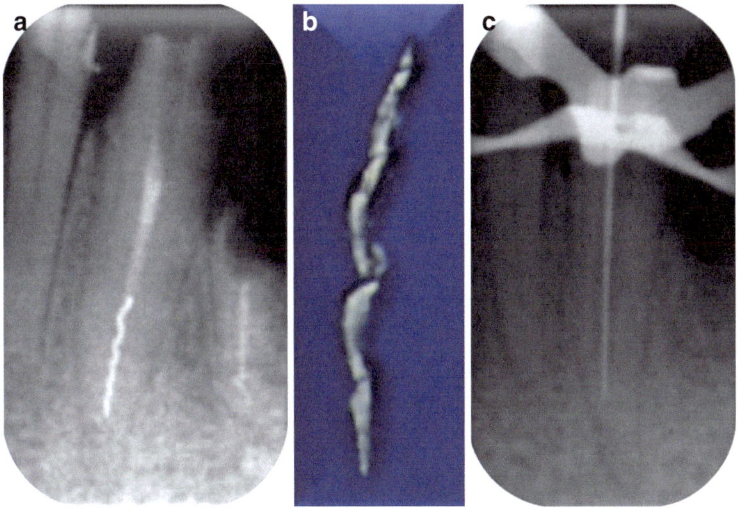

Fig. 7.10 (**a**) Fragment in the apical part of a mandibular canine. (**b**) Successfully removed fragment. (**c**) The control radiograph shows ledging at the outer side of the curvature, not allowing preparation and obturation to the apical terminus

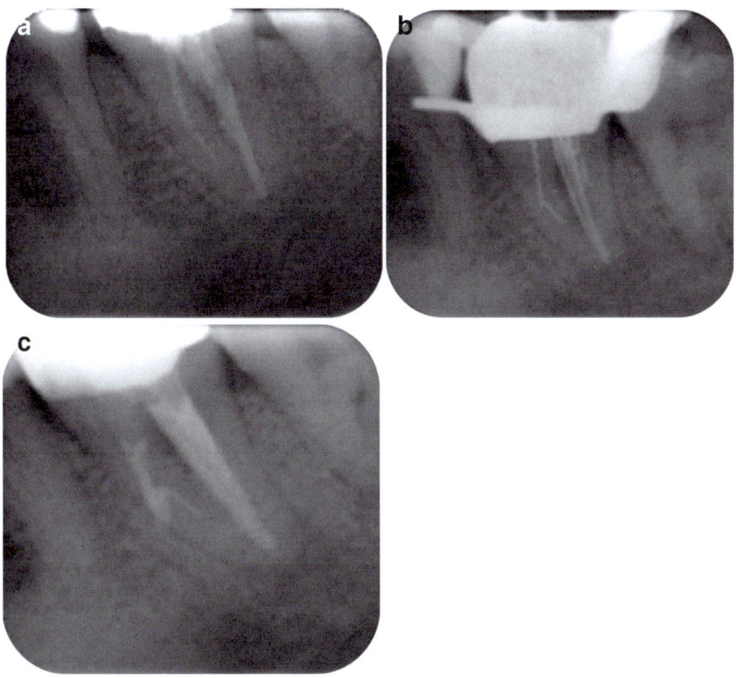

Fig. 7.11 (**a**) Preoperative radiograph. (**b**) Small ledge created during the attempt to bypass the fragment at the outer side of the curve. (**c**) Removal attempts were continued at the outer side of the curve, resulting in enlargement of the ledge and a small perforation

removal attempts for fragments located in the middle or apical third as these (attempts) significantly affect tooth strength (Souter and Messer 2005; Madarati et al. 2010) and consequently may predispose to vertical root fracture.

Ledges always occur at the outer side of a curved root canal when inflexible instruments are powerfully forced in an apical direction, preferably in a rotary, screwing motion. Also, the uncontrolled use of too large Gates Glidden burs, used with a cutoff safety tip for preparation of a staging platform, can create a ledge as well as the use of high-powered ultrasonic tips.

Prevention

The prevention of ledging basically follows the same recommendations given for the prevention of perforations. The use of low-power ultrasonics, careful use of Gates Glidden drills for preparation of a staging platform, careful use of instruments for bypassing, and permanent awareness of the risk of ledging at the outer side of the curvature are the most important steps for minimizing the incidence of ledging.

- Transportation

  Transportation is defined as an alteration of the original axis of the root canal. If transportation occurs over the complete length of the root canal, this includes enlargement and transportation of the apical foramen to the outer side of the root. Consequently, the outer side of the root canal is overprepared, with the inner side remaining underprepared and probably insufficiently cleaned and disinfected. Transportation during removal of fractured instruments occurs when bypassing is attempted with inflexible instruments at the outer side of the curvature (Fig. 7.12).

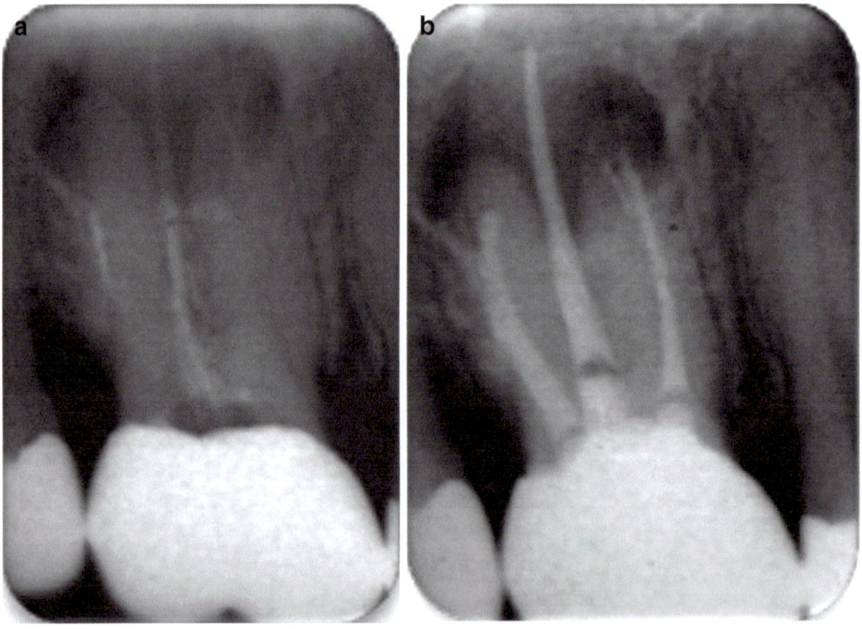

Fig. 7.12 (**a**) Fractured instrument in the distobuccal root canal of a maxillary molar. (**b**) Following initial bypassing of the fragment, severe transportation of the root canal occurred

Prevention

Before attempting to bypass a fractured instrument, the best route for bypassing should be thoroughly considered, seriously balancing the risk of strip perforation at the inner side and of ledging, transportation or perforation at the outer side of the curve. If feasible, bypassing via the more straight lateral aspects of the root can be attempted.

- Transportation of the instrument fragment deeper into the root canal

  This complication rarely occurs as it requires some space below the fragment larger in diameter than the fragment itself. Ultrasonic energy, when applied to a Ni-Ti instrument fragment tightly locked into the dentine wall, might break it up into fragments and, if applied to the coronal end of any relatively loose SS or Ni-Ti fragment, might "push" it deeper into the root canal (Fig. 7.13). This, of course, only can happen when the ultrasonic tip is placed on top of the fragment instead besides the fragment.

  Prevention

Applying pressure onto the top of the fragment in an apical direction should be avoided.

- Dislodgement of a fragment into another root canal

  Once loosened by ultrasonics, the motions of the fragment become uncontrollable, and it can be dislodged inadvertently into another open root canal of the same tooth (Fig. 7.14). Removal can be easily achieved by irrigation, suctioning, or tipping away with a moistened paper point as the fragment usually does have any friction in this new position. Great care has to be taken not to push the fragment deeper into the root canal.

  Prevention

To prevent the dislodgement of a loosened fragment into another root canal, blockage of all other root canal orifices during removal attempts is recommended.

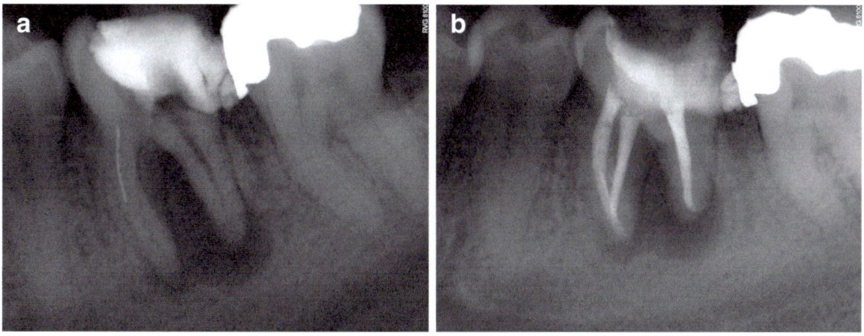

Fig. 7.13 Transportation of a fragment deeper into the root canal. (**a**) Preoperative radiograph. A 6 mm fragment of a #25 Hedstrom file can be seen at the coronal third of the mesiobuccal canal of the first mandibular molar. During retrieval attempts, a 1.5 mm segment of the original fragment was broken and removed, but the remaining part was inadvertently pushed apically. (**b**) The remaining portion was eventually bypassed with the file bypass technique and the root canal was instrumented and obturated up to the apex incorporating the fragment in the mass of gutta-percha

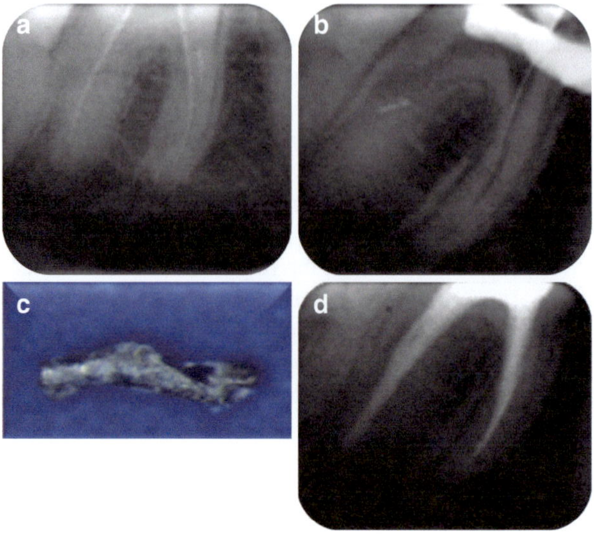

Fig. 7.14 (**a**) Preoperative radiograph showing a fragment in the coronal part of the mesial root canal. (**b**) The fragment has been removed but has been dislodged into the distal root canal. (**c**) Having no friction, the fragment could be removed using a moist paper point. (**d**) Removed fragment

Gutta-percha, cotton pellets, Cavit, Teflon band, and many more materials can be safely used for this purpose.

- Extrusion of the fragment beyond the apex

  The extrusion of a fractured instrument through the apical constriction into the periapical tissues is a rare complication of fragment removal attempts (Figs. 7.15, 7.16, and 7.17). It requires a foramen diameter, naturally present, created iatrogenically or induced by resorption, larger than the diameter of the fragment. Additionally, the fragment has to be pushed with some force in an apical direction, dissolving its friction inside the root canal. Once extruded, it can only be removed by apical surgery.

  Prevention

Applying pressure onto the top of the fragment in an apical direction should be avoided, especially when the fragment is located in the apical third of the root canal.

- Thermal injury of dental and periodontal tissues

  A major concern in the use of ultrasonic devices is the temperature rise on the external root surface and its potential effects on the adjacent periodontal ligament and the bone. It has been reported that a 10 °C temperature rise for 1 min could cause irreversible histologic changes in the periodontal tissues of rabbits (Eriksson and Albrektsson 1983). Cases of severe burn injuries during ultrasonic removal of posts that resulted in teeth extraction were also reported (Gluskin et al. 2005; Walters and Rawal 2007). This should be carefully considered if ultrasonics is used without a coolant to enhance visualization.

  It is advocated that ultrasonic tips should be activated with no coolant while removing broken instruments. The potential harmful temperature rise generated on the external root surface with ultrasonic removal of fractured instruments has

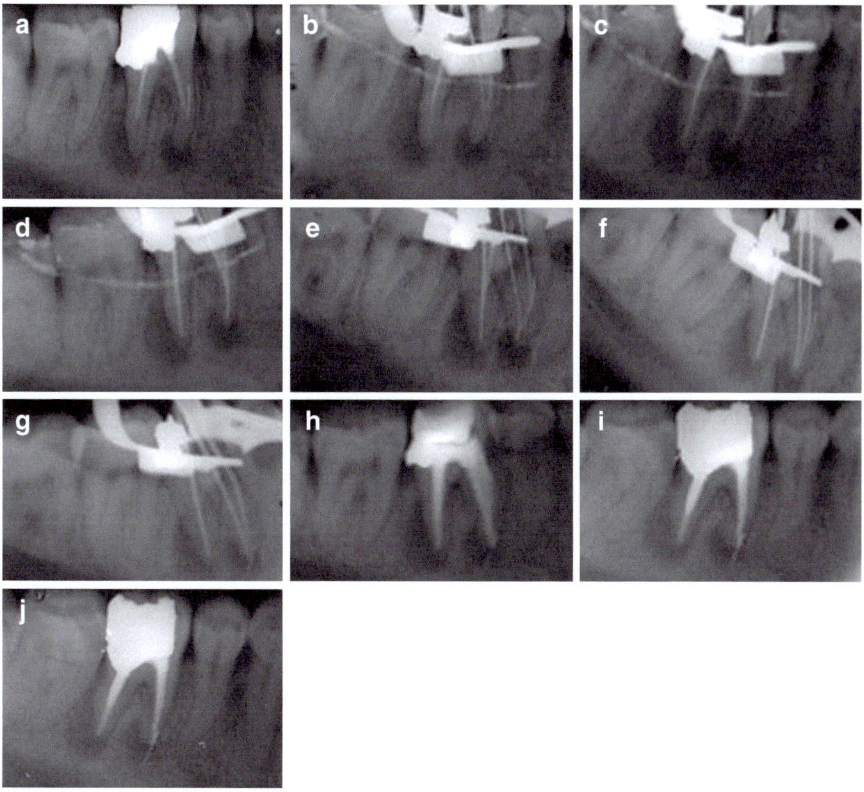

Fig. 7.15 (**a**) Preoperative radiograph. An approximately 4 mm long fragment of an SS file can be seen in the mesial root of an underobturated mandibular molar. (**b–g**) "Movement" of the fragment toward the apex and eventual extrusion into the periapex during efforts to bypass and retrieve it with the file bypass technique. (**h**) Immediate post-obturation radiograph. (**i**) One-year recall radiograph (Courtesy Dr. G. Alexandrou)

been investigated (Hashem 2007; Madarati et al. 2008b, 2009a, b). The temperature rise on the external root surface was found to be a function of root canal wall thickness, ultrasonic tip type, power setting, and application time (Madarati et al. 2008b). Large ultrasonic tips induce higher temperature rise than smaller tips, though overzealous prolonged use regardless of the size of the tip significantly increases the temperature rise at the external root surface (Hashem 2007). Thus, small-sized tips should be used at a reduced power setting with frequent irrigation and intermittent motion to prevent excessive generation of heat and at the same time disinfect the root canal (Hashem 2007; Madarati et al. 2008b).

The friction of the oscillating ultrasonic tip against the fractured instrument also generates a temperature rise greater than that resulting from friction against dentine (Madarati 2015). Therefore, the increase in temperature within the canal might be several times that noted on the external root surface with possible

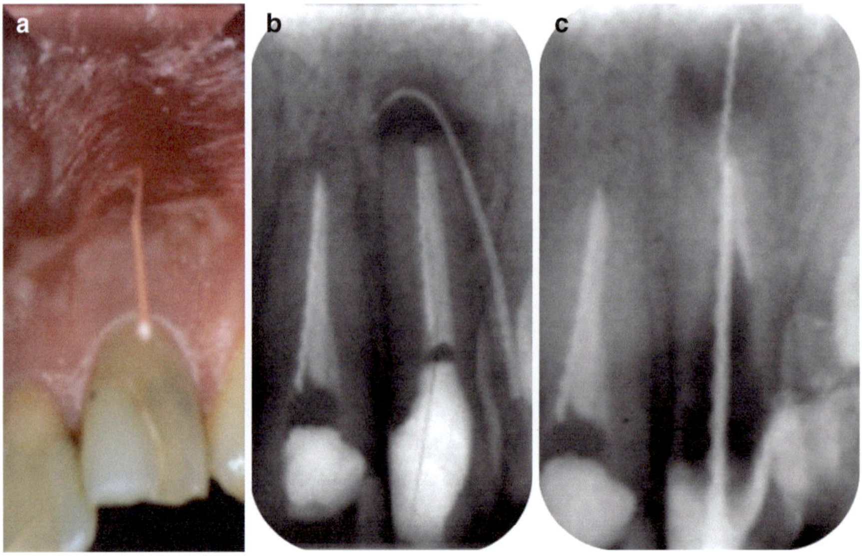

Fig. 7.16 (**a**) Gutta-percha point introduced into a sinus tract. (**b**) The gutta-percha point identifies the already apicected tooth 21 as the origin of the fistula. (**c**) A removal attempt resulted in massive loss of dentine, making the tooth unrestorable and in the apical extrusion of the fragment

implications on the dentine structure of the root canal walls. In an ex vivo study on the role of the type of the instrument fragment on heat generation during ultrasonic application with or without air-active function, it was concluded that significantly higher temperature rises were produced when ultrasonic tips were activated against Ni-Ti instruments as compared to SS fragments (Madarati 2015). The resulting temperature rise was related to the application time and power settings of the ultrasonic unit and was significantly decreased when activation of the ultrasonic tips was combined with the air-active function (Madarati 2015). The difference in temperature rise between Ni-Ti and SS instruments can be attributed to the mechanical and thermal properties of the alloys (Madarati 2015; O'Hanian 1985), but further investigation is required to verify the property which contributes most to this difference. The clinical relevance of temperature rise during attempts of instrument removal still needs to be clarified.

When laser irradiation is used within the root canal, the injurious consequences of temperature rise on root dentine (Fig. 7.18) are always considered. In a study using stereoscopy and SEM on removal effects of filling materials and broken files from root canal using pulsed Nd:YAG laser, the morphological changes of root canal walls were found to be greatly dependent on the irradiation power applied (Yu et al. 2000). Partial carbonization and recrystallization of dentine with some open dentinal tubules covered with burned debris were among the reported findings (Yu et al. 2000).

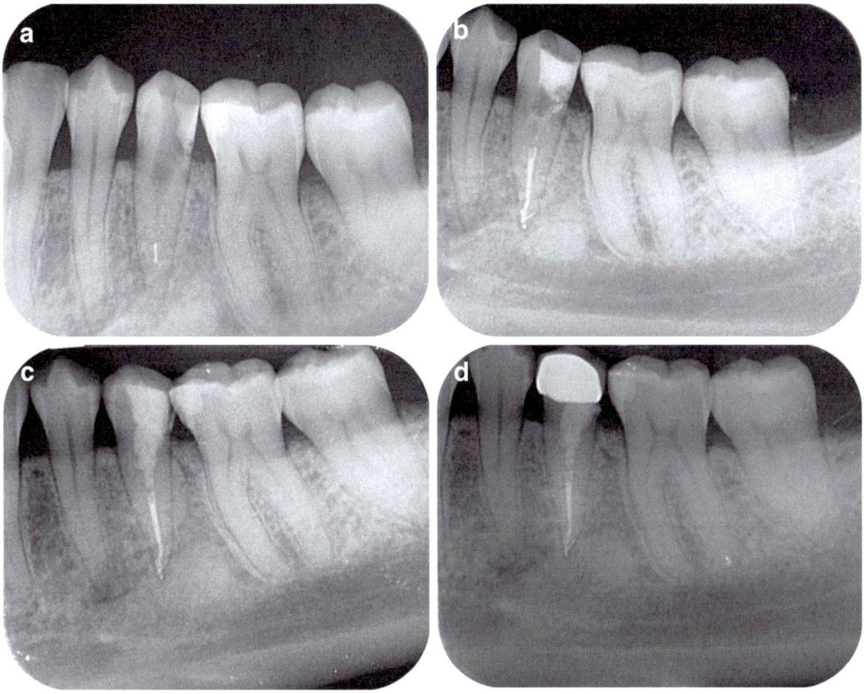

Fig. 7.17 (**a**) Preoperative radiograph as submitted by the referring dentist with extensive removal of tooth structure in the crown and in the coronal root third and a fragment in the apical third. (**b**) Unsuccessful efforts to retrieve it with the file bypass technique resulted in its extrusion to the periapical tissues, as can be seen in the immediate post-obturation radiograph. (**c**, **d**) The 3- and 12-month scheduled clinical and radiographic recall examinations revealed uneventful healing

Prevention

The prevention of excessive temperature rise includes the use of low ultrasonic power, the use of small-sized instruments in an intermittent mode, and frequent irrigation.

To reduce the harmful effects of laser energy with the resultant dentinal carbonization and temperature elevation on the external root surface, a welding method for removal of instrument fragments debris from root canals has been proposed (Hagiwara et al. 2013) (see Chap. 4). According to this, the optical fiber is inserted into a tube and energized while maintaining contact with the freed coronal portion of the fragment. Laser welding was performed (Hagiwara et al. 2013) on stainless steel or nickel titanium files using an Nd:YAG laser in order to evaluate the retention force between the files and metal extractor and the increase in temperature on the root surface during laser irradiation. They reported that the retention force on stainless steel was significantly greater than that on nickel titanium. The maximum temperature increase was 4.1 °C. The temperature increase on the root surface was

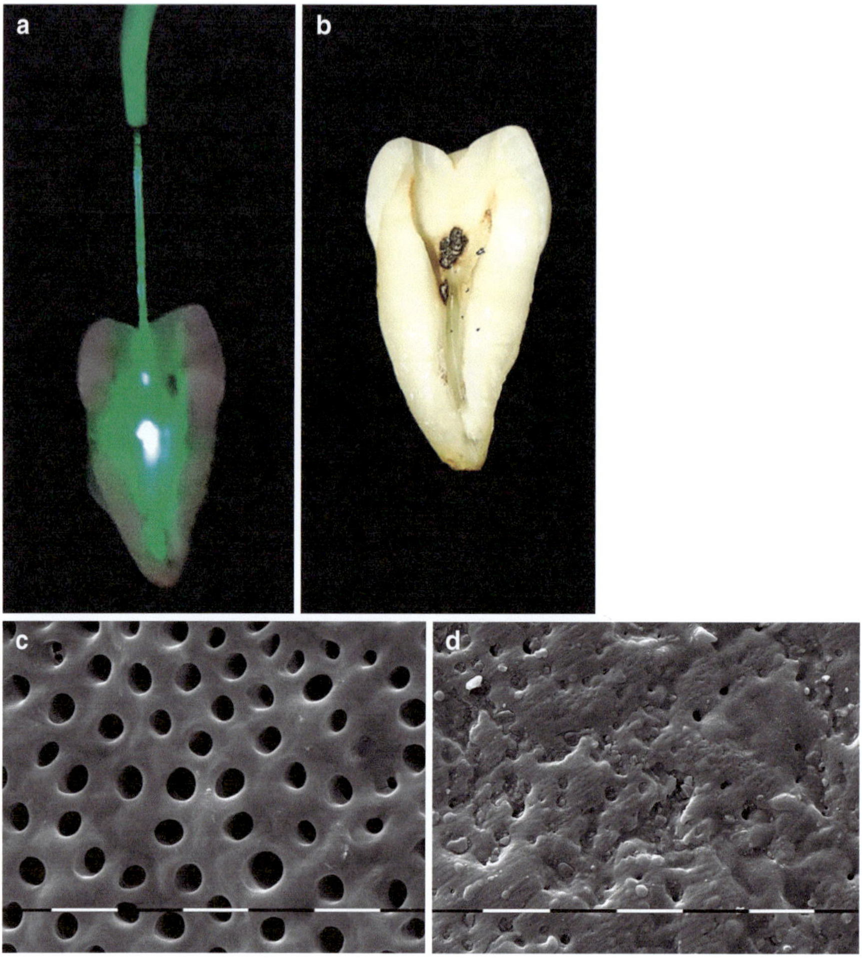

Fig. 7.18 Undesirable thermal effects of Nd:YAG irradiation in a dry root canal. (**a**) When the optical fiber comes into contact with the dentinal wall, it can cause (**b**) carbonization. (**c**, **d**) SEM image of an unirradiated dentine surface and of dentine irradiated with Nd:YAG laser (dry canal, 3 W, 300 mJ/10 Hz); areas of melted dentine and closed dentinal tubules can be seen in the irradiated dentine (Courtesy Prof. G. Tomov)

greater in the vicinity of the welded area than that at the apical area. Scanning electron microscopy revealed that the files and extractors were welded together.

7.2 Complications During and Following Surgical Attempts of Fragment Removal

The introduction of magnification and particularly of the dental operating microscope has widened the range of conditions that can be treated by surgical endodontics. Certain conditions are commonly encountered during or after surgical endodontics and are not considered complications. These include pain, swelling, ecchymosis, and lacerations. Additionally, all postoperative complications related to surgical endodontics might also occur during the surgical management of fractured instruments. These include:

- Anesthesia-related complications
- Soft tissue and esthetic complications
- Surgical site infection
- Complications related to the vicinity/injury of anatomical structures such as maxillary sinus, nerves (sinusitis, paresthesia, dysesthesia)
- Complications related to root-end management (root resection, retrograde cavity preparation, sealing material)
- Periodontal complications most of the time related to improper hemisection at the expense of the root to be retained as opposed to correct sectioning at the expense of the root to be removed
- Periodontal complications related to root amputation
- Periodontal complications due to excessive apical resection during apicoectomy

A detailed presentation of these complications is far beyond the scope of this chapter. They are thoroughly described in books on surgical endodontics (Kim et al. 2001; Merino 2009; Tsesis 2014). Nevertheless, some characteristic cases with complications related to surgical attempts to manage fractured endodontic instruments will be presented (Fig. 7.19).

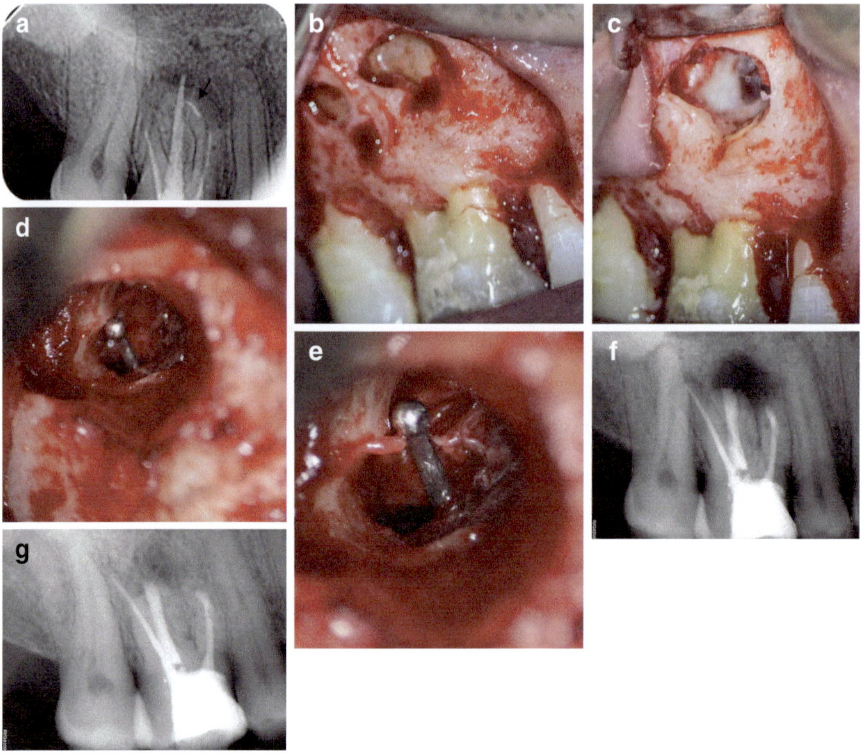

Fig. 7.19 (**a**) Fragment of a small-sized Ni-Ti instrument beyond the nearly 90° curvature in the mesiobuccal canal of the first maxillary molar. (**b**) Immediate post-obturation radiograph short of the working length with transportation in the mesiobuccal canal. The instrument was not removed or bypassed. (**c**) Reflection of a full mucoperiosteal flap. Buccal bone dehiscence and root curvature can clearly be seen. (**d**) Apicoectomy. (**e**, **f**) Fracture of a micro-burnisher during retrograde cavity preparation. (**g**) Immediate postoperative radiograph. Note the MTA retofillings in the palatal and mesiobuccal roots. (**h**) The 12-month recall examination revealed healing process of the periapical tissues (Courtesy Dr. Ch. Beltes)

References

Eriksson AR, Albrektsson T. Temperature threshold levels for heat-induced bone tissue injury: a vital-microscopic study in the rabbit. J Prosthet Dent. 1983;50(1):101–7.

Fu M, Zhang Z, Hou B. Removal of broken files from root canals by using ultrasonic techniques combined with dental microscope: a retrospective analysis of treatment outcome. J Endod. 2011;37(5):619–22.

Gerek M, Baser ED, Kayahan MB, Sunay H, Kaptan RF, Bayirli G. Comparison of the force required to fracture roots vertically after ultrasonic and Masserann removal of broken instruments. Int Endod J. 2012;45(5):429–34.

Gluskin AH, Ruddle CJ, Zinman EJ. Thermal injury through intraradicular heat transfer using ultrasonic devices: precautions and practical preventive strategies. J Am Dent Assoc. 2005;136(9):1286–93.

Hagiwara R, Suehara M, Fujii R, Kato H, Nakagawa K, Oda Y. Laser welding method for removal of instruments debris from root canals. Bull Tokyo Dent Coll. 2013;54:81–8.

Hashem AA. Ultrasonic vibration: temperature rise on external root surface during broken instrument removal. J Endod. 2007;33(9):1070–3.

Hülsmann M. [Removal of fractured root canal instruments using the Canal Finder System]. Dtsch Zahnärztl Z. 1990;45(4):229–32.
Hülsmann M, Schäfer E. Problems in endodontics. etiology, diagnosis and treatment. London: Quintessence; 2009.
Hülsmann M, Schinkel I. Influence of several factors on the success or failure of removal of fractured instruments from the root canal. Endod Dent Traumatol. 1999;15(6):252–8.
Kim S, Pecora G, Rubinstein R. Color atlas of microsurgery in endodontics. Philadelphia: Saunders; 2001.
Lambrianidis T. Risk management in root canal treatment. Thessaloniki: University Studio Press; 2001. p. 199–247.
Lertchirakarn V, Palamara JE, Messer HH. Patterns of vertical root fracture: factors affecting stress distribution in the root canal. J Endod. 2003;29(8):523–8.
Madarati AA. Temperature rise on the surface of NiTi and stainless steel fractured instruments during ultrasonic removal. Int Endod J. 2015;48(9):872–7.
Madarati AA, Watts DC, Qualtrough AJ. Opinions and attitudes of endodontists and general dental practitioners in the UK towards the intra-canal fracture of endodontic instruments. Part 2. Int Endod J. 2008a;41(12):1079–87.
Madarati AA, Qualtrough AJ, Watts DC. Factors affecting temperature rise on the external root surface during ultrasonic retrieval of intracanal separated files. J Endod. 2008b;34(9):1089–92.
Madarati AA, Qualtrough AJ, Watts DC. Efficiency of a newly designed ultrasonic unit and tips in reducing temperature rise on root surface during the removal of fractured files. J Endod. 2009a;35(6):896–9.
Madarati AA, Qualtrough AJ, Watts DC. A microcomputed tomography scanning study of root canal space: changes after the ultrasonic removal of fractured files. J Endod. 2009b;35(1):125–8.
Madarati AA, Qualtrough AJ, Watts DC. Vertical fracture resistance of roots after ultrasonic removal of fractured instruments. Int Endod J. 2010;43(5):424–9.
Merino E. Endodontic microsurgery. London: Quintessence; 2009.
Nagai O, Tani N, Kayaba Y, Kodama S, Osada T. Ultrasonic removal of broken instruments in root canals. Int Endod J. 1986;19(6):298–304.
Nevares G, Cunha RS, Zuolo ML, Bueno CE. Success rates for removing or bypassing fractured instruments: a prospective clinical study. J Endod. 2012;38(4):442–4.
O'Hanian H. Physics. WW Norton: New York; 1985.
Shahabinejad H, Ghassemi A, Pishbin L, Shahravan A. Success of ultrasonic technique in removing fractured rotary nickel-titanium endodontic instruments from root canals and its effect on the required force for root fracture. J Endod. 2013;39(6):824–8.
Souter NJ, Messer HH. Complications associated with fractured file removal using an ultrasonic technique. J Endod. 2005;31(6):450–2.
Suter B, Lussi A, Sequeira P. Probability of removing fractured instruments from root canals. Int Endod J. 2005;38(2):112–23.
Tsesis I. Complications in endodontic surgery, prevention, identification and management. Heidelberg: Springer; 2014.
Walters JD, Rawal SY. Severe periodontal damage by an ultrasonic endodontic device: a case report. Dent Traumatol. 2007;23(2):123–7.
Ward JR, Parashos P, Messer HH. Evaluation of an ultrasonic technique to remove fractured rotary nickel-titanium endodontic instruments from root canals: an experimental study. J Endod. 2003a;29(11):756–63.
Ward JR, Parashos P, Messer HH. Evaluation of an ultrasonic technique to remove fractured rotary nickel-titanium endodontic instruments from root canals: clinical cases. J Endod. 2003b;29(11):764–7.
Yoldas O, Oztunc H, Tinaz C, Alparslan N. Perforation risks associated with the use of Masserann endodontic kit drills in mandibular molars. Oral Surg Oral Med Oral Pathol Oral Radiol Endod. 2004;97(4):513–7.
Yu DG, Kimura Y, Tomita Y, Nakamura Y, Watanabe H, matsumoto K. Study on removal effects of filling materials and broken files from root canals using pulsed nd:YAG laser. J Clin Laser Med Surg. 2000;18(1):23–8.

8 Prognosis of Root Canal Treatment with Retained Instrument Fragment(s)

Peter Parashos

8.1 Introduction

The use of rotary nickel-titanium (NiTi) root canal instruments is commonplace for endodontists and many general dentists across the world (Parashos and Messer 2004; Madarati et al. 2008; Bird et al. 2009; Locke et al. 2013; Thomas et al. 2013; Savani et al. 2014). It has been shown that a sensible approach has been adopted in the incorporation of rotary NiTi instruments into both general dental practice and specialist endodontic practice (Parashos and Messer 2004). Since the introduction of NiTi alloy in 1960, many innovative improvements and alterations to the metallurgical properties of the alloy have been introduced, aiming to improve the quality and efficiency of root canal instruments (Singh et al. 2016). However, fracture of rotary NiTi instruments is a known clinical complication (Parashos and Messer 2006) that can occur without warning (Pruett et al. 1997; Parashos et al. 2004; Alapati et al. 2005) and even single-use of the instruments will not eliminate the chances of fracture (Arens et al. 2003).

Historically, the fracture of a root canal instrument was recognized and accepted as being sufficiently common that "any clinician who is yet to experience the pang, anguish and mortification" of fracture "has not treated many root canals" (Grossman 1969). Most dentists and endodontists surveyed have experienced endodontic instrument fracture, whether it was a stainless steel (SS) file or a rotary NiTi instrument (Parashos and Messer 2004; Madarati et al. 2008). A number of studies have attempted to investigate the incidence and prevalence of instrument fracture through a variety of different research designs. One simple method involves the collection of

P. Parashos, MDSc, PhD, FRACDS
Faculty of Medicine, Dentistry and Health Sciences, Endodontic Unit,
Melbourne Dental School, University of Melbourne,
720 Swanston Street, Melbourne, VIC 3010, Australia
e-mail: parashos@unimelb.edu.au

T. Lambrianidis (ed.), *Management of Fractured Endodontic Instruments*,
DOI 10.1007/978-3-319-60651-4_8

discarded instruments with subsequent assessment for signs of deformation or fracture. The largest such study involved four countries and 7159 discarded rotary NiTi instruments finding an overall defect rate of 17%, 5% of which were fractures (Parashos et al. 2004). Similarly, Alapati et al. (2005) found fractures in 5.1% of 822 instruments. However, two earlier studies reported quite different fracture prevalences, with Arens et al. (2003) only noting a 0.9% fracture rate in single-use of ProFile Series 29 rotary NiTi instruments, while with multi-use of rotary NiTi instruments, Sattapan et al. (2000) found a 21% fracture rate among discarded Quantec instruments. Importantly, the former study involved pre-flaring with a series of three Gates Glidden burs, while the latter involved use of each instrument to full working length after only glide-path preparation with a size 15 SS file. Hence, differences in fracture prevalence will depend not only on instrument design (Parashos et al. 2004) but also clinical protocol. However, it is also important to remember that fracture incidence is independent of number of uses (Arens et al. 2003; Parashos et al. 2004; Spanaki-Voreadi et al. 2006; Wolcott et al. 2006) and that root canal instrument fracture is realistically due to many factors (Alapati et al. 2005; Parashos and Messer 2006; Spanaki-Voreadi et al. 2006; Shen et al. 2009; Cheung 2009).

Importantly, caution must be exercised when interpreting the information from discarded instrument studies because they offer no information about whether or not the fractured fragment was still present and interfering with treatment, which is arguably the most relevant outcome rather than simply the fracture of the instrument (Parashos and Messer 2006). On the other hand, discarded instrument studies are far more valuable in their ability to indicate why instruments fracture rather than how often they do so.

Several clinical studies, with either prospective or retrospective designs, have attempted to establish the incidence of fractured SS instruments that are actually retained within teeth. With the exception of Crump and Natkin (1970), most of the early information available about the incidence of SS file fracture is extrapolated from outcome studies (Strindberg 1956; Engström and Lundberg 1965; Kerekes and Tronstad 1979; Sjögren et al. 1990). When the information from these papers is combined, an overall prevalence of approximately 1.6% (0.7–7.4%) can be deduced. Ramirez-Salomon et al. (1997), evaluating rotary NiTi instruments, used a small sample size of 52 teeth and found that a fracture occurred in 11.5% of teeth or 3.7% of roots, the majority of which could then be bypassed. A much larger study (Iqbal et al. 2006) found a prevalence of 1.68% for the fracture of rotary NiTi instruments and 0.25% for hand instruments. It should be noted that because of the retrospective nature of this study, it did not account for fragments too small to be seen radiographically or those that were bypassed or removed.

Probably the largest study offering insight into the prevalence of instrument fracture was by Spili et al. (2005) in which 8460 teeth were retrospectively examined, with 277 having one or more instrument fragments present, amounting to 3.3%; fractured instruments included NiTi, SS, paste fillers, and lateral spreaders. Subsequently, two other large-scale studies have been published, each with just under 5000 canals (Wolcott et al. 2006; Tzanetakis et al. 2008). Wolcott et al. (2006)

investigated the number of times that ProTaper instruments could be safely used and reported a fracture prevalence of 2.4%, whereas Tzanetakis et al. (2008) found that postgraduate students experienced fracture in 1.83% of canals.

From the available literature, it would appear that instrument fracture is a significant albeit uncommon complication of root canal treatment (RCT). Overall, it can be concluded that instrument fracture, and particularly rotary NiTi fracture, is an event with a multifactorial etiology, which can occur unexpectedly even when all predisposing factors have been taken into consideration.

8.2 Effect of Fractured Instrument on Prognosis

Evidence-based clinical decision making requires the availability of high-quality clinical evidence (Kim et al. 2001). This has prompted clinicians and researchers to focus more on the validity of all the available evidence—in particular, the "current best evidence" (Sackett et al. 1997)—to support clinical decisions. This evidence-based approach also allows a more definitive prognosis or decision on outcome for such treatment. According to Friedman (2002), "prognosis is the forecast of the course of a disease," and as far as apical periodontitis (AP) is concerned, it "applies to both the time course and chances of healing." He clearly distinguishes this from a closely related term, "treatment outcome," which "may be used to describe the short-term consequences of treatment, as well as the long-term healing or development of AP" (Friedman 2002).

A generally recognized hierarchy in levels of evidence in clinical studies, in decreasing order of importance, includes randomized controlled trials, cohort studies, case-control studies, case series, and case reports (Sackett et al. 1997; Concato et al. 2000). The overall level of evidence available concerning the impact of retained instrument fragments on endodontic prognosis is low (Panitvisai et al. 2010). Considering that instrument fracture is a relatively uncommon complication of treatment, this contributes to it being difficult to study. Any prospective study design would have to have an unrealistically large sample population in order to show any statistically significant effects and has obvious ethical implications. Hence, realistically, the highest achievable level of evidence would be retrospective case-controlled studies of which only two exist (Crump and Natkin 1970; Spili et al. 2005). While these two investigations should be the focus of any discussion on prognosis, some thought must also be given to lower-level evidence (case series and cohort studies).

A direct comparison among the numerous published outcome studies is meaningless, ineffective, and misleading owing to their diversity (Molven and Halse 1988; Smith et al. 1993; Friedman 1998, 2002). This is a consequence of their lack of standardization due to variations in material composition, treatment procedures, and methodology (Friedman 1998, 2002). Importantly, the old concepts of "success" and "failure" (Huumonen and Ørstavik 2002) have been challenged with the contemporary emphasis on "healing," "disease," and "functionality" (Friedman 2002; Farzaneh et al. 2004a, b). Consequently, the evidence concerning prognosis/

outcome with retained instrument fragments must be considered in this context. Clinical experience gained from conducting these studies (Spili et al. 2005) alludes to the fact that many radiographically uncertain or failed cases may still be asymptomatic and functional.

8.3 Lower-Level Evidence

Spili et al. (2005) listed 13 studies between 1956 and 2001 reporting the outcome of clinical cases following fracture of an endodontic instrument, all of which were either carbon steel or stainless steel (Strindberg 1956; Grahnén and Hansson 1961; Engström et al. 1964; Ingle and Glick 1965; Engström and Lundberg 1965; Grossman 1969; Crump and Natkin 1970; Fox et al. 1972; Bergenholtz et al. 1979; Kerekes and Tronstad 1979; Cvek et al. 1982; Sjögren et al. 1990; Molyvdas et al. 2001). Of these, four studies (Strindberg 1956; Grossman 1969; Crump and Natkin 1970; Molyvdas et al. 2001) differentiated cases with preoperative lesions from those without, but Engström·and Lundberg (1965) and Cvek et al. (1982) only had five "no-lesion" and four "lesion" cases, respectively, so comparison was not possible. Subsequently, after Spili et al. (2005), several other papers have been published adding to this database (Table 8.1). Overall, a total of 508 cases were represented by these studies, of which 308 made the distinction between cases with a preoperative PA lesion and those without (Table 8.1). Interestingly, there is no overall statistically significant difference in outcome between these two groups ($\chi^2 = 0.56$, $p = 0.45$).

The landmark outcome-based paper by Strindberg (1956) was the earliest research to look at the impact of fractured files on clinical and radiographic outcomes. This comprehensive long-term follow-up study of factors related to the results of pulp therapy was the first published work to report the influence of retained fractured instruments (or what he referred to as "file breakage") on the prognosis of endodontic treatment. Using strict criteria for healing (i.e., "incomplete" or "uncertain" healing were categorized as "failure") and observation periods of 4–10 years of his own cases, Strindberg (1956) included 15 cases with fractured instruments (five in single-rooted teeth *without* apical periodontitis, two in single-rooted teeth *with* apical periodontitis, six in multi-rooted teeth *without* apical periodontitis, and two in multi-rooted teeth *with* apical periodontitis). Four failures occurred among the 15 teeth with fractured instruments present (27%) compared with 42 of 453 (9%) teeth without fractured files. Despite the small numbers of fractured instruments associated with periapical lesions, Strindberg (1956) concluded that, while the presence of fractured files would always reduce the prognosis of RCT, the effect would be more profound if there was a preoperative lesion present. Strindberg (1956) considered instrument fracture a serious problem, and although he was usually unaware of the bacterial status of the root canal prior to file breakage, he surmised that prognosis would be poorer in the presence rather than in the absence of infection (i.e., a periapical radiolucency). Further, he speculated that in cases where there was intracanal infection apical to the retained fragment, subsequent conservative therapy alone would probably not eradicate such infection or eliminate its potential consequences.

Table 8.1 Studies reporting the effect of a retained fractured instrument on the outcome of endodontic treatment

Study	Lesion[a]	No lesion	Healing (%)	Effect on healing
Strindberg (1956)	2/4	9/11	11/15 (73%)	Overall 19% reduction (although lower when lesion is present)
Grahnén and Hansson (1961)	NR	NR	NR	No effect
Ingle and Glick (1965)	NR	NR	NR	No effect
Engström et al. (1964)	NR	NR	6/9 (67%)	No effect
Engström and Lundberg (1965)	0/0	5/5	5/5 (100%)	No effect
Grossman (1969)	9/19	42/47	51/66 (77%)	Reduced only when lesion is present
Crump and Natkin (1970)	27/29	21/24	48/53 (91%)	No effect
Fox et al. (1972)	NR	NR	93/100 (93%)	Reduced only when lesion is present
Bergenholtz et al. (1979)	NR	NR	NR	Reduced only when lesion is present
Kerekes and Tronstad (1979)	NR	NR	9/11 (82%)	Reduced only in teeth with necrotic pulps
Cvek et al. (1982)	3/4	NA	3/4 (75%)	Not stated specifically for fractured files
Sjögren et al. (1990)	NR	NR	9/11 (82%)	Not discussed
Molyvdas et al. (2001)	8/11	32/35	40/46 (87%)	Reduced only when lesion is present
Spili et al. (2005)	51/56	62/63	113/119 (95%)	No effect
Imura et al. (2007)	NR	NR	8/11 (73%)	Not discussed
Fu et al. (2011)	NR	NR	3/8 (38%)	Reduced due to perforation
Ng et al. (2011)	NR	NR	18/27 (67%)	Not reported
Ungerechts et al. (2014)	NR	NR	13/23 (57%)	No effect
Total (%)	100/123 (81%)	171/185 (92%)	430/508 (85%)	

[a]Number of cases judged to be successful over total number of cases. *NR* not reported

Using the clinical and radiographic methods described by Strindberg (1956), Grahnén and Hansson (1961) calculated the failure frequency of pulp and root canal therapy on adult patients treated by students. They analyzed 763 teeth (1277 roots) with a review period of 4–5 years and claimed that the failure rate of cases with fractured files was no different from that of cases without retained file fragments even when the preoperative periradicular status was considered. However, they did not actually specify the number of fractured file cases, although the overall failure rate was 12%. The 4–5-year follow-up investigation by Engström et al. (1964) of 306 conservatively root-filled teeth revealed no statistically significant difference between fractured instrument cases with (2 of 4 failures) or without (1 of 5 failures) pretreatment positive bacterial culture. The following year, Engström and Lundberg (1965) also published a 3.5–4-year radiographic follow-up study of teeth conservatively root-filled following pulpectomy; hence, there were no cases with lesions. All five fractured instrument cases, which yielded negative cultures before obturation, were classified as successes. However, contemporary concepts question the validity of culturing (Sathorn et al. 2007).

The classic "Washington study" described (but not actually published) by Ingle and Glick (1965) in the first edition of Ingle's textbook also concluded that treatment outcome was unaffected by a retained fractured instrument. During the eight years of the study, which also provided the caseload for Crump and Natkin (1970), a great number of instruments were fractured, yet only one case out of the 104 failures from 1229 cases at the 2-year recall could be attributed to a broken instrument. The authors hypothesized that a broken instrument itself could serve as "an adequate root canal filling," which was to be later supported by Fox et al. (1972). Ingle and Glick (1965) concluded that even though fractured instruments were not "favored," they were unlikely to affect prognosis and were amenable to surgical treatment if found in the apical third.

Grossman (1968, 1969) conducted a 5-year survey of patients in a university clinic to assess the effect of fractured files on prognosis. With an average follow-up period of 2 years, the data ($n = 66$) included 19 cases with lesions and 47 without (31 of the latter having vital pulps). The outcomes were then compared with a sample of "normal" controls (presumably cases without fractured files, although this was not specified). No difference was found between vital cases and necrotic cases without preoperative periapical lesions; however, there was a 39% reduction in success (47% vs. 86%) when "rarefaction" was present; if "doubtful" the cases were considered failures. Grossman (1968, 1969) claimed this to be a significant difference compared with vital cases and cases without a periapical lesion; however, he did not provide any statistical analysis or further details on the "normal" cases. Additionally, an unspecified number of teeth in this study were obturated with silver cones. The study design of this investigation could be considered a case series. Like most other outcome studies, including those that evaluated the prognostic impact of a retained fractured instrument, it highlights the limitations or weaknesses inherent with such a research design. This view that the presence of periapical pathosis rather than the fractured instrument per se was of greater impact was supported in subsequent papers by Fox et al. (1972) and Molyvdas et al. (1992), finding that fractured files had reduced prognosis in the presence of a periapical radiolucency.

The interesting study by Fox et al. (1972) reported similar conclusions to those of Grossman (1968, 1969). In their case series, of 304 teeth with retained carbon steel or SS files, fractured either accidentally ($n = 100$; 32.9%) or intentionally ($n = 204$; 67.1%), the overall "failure" rate noted was 6.25% ($n = 19$). However, for the accidentally fractured cases, the failure rate was 7%. Interestingly, these authors described a technique of intentionally filling root canals with SS instruments that were cemented in place with root canal sealer. On the other hand, in the case of accidental fracture, no attempt was made to bypass or remove the instruments; rather the remainder of the canal was filled with gutta-percha and sealer. Teeth with preoperative periapical radiolucencies increased the probability of failure by threefold. Similarly, Molyvdas et al. (1992) found that all cases ($n = 23$) with preoperative diagnosis of pulpitis were categorized as successes, whereas only 75% of 12 necrotic cases and 73% of 11 teeth with periapical pathosis were successes; "compromised" cases were considered failures. Importantly, the latter authors found that bypassing the instrument fragment in 22 cases resulted in 95% success.

Kerekes and Tronstad (1979) investigated the outcome of a standardized treatment protocol performed by dental students on 647 roots (in 478 teeth). There were only 11 instances of instrument fractures with six occurring in vital cases and five in necrotic cases. Of these cases, all of the vital teeth were considered to have successful outcomes, while two of the necrotic cases resulted in failure. The criteria used to analyze the radiographs were such that anything larger than a "slight" radiolucent zone around the gutta-percha was considered uncertain or failure. Although the low prevalence of instrument fracture did not allow statistical analysis, the data did support the finding of the other studies described above. Bergenholtz et al. (1979) conducted a radiographic follow-up to assess the effect of over-instrumentation and over-filling only on retreated root canals. They observed 11 retained file fragments that were fractured during the retreatment of 660 cases subsequently followed up for 2 years. They concluded that file fracture did not seem to influence prognosis in those cases retreated purely for technical reasons but did reduce prognosis for retreated cases with preoperative periapical pathosis.

Cvek et al. (1982) evaluated the treatment outcome of 54 endodontically treated non-vital maxillary and mandibular incisors with post-traumatically reduced pulpal lumens and preoperative periapical lesions. In this study, four file fractures were noted, all of which occurred when the smallest observable lumen diameter was 0–0.1 mm, which was measured by comparing with an orthodontic wire of 0.1 mm diameter; 0.1 mm was found to be the smallest width discernible in the radiograph with acceptable precision. Of these four teeth only one showed signs of "osteitis" at 4 years following treatment. In the Sjögren et al. (1990) outcome-based study of 356 teeth, retained instruments were present in 11 roots, two of which subsequently showed periapical lesions. However, there was no information on the preoperative status of these teeth, and as with Kerekes and Tronstad (1979), they considered roots rather than teeth. In a study of the outcome of endodontic retreatment, Van Nieuwenhuysen et al. (1994) reported 10 (1.6%) cases of fractured instruments from 612 retreated roots but did not clarify whether these instruments were retained or retrieved following fracture. Their findings indicated that complications during retreatment, such as file fracture, resulted in a reduced retreatment outcome, but no further details were provided.

More recently, a retrospective study of 2000 cases (Imura et al. 2007) treated in a single private practice over 30 years found that teeth without intraoperative complications (instrument fracture, perforation, and flare-up) healed at a higher rate than those with such complications (91.9% vs. 72.6%). Complications occurred in 51 cases, but file fractures only accounted for 11, of which only three resulted in failure; the actual type of instruments was not specified. With such a low-fracture prevalence, statistical analysis was not feasible without being combined with other complications. This is a common theme in much of the outcome literature with the earlier pooled phases of the Toronto study (de Chevigny et al. 2008) also encountering 11 fractured files (in 373 teeth), but the authors only reported the change in healing between teeth with and without complications (including pulp chamber cracks, aberrant anatomy, perforation, and non-negotiable canals) rather than specifically for fractured files alone.

Another more recent study that attempted to report the effect of fractured files on treatment outcome (Fu et al. 2011) reexamined 102 teeth with fractured instruments present 12–68 months after treatment. Using PAI scores to measure periapical disease and a dichotomized description of root fillings as either adequate (including fractured instruments in the apical third) or inadequate (nonhomogeneous appearance or not ending at either the point of obstruction or within 2 mm of the apex), they were able to follow up 66 cases, of which 58 had the fragments successfully removed and eight still had the fractured instrument present at the time of review. Of these eight cases, five were deemed failures. In these five cases, two instrument fragments were pushed through the apex during the attempt at removal. Though the authors concluded that a failure to remove a fractured instrument reduced prognosis, it is difficult to establish whether the attempted removal (which resulted in perforation in three of the five teeth) may have actually contributed to the rate of failure. Interestingly, the only other factor that significantly impacted the prognosis of these teeth was the quality of the root canal filling, which may be interpreted to suggest that control of intraradicular infection rather than file removal per se is the key to obtaining favorable outcomes as indicated by Fox et al. (1972). Interestingly, one of the more robust prospective outcome studies of recent times (Ng et al. 2011) did analyze the impact of fractured instruments on prognosis as an independent variable, recording 15 instrument fractures (of 1155 roots) in primary treatment and 12 (of 1302) in retreatment cases. There was only a significant difference in healing in the retreatment cases (50% healing vs. 80% in primary treatment cases). However, despite this finding, the authors pointed out that the type of fractured instrument as well as its fate was in the same confounding pathway as the ability to obtain patency. Hence, the inference was that the presence of the fractured file itself was unlikely to be the true cause of persistent disease but rather has a negative impact because of its interference with the ability to gain patency.

A very recent study (Ungerechts et al. 2014) analyzed the outcome of treatment by students at a Norwegian university dental clinic focusing on the impact of instrument fracture. Fractured instruments occurred in 38 of 3854 treated teeth and mostly comprised SS hand files and lentulo-spiral burs (81.6%) as well as several NiTi instruments (18.4%). Ten of these instruments were removed prior to obturation, and the other 28 were left in situ. As with Fu et al. (2011), the authors found higher rates of success associated with teeth that had the fragments removed prior to obturation (71.4% vs. 56.5%) as well as those teeth with preoperative diagnosis of vital pulps compared with those that were necrotic or previously treated (72.7% vs. 58.3% vs. 42.9%, respectively). However, none of these findings reached statistical significance, likely because eight of the 38 fractured instrument cases could not be followed up. Unfortunately, the fractured instrument cases were not matched to "normal" controls nor was any information provided about the periapical status of the teeth in question. As a result, limited information can be gathered from this paper about the impact of fractured instruments on prognosis.

In summary, the lower-level evidence on the prognosis for fractured instruments seems to suggest that, in cases without preoperative lesions, the presence of a fractured instrument has no impact on prognosis. However, most of these early papers offer little insight into the actual impact of instrument fracture on the prognosis of modern endodontic treatment. This is because of the inherent issues in study design, including a lack of matched controls and a small sample size of fractured instruments, and the questionable relevance of the techniques and instruments to contemporary practices. Consequently, the conclusions of the authors of many of these papers were often subjective, contradictory, and made unsubstantiated statements based on insufficient sample size, inappropriate or no control groups, poor or no inclusion/exclusion criteria, lack of blinding leading to observer bias, unsatisfactory or undefined outcome measures and criteria, uncontrolled confounding factors, and especially unsatisfactory statistical analyses. Further, a major shortcoming of most of these studies was recognized by Strindberg (1956), who stated the following when summarizing the limitations of the published studies in his survey of the literature: "The effect of any one factor on the results has been studied without regard for other factors"—in other words, most studies failed to perform logistic regression analysis to account for possible associations among various potential prognostic (independent) variables and treatment outcome (the dependent variable).

8.4 Case-Controlled Studies

Case-controlled studies offer the greatest level of insight into the impact of instrument fracture on prognosis by allowing comparison of outcomes in teeth which differ only in the presence or absence of a retained instrument but are similar in all other respects. Crump and Natkin (1970) provided the first of such studies, searching through 8500 cases treated by dental students at the University of Washington between 1955 and 1965. They identified 178 retained fractured instrument (carbon steel or SS) cases and matched them to a selection of 400 controls by tooth type, canal number, material, and the presence of absence of a lesion (but not pretreatment pulpal status, medicament used, or quality of root filling). All teeth were required to have had at least a 2-year review, and new recalls were made for study patients and matched controls for clinical and radiographic evaluation. Clinically, the presence of signs or symptoms of persistent periapical disease was assessed, and radiographs were taken to categorize the teeth as either "success" (the complete absence of any discernible periapical lesion), "uncertain" (a questionable clinical sign or a periapical lesion reduced in size by more than 75% or the presence of PDL thickening up to 1 mm where there was an initial diagnosis of normal apical tissues), or "failure" (the presence of definitive clinical signs or symptoms, less than 75% reduction in lesion size, or appearance of a new lesion). A total of 53 matched pairs could be recalled and reviewed. No significant differences could be found between the outcomes of teeth with and without fractured instruments whether they were analyzed in three groups (success, failure, uncertain) or two groups (with uncertain considered as success or failure). In order to show that the negative result was not a consequence of unmatched variables, the authors analyzed the distribution of these variables (including lateral canals, voids, unfilled canals, root resorption, and root perforation) and showed they were evenly distributed among controls and fractured instrument cases as well as between successes and failures. Based on these findings, Crump and Natkin (1970) suggested a conservative approach to the management of fractured files.

Spili et al. (2005) conducted a more recent, and the only other, case-controlled study. The study itself consisted of two distinct parts with the first assessing the incidence of instrument facture over a 13.5-year period and the second part comparing the outcome of treatment in cases with retained instruments with matched controls in order to determine the impact of instrument retention on prognosis. A total of 8460 cases treated between 1990 and 2003 were screened (with the transition from hand to rotary instruments occurring between 1996 and 1997) and coded for various variables with all cases, which had both the presence of a retained instrument and at least a 1-year clinical and radiographic follow-up identified. Teeth with previously fractured instruments, obviously defective restorations, or insufficient clinical or radiographic documentation were excluded. The radiographic observations were separated into signs of complete healing, incomplete healing, uncertain healing, and no healing, while the teeth were judged clinically as either having the presence or absence of clinical signs or symptoms. Success was then determined to be complete or incomplete healing in the absence of clinical signs or symptoms.

The results reported by Spili et al. (2005) showed 277 teeth with fractured instruments of which 146 had a greater than 1-year recall available. The total number of fractures accounted for 5.1% of the teeth with 4.4% being rotary NiTi instruments and 0.7% being SS files (in the period between 1997 and 2003 where hand instruments were used exclusively as pathfinders). For the case-control portion of the study, the overall rates of healing were 91.8% and 94.5% for cases and controls, respectively. When these results were divided according to the absence or presence of a radiographic lesion prior to treatment, the results were 96.8% compared with 98.4% for controls (without a lesion) and 86.7% compared with 92.9% for controls (with a lesion). These differences were not statistically significant, with the 95% confidence interval for the reduction in healing rate in the presence of a periapical lesion ranging from −3.0 to 15.3%. In fact, the only factor that was shown to have a statistically significant impact on prognosis was the presence or absence of a preoperative lesion. Like previous authors (Molyvdas et al. 2001), Spili et al. (2005) hypothesized that despite the positive results, the true impact of fractured instruments may depend on the stage of root canal preparation at which the fracture occurred, although the information required to be able to confirm this was not available from the study sample. Spili et al. (2005) concluded that, based on the results of the study, instrument fracture, when occurring in the hands of experienced endodontists, does not in itself affect prognosis.

8.5 Meta-Analysis

A literature review and meta-analysis was performed by Panitvisai et al. (2010), to answer the question "in adult patients who have had nonsurgical RCT, does the retention of a separated instrument, compared with no retained fractured instrument, result in a poorer clinical outcome?" Of the 17 studies retrieved, all but two were excluded for various reasons, mostly due to the fact that they were not case controlled. The two included studies were those already discussed above (Crump and Natkin 1970; Spili et al. 2005). Despite several differences between the two studies, namely, the different instruments and techniques employed in treatment as well as the difference in treatment setting, Panitvisai et al. (2010) combined the data through meta-analysis, with the main justifications being the similarity in study design and the fact that endodontic outcomes have not changed considerably in preceding three decades. When the data from the two case-controlled studies were combined, no significant difference was found in healing with or without the presence of a retained instrument, with a 95% confidence interval of −0.05 to 0.06. The authors pointed out that despite the relatively small sample size, due to the review being based on only two articles, the narrow confidence interval would suggest that larger samples would not alter the results. The authors concluded that, based on these findings, there was no significant reduction in prognosis when fractured endodontic instruments were retained in canals, although this may not be fully applicable to general practice dentistry.

However, a controversy concerning this review and meta-analysis is the decision to pool the results from the two studies despite their differences. While the authors' justification was logical, some authors (Murad and Murray 2011) have expressed some uneasiness given the vastly different materials, instruments, treating clinicians (students vs. endodontists), and even caliber of patients (the authors suggested that patients suitable for treatment by dental students would theoretically present with more straightforward cases than those referred for specialist treatment). Other issues have been pointed out about the quality of the analyzed studies themselves including not using power calculations to determine sample size and, in the case of Spili et al. (2005), not matching for variables such as voids, level of canal filling, root resorptions, and perforations. Importantly, both these issues are a direct consequence of the infrequency of retained fractured instruments, which makes achieving large sample sizes incredibly difficult and unrealistic; indeed case-controlled studies are ideal for such rare occurrences (Haapasalo 2016). The other issue was the applicability of the finding regarding treatment provided by two specific subgroups (students and specialists) to everyday dental practice. Murad and Murray (2011) recommended that a randomized controlled trial would be possible given that "most fractured instrument" cases make their way to private endodontists or specialist units and cite one paper (Cujé et al. 2010) as support for their opinion. Unfortunately, such opinions ignore the fact that lower levels of evidence are not weak evidence, merely one step toward best evidence (Haapasalo 2016). In fact, Cujé et al. (2010) made no such claim and actually stated that "the results should not be generalized and may not be valid for other groups or communities of general dental practitioners"; this paper only reported the success rate of removal of retained fractured instrument fragments but did not present healing outcomes. Further, that opinion of "most fractured instruments" is not based on the evidence concerning fracture prevalence as reported in detail above. Consequently, to even consider a randomized controlled trial for deriving evidence concerning outcome of cases with retained fractured instruments is unrealistic, and the ethical issues alone would make such a study impossible (Haapasalo 2016).

However, an important observation by Cujé et al. (2010) was that attempting to remove fractured instruments carries risks of root and root canal damage as has been convincingly confirmed in the literature (Hülsmann and Schinkel 1999; Ward et al. 2003a, b; Souter and Messer 2005; Suter et al. 2005; Parashos and Messer 2006; Rhodes 2007; Cheung 2009; Nevares et al. 2012). Hence, case-controlled studies realistically and ethically provide the highest level of evidence possible in such investigations.

8.6 Practical Considerations

An interesting way of looking at the problem of fractured instruments is assessing the effect of fractured instruments on bacterial penetration. Saunders et al. (2004) performed an ex vivo study to assess whether a fluted rotary NiTi instrument that was fractured in a root canal would allow quicker penetration of bacteria than the same length of gutta-percha and sealer. A size 40 ProFile instrument was fractured in such a way that a 3 mm segment remained in the apical third of the root. The root canals were subsequently filled with gutta-percha and Roth sealer using lateral compaction up to the level of the fractured instrument. The study found that the presence of a 3 mm fragment of a NiTi instrument did not enhance or slow the penetration of bacteria when compared with the normally obturated group. These findings were confirmed by a later study using K3 rotary NiTi instruments and AH26 sealer, in which no significant difference in bacterial penetration could be observed (Mohammadi and Khademi 2006). Such studies may go some way in explaining the findings of Fox et al. (1972) with their intentionally fractured files. However, the variety of contemporary instruments and techniques would make such an approach obsolete except perhaps in the most unusual anatomical complexities.

There are no studies in the literature that record fractured instrument outcomes in relation to the size of instrument fractured or the stage of treatment in which an instrument is fractured relative to the overall treatment sequence. Logically, clinical reality is that a retained fractured instrument that cannot be bypassed will limit access to the apical part of the canal, which will not allow appropriate canal shaping and disinfection (Lin et al. 2005; Simon et al. 2008). In some instances, there is almost no choice other than to attempt instrument removal (Fig. 8.1). Persistence of microorganisms in this critical apical part of the root canal system will result in persistence of disease (Siqueira 2001). Therefore, an important consideration is the stage of the RCT that the instrument fractured (Molyvdas et al. 2001; Spili et al. 2005; Madarati et al. 2013; Torabinejad and Johnson 2015). However, if an

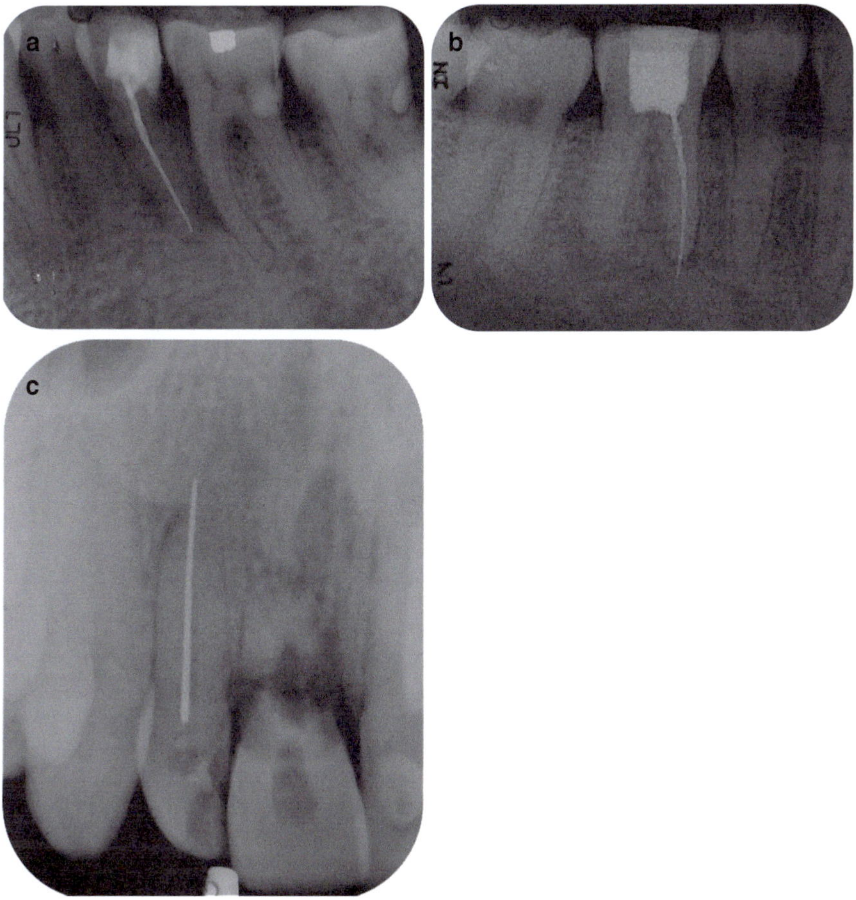

Fig. 8.1 Examples where the entire length of a 35/0.04 rotary NiTi instrument (**a**, **b**) and a SS hand file (**c**) have been fractured and retrieval is essentially mandatory but fortunately not too complicated (**a**, **b**, Courtesy Dr. J. Brichko)

instrument is fractured in the final stages of canal shaping (Figs. 8.2 and 8.3), at which point the apical canal has, for all intents and purposes, been adequately shaped and disinfected, then prognosis can be presumed to be better than the case in which there is a preoperative periapical radiolucency and a small instrument fractures during glide path preparation. Further, where the RCT is completed to a high technical standard in a tooth with no evidence of apical periodontitis, then the retained fractured instrument will not significantly reduce prognosis (Saunders et al. 2004; Spili et al. 2005; McGuigan et al. 2013). Hence, for instrument fracture in cases of vital pulps or in cases of infected necrotic pulps before radiographic evidence of apical periodontitis indicates long-standing infection (Fig. 8.4), the outcomes can be predicted to be favorable (Seltzer et al. 1967; Lin et al. 2005).

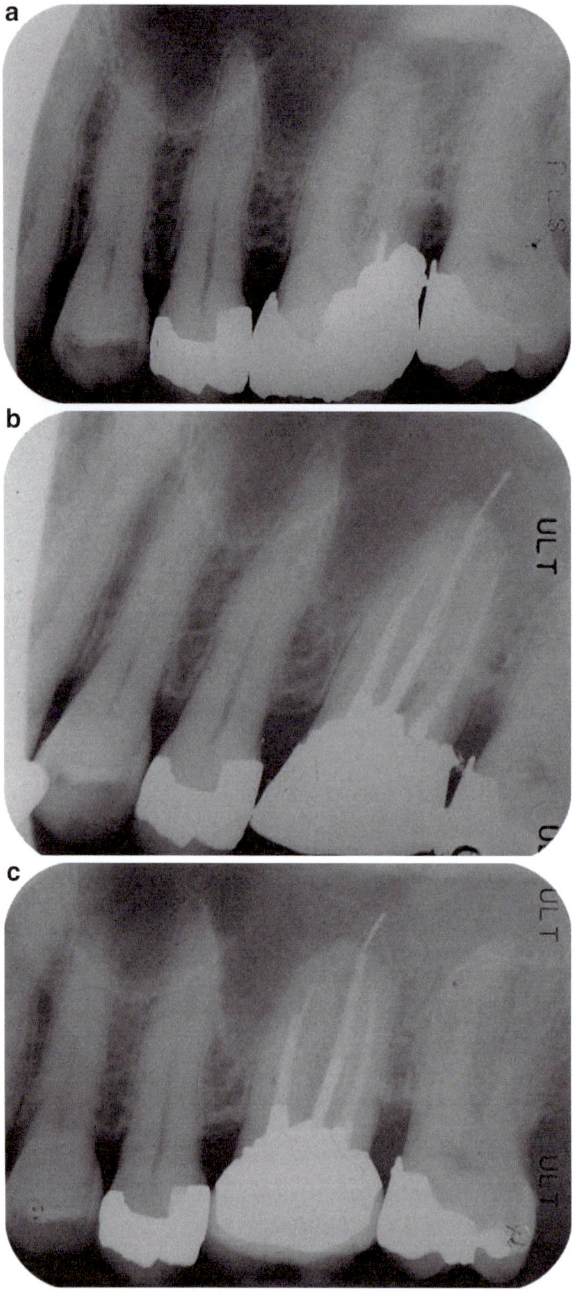

Fig. 8.2 (**a**) Preoperative radiograph of tooth 26 with calcified root canals and evidence of apical periodontitis around the palatal root. (**b**) During endodontic treatment, a 25/0.04 taper rotary NiTi instrument was fractured in the mesiobuccal canal. An attempt to remove the fractured instrument with ultrasonics resulted in part of the fragment fracturing off and relocating in the palatal canal and extending beyond the apex. The palatal canal had previously been prepared to a size 60/0.04 taper. (**c**) Four-year review showed healing

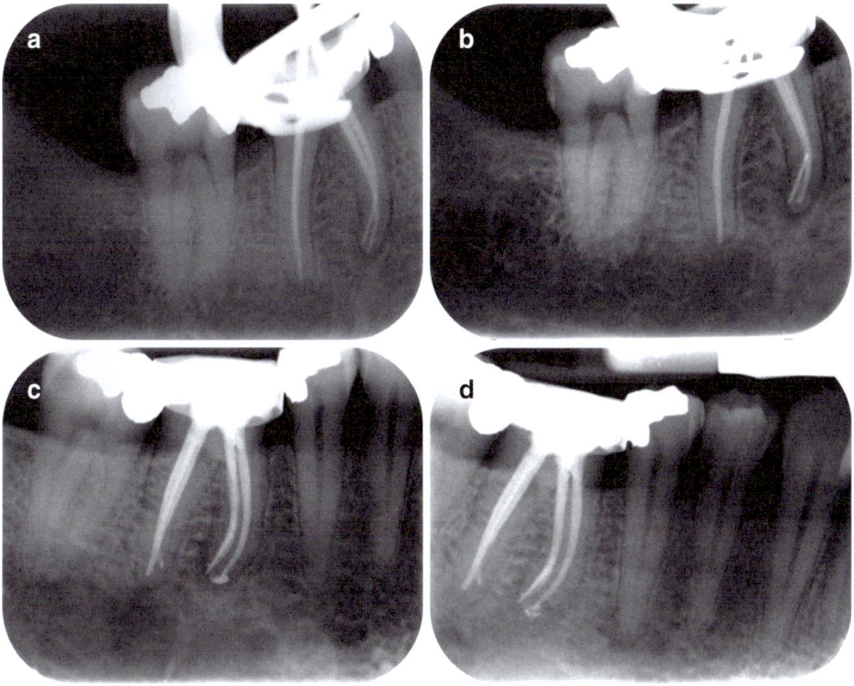

Fig. 8.3 (**a**) Tooth 46 with three canals prepared and master gutta point selection. (**b**) One month later at the second visit, a 35/0.04 taper instrument fractured in the mesiobuccal canal while being used by hand to remove the intracanal dressing. (**c**) The instrument was unable to be removed but was bypassed and the root filling completed. (**d**) One-year review shows apical healing (Courtesy Dr. P. Spili)

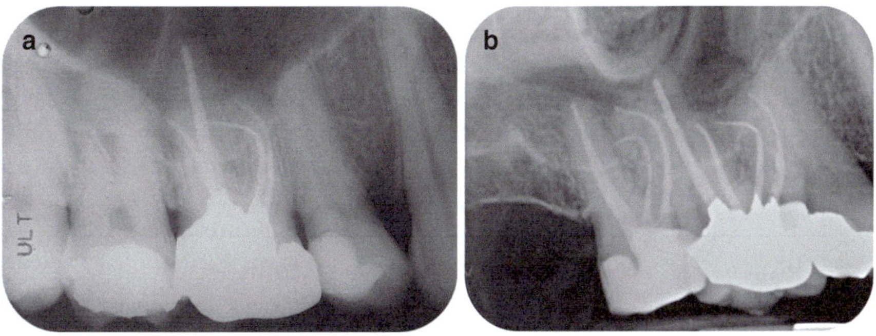

Fig. 8.4 (**a**) Tooth 16 endodontically treated subsequent to a diagnosis of irreversible pulpitis. A 25/0.4 taper rotary NiTi instrument was fractured at working length in the accessory mesiobuccal canal which appears to be a separate root. (**b**) Pathosis-free after 15 years; note tooth 17 had a similar anatomy

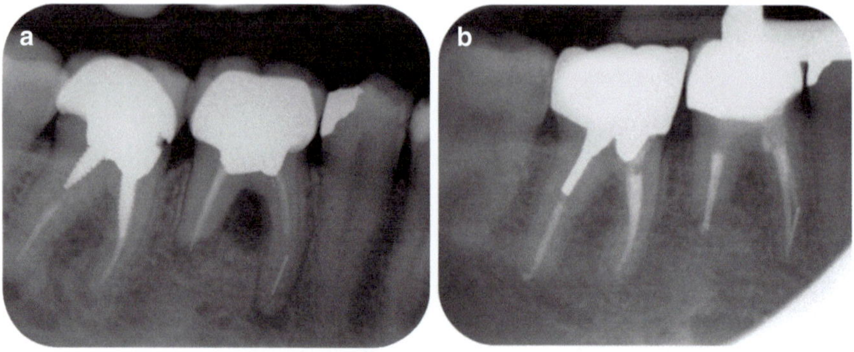

Fig. 8.5 (**a**) Fractured instrument in the mesiobuccal root of tooth 46 which was too deep to justify further dentine removal in an already compromised tooth. Location and negotiation of the mesiolingual canal allowed access to the apical root canal system below the point at which the canals joined. (**b**) The 5-year review shows apical healing. NB: an original furcal perforation was sealed with MTA (Courtesy Dr. M. Rahimi)

However, in cases with preoperative apical periodontitis where instrument fracture occurs very early in the RCT, then the apical portion of the root canal system has likely not been adequately disinfected (Kerekes and Tronstad 1979; Simon et al. 2008). In such situations the logical and most conservative option is to attempt to bypass the instrument (Figs. 8.5 and 8.6), followed by obturating the canal to the level of the fractured instrument (Fors and Berg 1986; Al-Fouzan 2003; Parashos and Messer 2006; Altundasar et al. 2008; Taneja et al. 2012; Shahabinejad et al. 2013; Brito-Junior et al. 2014). However, the type of instrument fragment retained and form of obturation may influence the seal (Altundasar et al. 2008; Taneja et al. 2012). Instrument designs that lead to compaction of dentinal debris within the flutes may be more likely to allow microleakage (Altundasar et al. 2008), although this may be partially countered by using thermoplasticized gutta-percha techniques above the instrument fragment (Altundasar et al. 2008; Taneja et al. 2012). Despite the advances in techniques and equipment to remove instrument fragments from root canals (Ruddle 2004; Yang et al. 2017), the aim should be to avoid any attempts to remove the instrument fragments that require sacrificing dentine (Fig. 8.7) leading to increased fracture susceptibility (Hülsmann and Schinkel 1999; Ward et al. 2003a, b; Souter and Messer 2005; Suter et al. 2005; Rhodes 2007; Nevares et al. 2012; Garg and Grewal 2016). While newer technologically advanced burs and techniques continue to be developed, by definition they require the removal of sound dentine (Yang et al. 2017).

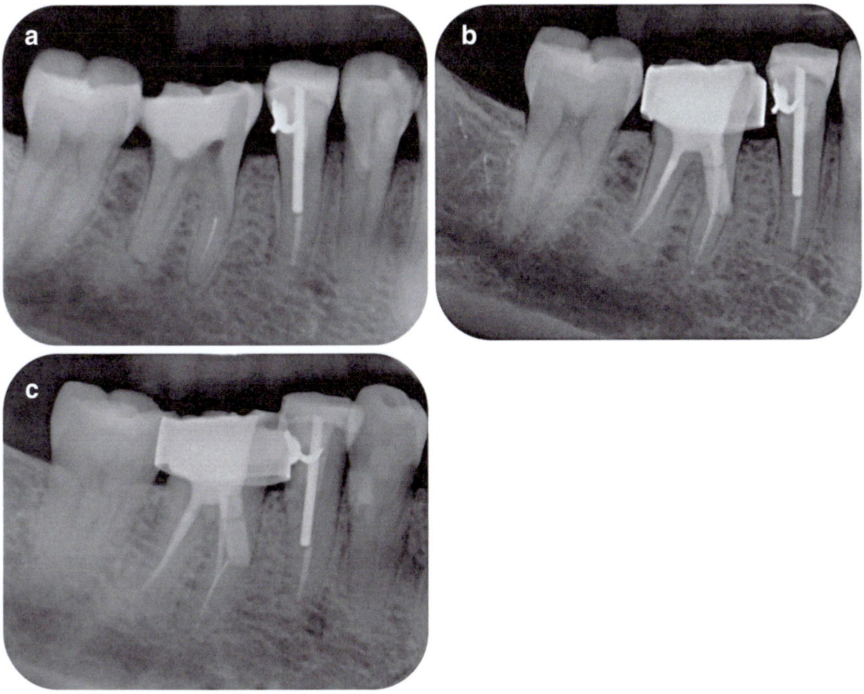

Fig. 8.6 (**a**) Preoperative radiograph of tooth 46 with fractured rotary NiTi instrument in the mesiolingual canal. The referring practitioner attempted to remove the fragment. (**b**, **c**) The instrument was able to be bypassed via the mesiobuccal canal which merged with the mesiolingual. While structural prognosis is very compromised, endodontic prognosis is favorable (Courtesy Dr. M. Weis)

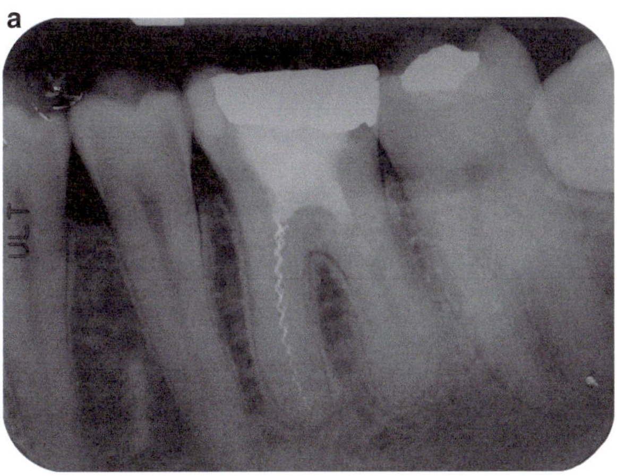

Fig. 8.7 (**a**) Lower molar with several lentulo-spiral burs fractured in both mesial canals, which had been there for some 10 years. While some of the smaller, more coronal fragments were retrieved, conservative attempts at removal of the full-length fragments were unsuccessful. The remaining fragments were bypassed up to a size 25 Hedström file; the mesiolingual canal was prepared to a size 35/0.04 NiTi by hand and the mesiobuccal to 25/0.04. (**b**) Canals obturated with gutta-percha and a thick mix of AH26 sealer. (**c**) Five-year review showing normal apical tissues (Courtesy Dr. O. Pope)

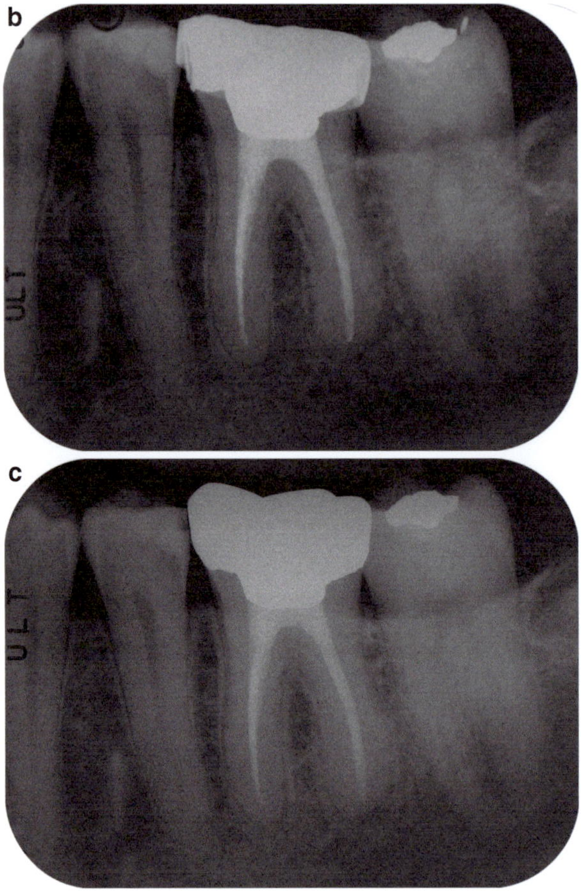

Fig. 8.7 (continued)

8.7 Recommendations

Overall, the current best evidence would suggest that there is no difference in outcome between cases with and without fractured instruments. However, it must be acknowledged that almost all the evidence on the impact of fractured instruments on prognosis looks at instruments which remain in canals presumably after at least some attempt to bypass them or to remove them. Therefore, if an attempt at fractured instrument bypass or removal will not structurally compromise the tooth (Parashos and Messer 2006), then it should be attempted because often the circumstances applicable to a particular case, concerning intraradicular infection, are unpredictable. However, on the other hand, given the overall lack of convincing evidence to condemn teeth with retained fractured instruments and that higher-level evidence strategies for this particular clinical complication are unrealistic, it seems prudent to adopt a conservative approach as suggested by Crump and Natkin (1970) and Fox et al. (1972). Such a conservative approach should consist of filling the root canal to the level of the fractured instrument and standard periodic review to follow progress.

Despite the obvious but probably unfounded anxiety caused by the unintentional fracturing of an endodontic instrument in a root canal system (Frank 1983; Torabinejad and Johnson 2015), the implications of a fractured instrument are realistically no different and, if anything, less significant than those of any other intraoperative complication (Parashos and Messer 2006). A far greater clinical crime is producing technically poor endodontic treatment overall with its attendant poor outcomes (Friedman 2002; Farzaneh et al. 2004a, b). An instrument fragment, in itself, is rarely the direct cause of the problem; it does, however, limit access to the apical part of the canal, compromising disinfection and obturation (Panitvisai et al. 2010). The clinical situation (existence of periapical lesion), stage of canal preparation when the instrument fracture occurred (canal infection) (Fors and Berg 1986), canal anatomy, fragment position, and type of fractured instrument can significantly influence prognosis and the approach to management (Parashos and Messer 2006). The presence of a preoperative periapical lesion, rather than the instrument per se, is a more clinically significant prognostic indicator (Spili et al. 2005). Should access apical to the instrument be required, an attempt to bypass the instrument should initially be considered. If this is unsuccessful, consideration should be given to various biological and biomechanical factors (Solomonov et al. 2014) including loss of root dentine and presence or otherwise of signs and symptoms, before undertaking more invasive measures. Importantly, as clinicians, we must recognize that the biology of the instrument fracture is one thing, but quite another is the psychological aspects that can affect both dentist and patient (Frank 1983; Torabinejad and Johnson 2015). Furthermore, as clinicians, it is incumbent upon us to remind patients that we treat dental diseases and we do not, and cannot, "fix" teeth.

Finally, "It's a pity that it happens, but it doesn't really matter" (Dr Peter Spili, personal communication).

References

Alapati SB, Brantley WA, Svec TA, Powers JM, Nusstein JM, Daehn GS. SEM observations of nickel-titanium rotary endodontic instruments that fractured during clinical use. J Endod. 2005;31(1):40–3.

Al-Fouzan KS. Incidence of rotary ProFile instrument fracture and the potential for bypassing in vivo. Int Endod J. 2003;36(12):864–7.

Altundasar E, Sahin C, Ozcelik B, Cehreli ZC. Sealing properties of different obturation systems applied over apically fractured rotary nickel-titanium files. J Endod. 2008;34(2):194–7.

Arens FC, Hoen MM, Steiman HR, Dietz GC Jr. Evaluation of single-use rotary nickel-titanium instruments. J Endod. 2003;29(10):664–6.

Bergenholtz G, Lekholm U, Milthon R, Heden G, Ödesjö B, Engström B. Retreatment of endodontic fillings. Scand J Dent Res. 1979;87(3):217–24.

Bird DC, Chambers D, Peters OA. Usage parameters of nickel-titanium rotary instruments: a survey of endodontists in the United States. J Endod. 2009;35(9):1193–7.

Brito-Junior M, Silva-Sousa YTC, Bruniera JFB, Camilo CC, Faria-e-Silva AL, Saquy PC. Obturation over an S1 ProTaper instrument fragment in a mandibular molar with three years follow-up. Braz Dent J. 2014;25(6):571–4.
Cheung GSP. Instrument fracture: mechanisms, removal of fragments, and clinical outcomes. Endod Top. 2009;16(1):1–26.
Concato J, Shah N, Horwitz RI. Randomized, controlled trials, observational studies, and the hierarchy of research designs. N Engl J Med. 2000;342(25):1887–92.
Crump MC, Natkin E. Relationship of broken root canal instruments to endodontic case prognosis: a clinical investigation. J Am Dent Assoc. 1970;80(6):1341–7.
Cujé J, Bargholz C, Hülsmann M. The outcome of retained instrument removal in a specialist practice. Int Endod J. 2010;43(7):545–54.
Cvek M, Granath L, Lundberg M. Failures and healing in endodontically treated non-vital anterior teeth with posttraumatically reduced pulpal lumen. Acta Odontol. 1982;40(4):223–8.
de Chevigny C, Dao TT, Basrani BR, Marquis V, Farzaneh M, Abitbol S, Friedman S. Treatment outcome in endodontics: the Toronto study--phase 4: initial treatment. J Endod. 2008;34(3):258–63.
Engström B, Lundberg M. The correlation between positive culture and the prognosis of root canal therapy after pulpectomy. Odontol Revy. 1965;16(3):193–203.
Engström B, Hård L, Segerstad AF, Ramström G, Frostell G. Correlation of positive cultures with the prognosis for root canal treatment. Odontol Revy. 1964;15:257–70.
Farzaneh M, Abitbol S, Lawrence HP, Friedman S. Treatment outcome in endodontics – The Toronto Study. Phase II: initial treatment. J Endod. 2004a;30(5):302–9.
Farzaneh M, Abitbol S, Friedman S. Treatment outcome in endodontics: The Toronto Study. Phases I and II: orthograde retreatment. J Endod. 2004b;30(9):627–33.
Fors UGH, Berg JO. Endodontic treatment of root canals obstructed by foreign objects. Int Endod J. 1986;19(1):2–10.
Fox J, Moodnik R, Greenfield E, Atkinson J. Filing root canals with files radiographic evaluation of 304 cases. N Y State Dent J. 1972;38(3):154–7.
Frank A. The dilemma of the fractured instrument. J Endod. 1983;9(12):515–6.
Friedman S (1998) Treatment outcome and prognosis of endodontic therapy. In: Ørstavik D, Pitt Ford TR, eds. Essential endodontology – prevention and treatment of apical periodontitis. Oxford: Blackwell Science, pp 367–91.
Friedman S. Prognosis of initial endodontic therapy. Endod Top. 2002;2:59–88.
Fu M, Zhang Z, Hou B. Removal of broken files from root canals by using ultrasonic techniques combined with dental microscope: a retrospective analysis of treatment outcome. J Endod. 2011;37(5):619–22.
Garg H, Grewal MS. Cone-beam computed tomography volumetric analysis and comparison of dentin structure loss after retrieval of separated instrument by using ultrasonic EMS and ProUltra tips. J Endod. 2016;42(11):1693–8.
Grahnén H, Hansson L. The prognosis of pulp and root canal therapy. Odontol Revy. 1961;12:146–65.
Grossman LI. Fate of endodontically treated teeth with fractured root canal instruments. J Br Endod Soc. 1968;2(3):35–7.
Grossman LI. Guidelines for the prevention of fracture of root canal instruments. Oral Surg Oral Med Oral Pathol. 1969;28(5):746–52.
Haapasalo M. Level of evidence in endodontics: what does it mean? Endod Top. 2016;34(1):30–41.
Hülsmann M, Schinkel I. Influence of several factors on the success or failure of removal of fractured instruments from the root canal. Endod Dent Traumatol. 1999;15(6):252–8.
Huumonen S, Ørstavik D. Radiological aspects of apical periodontitis. Endod Top. 2002;1(1):3–25.
Imura N, Pinheiro ET, Gomes BP, Zaia AA, Ferraz CC, Souza-Filho FJ. The outcome of endodontic treatment: a retrospective study of 2000 cases performed by a specialist. J Endod. 2007;33(11):1278–82.
Ingle JI, Glick D. The Washington study. In: Ingle JI, editor. Endodontics. 1st ed. Philadelphia: Lea and Febiger; 1965. p. 54–77.

Iqbal MK, Kohli MR, Kim JS. A retrospective clinical study of incidence of root canal instrument separation in an endodontics graduate program: a Penn Endo database study. J Endod. 2006;32(11):1048–52.
Kerekes K, Tronstad L. Long-term results of endodontic treatment performed with a standardized technique. J Endod. 1979;5(3):83–90.
Kim MY, Lin J, White R, Niederman R. Benchmarking the endodontic literature. J Endod. 2001;27(7):470–3.
Lin LM, Rosenberg PA, Lin J. Do procedural errors cause endodontic treatment failure? J Am Dent Assoc. 2005;136(2):187–93, quiz 231.
Locke M, Thomas MB, Dummer PMH. A survey of adoption of endodontic nickel-titanium rotary instrumentation part 1: general dental practitioners in Wales. Br Dent J. 2013;214(3):E6(1–10).
Madarati AA, Watts DC, Qualtrough AJE. Opinions and attitudes of endodontists and general dental practitioners in the UK towards the intracanal fracture of endodontic instruments: part 1. Int Endod J. 2008;41(8):693–701.
Madarati AA, Hunter MJ, Dummer PMH. Management of intracanal separated instruments. J Endod. 2013;39(5):569–81.
McGuigan M, Louca C, Duncan HF. The impact of fractured endodontic instruments on treatment outcome. Br Dent J. 2013;214(6):285–9.
Mohammadi Z, Khademi AA. Effect of a separated rotary instrument on bacterial penetration of obturated root canals. J Clin Dent. 2006;17(5):131–3.
Molven O, Halse A. Success rates for gutta-percha and Kloroperka N-Ø root fillings made by undergraduate students: radiographic findings after 10-17 years. Int Endod J. 1988;21(4):243–50.
Molyvdas I, Lambrianidis T, Zervas P, Veis A. Clinical study on the prognosis of endodontic treatment of teeth with broken endodontic instruments. Stoma. 1992;20:63–72 (in Greek). Cited in Lambrianidis TP "Fractured instrument" in Risk management of root canal treatment. Thessaloniki: University Studio Press; 2001. p. 228–37.
Murad M, Murray C. Impact of retained separated endodontic instruments during root canal treatment on clinical outcomes remains uncertain. J Evid Based Dent Pract. 2011;11(2):87–8.
Nevares G, Cunha RS, Zuolo ML, Bueno CE. Success rates for removing or bypassing fractured instruments: a prospective clinical study. J Endod. 2012;38(4):442–4.
Ng YL, Mann V, Gulabivala K. A prospective study of the factors affecting outcomes of nonsurgical root canal treatment: part 1: periapical health. Int Endod J. 2011;44(7):583–609.
Panitvisai P, Parunnit P, Sathorn C, Messer HH. Impact of a retained instrument on treatment outcome: a systematic review and meta-analysis. J Endod. 2010;36(5):775–80.
Parashos P, Messer HH. Questionnaire survey on the use of rotary nickel-titanium endodontic instruments by Australian dentists. Int Endod J. 2004;37(4):249–59.
Parashos P, Messer HH. Rotary NiTi instrument fracture and its consequences. J Endod. 2006;32(11):1031–43.
Parashos P, Gordon I, Messer HH. Factors influencing defects of rotary nickel-titanium endodontic instruments after clinical use. J Endod. 2004;30(10):722–5.
Pruett JP, Clement DJ, Carnes DL Jr. Cyclic fatigue testing of nickel-titanium endodontic instruments. J Endod. 1997;23(2):77–85.
Ramirez-Salomon M, Soler-Bientz R, de la Garza-Gonzalez R, Palacios-Garza CM. Incidence of Lightspeed separation and the potential for bypassing. J Endod. 1997;23(9):586–7.
Rhodes JS. Essential elements of endodontic treatment: removal of fractured instruments. Endod Prac. 2007;9:6–12.
Ruddle CJ. Nonsurgical retreatment. J Endod. 2004;30(12):827–45.
Sackett D, Richardson W, Rosenberg W, Haynes R. Evidence-based medicine: how to practice and teach EBM. London: Churchill Livingstone; 1997.
Sathorn C, Parashos P, Messer HH. How useful is root canal culturing in predicting treatment outcome? J Endod. 2007;33(3):220–5.

Sattapan B, Nervo GJ, Palamara JE, Messer HH. Defects in rotary nickel-titanium files after clinical use. J Endod. 2000;26(3):161–5.
Saunders JL, Eleazer PD, Zhang P, Michalek S. Effect of a separated instrument on bacterial penetration of obturated root canals. J Endod. 2004;30(3):177–9.
Savani GM, Sabbah W, Sedgley CM, Whitten B. Current trends in endodontic treatment by general dental practitioners: report of a United States national survey. J Endod. 2014;40(5):618–24.
Seltzer S, Bender IB, Smith J, Freedman I, Nazimov H. Endodontic failures: an analysis based on clinical, roentgenographic and histologic findings. Part II. Oral Surg Oral Med Oral Pathol. 1967;23(4):517–30.
Shahabinejad H, Ghassemi A, Pishbin L, Shahravan A. Success of ultrasonic technique in removing fractured rotary nickel-titanium endodontic instruments from root canals and its effect on the required force for root fracture. J Endod. 2013;39(6):824–8.
Shen Y, Cheung GS, Peng B, Haapasalo M. Defects in nickel-titanium instruments after clinical use: part 2—fractographic analysis of fractured surface in a cohort study. J Endod. 2009;35(1):133–6.
Simon S, Machtou P, Tomson P, Adams N, Lumley P. Influence of fractured instruments on the success rate of endodontic treatment. Dent Update. 2008;35(3):172–9.
Singh K, Aggarwal A, Gupta SK. Root canal instrument materials – metallurgical prospective: a mini review. J Adv Med Dent Sci Res. 2016;4:69–73.
Siqueira JF Jr. Aetiology of root canal treatment failure: why well-treated teeth can fail (literature review). Int Endod J. 2001;34(1):1–10.
Sjögren U, Hagglund B, Sundqvist G, Wing K. Factors affecting the long-term results of endodontic treatment. J Endod. 1990;16(10):498–504.
Smith CS, Setchell DJ, Harty FJ. Factors influencing the success of conventional root canal therapy – a five-year retrospective study. Int Endod J. 1993;26(6):321–33.
Solomonov M, Webber M, Keinan D. Fractured endodontic instrument: a clinical dilemma. Retrieve, bypass or entomb? N Y State Dent J. 2014;80(5):50–2.
Souter NJ, Messer HH. Complications associated with fractured file removal using an ultrasonic technique. J Endod. 2005;31(6):450–2.
Spanaki-Voreadi AP, Kerezoudis NP, Zinelis S. Failure mechanism of ProTaper Ni-Ti rotary instruments during clinical use: fractographic analysis. Int Endod J. 2006;39(3):171–8.
Spili P, Parashos P, Messer HH. The impact of instrument fracture on outcome of endodontic treatment. J Endod. 2005;31(12):845–50.
Strindberg LZ. The dependence of the results of pulp therapy on certain factors – an analytical study based on radiographic and clinical follow-up examinations. Acta Odont Scand. 1956;14(Suppl. 21):1–175.
Suter B, Lussi A, Sequeira P. Probability of removing fractured instruments from root canals. Int Endod J. 2005;38(2):112–3.
Taneja S, Chadha R, Gupta R, Gupta A. Comparative evaluation of sealing properties of different obturation systems placed over apically fractured rotary NiTi files. J Conserv Dent. 2012;15(1):36–40.
Thomas MB, Locke M, Dummer PMH. A survey of adoption of endodontic nickel-titanium rotary instrumentation part 2: community and hospital dental practitioners in Wales. Br Dent J. 2013;214(3):E7(1–5).
Torabinejad M, Johnson JD. Procedural accidents. In: Torabinejad M, Walton RE, Fouad AF, editors. Endodontics, principles and practice. 5th ed. St. Louis: Elsevier Saunders; 2015. p. 338–54.
Tzanetakis GN, Kontakiotis EG, Maurikou DV, Marzelou MP. Prevalence and management of instrument fracture in the postgraduate endodontic program at the Dental School of Athens: a five-year retrospective clinical study. J Endod. 2008;34(6):675–8.
Ungerechts C, Bårdsen A, Fristad I. Instrument fracture in root canals-where, why, when and what? A study from a student clinic. Int Endod J. 2014;47(2):183–90.
Van Nieuwenhuysen J-P, Aouar M, D'Hoore W. Retreatment or radiographic monitoring in endodontics. Int Endod J. 1994;27(2):75–81.

Ward JR, Parashos P, Messer HH. Evaluation of an ultrasonic technique to remove fractured rotary nickel-titanium endodontic instruments from root canals: an experimental study. J Endod. 2003a;29(11):756–63.

Ward JR, Parashos P, Messer HH. Evaluation of an ultrasonic technique to remove fractured rotary nickel-titanium endodontic instruments from root canals: clinical cases. J Endod. 2003b;29(11):764–7.

Wolcott S, Wolcott J, Ishley D, Kennedy W, Johnson S, Minnich S, Meyers J. Separation incidence of protaper rotary instruments: a large cohort clinical evaluation. J Endod. 2006;32(12):1139–41.

Yang Q, Shen Y, Huang D, Zhou X, Gao Y, Haapasalo M. Evaluation of two trephine techniques for removal of fractured rotary nickel-titanium instruments from root canals. J Endod. 2017;43(1):116–20.

Prevention

9

Theodor Lambrianidis

9.1 Introduction

Several nonsurgical and surgical techniques have been proposed and clinically applied for the management of instrument fragments. These management attempts can be considered as unpredictable and may include the possibility of further iatrogenic complications. Thus, clinicians must consistently take all necessary precautions during root canal treatment (RCT) or retreatment procedures to prevent instrument fracture. Since prevention is the best key to avoid iatrogenic errors, it should be emphasized that instrument fracture in the root canal could be reduced if the following guidelines are carefully considered and adopted in clinical practice.

Recommended guidelines to be carefully considered:

- Thorough preoperative clinical and radiographic examination of the anatomy of the tooth to be treated must be performed.
- Assessment of the "difficulty level" in endodontic instrumentation to enable the selection and use of the most appropriate instruments and root canal preparation technique(s). Particular attention should be paid to teeth with a challenging anatomy (S-shaped curves, calcifications, and dilacerations). In this assessment line, it should be kept in mind that the location of the curvature is as important as the severity of the curvature (McSpadden 2007) and that the radius of the curvature is the most significant factor in rotary file failure (Booth et al. 2003). In abruptly curved or dilacerated canals, instrumentation with rotary files should be avoided (McGuigan et al. 2013).
- Adequate/appropriate access cavity should be prepared to ensure unhindered straight-line access of the endodontic instruments to the apex.

T. Lambrianidis, D.D.S., Ph.D.
Department of Endodontology, Dental School, Aristotle University of Thessaloniki, Thessaloniki, Greece
e-mail: thlampri@dent.auth.gr

T. Lambrianidis (ed.), *Management of Fractured Endodontic Instruments*,
DOI 10.1007/978-3-319-60651-4_9

- Establishment of secure and comfortable finger rests is essential prior to any manipulations.
- Endodontic instruments should be carefully inspected prior to, during, and after use, preferably under magnification, for any signs of fracture or plastic deformation. Defects that have been observed after use under clinical conditions include fracture, unwinding, reverse winding, reverse winding with tightening of the spirals, bending, or a combination of the above (Sattapan et al. 2000). However, visual inspection is not a reliable method for evaluating whether to continue using a nickel titanium (NiTi) instrument or discard it. This is because there are studies where a low percentage of instruments ranging from 3.8 up to 24% withdrawn after use under clinical conditions presented fracture with signs of plastic deformation (Zinelis and Margelos 2003; Parashos et al. 2004a; Alapati et al. 2005; Kosti et al. 2011). These findings, combined with a fractographic analysis of the fractured surfaces under SEM, lead to the conclusion that fracture in in vivo conditions is most probably caused by a single overloading of the rotating instrument and not related to a gradual degradation caused by fatigue (Zinelis and Margelos 2003; Parashos et al. 2004a; Kosti et al. 2011).
- The incorporation of new types of instruments and, in particular, new rotary NiTi file systems and/or new techniques requires a learning curve. Recognition of the properties and limitations of the series of instruments to be used is required. Additionally, extensive practice on plastic blocks and/or preferably on extracted human teeth before clinical application is absolutely essential. This applies even to the most experienced clinician. Proper tuition and ex vivo training for mastering operators' competence are crucial for avoiding or minimizing the incidence of instrument locking, deformation, and fracture (Barbakow and Lutz 1997; Mandel et al. 1999; Yared et al. 2002, 2003; Zinelis and Margelos 2003). Each instrument is used only for the purpose it has been designed and manufactured for, always in the right way conforming to its specifications.
- NiTi systems should be used within safe torque and speed limits for optimal performance, provided by the manufacturer.
- NiTi instruments should be used exerting very slight apical pressure and always for a few seconds only (Machtou and Martin 1997). A prolonged use of the file would increase the contact surface with the canal walls. The instrument would then be subjected to high-level torque and fracture may occur (Machtou and Martin 1997).
- The clinician should grip the contra-angle firmly to prevent screwing of the tip of the NiTi instrument into the root canal walls. This precaution should be taken even when instruments rotate at low speed.
- Rotary endodontic instruments have non-cutting tips; thus, they should be advanced only into an explored and patent canal section. This is particularly recommended for the apical third of narrow and/or calcified canals. In these areas the tip of the NiTi instrument might encounter a root canal smaller than its diameter and lock leading to increased risk of fracture. In cases where resistance is encountered, rotary instrumentation should stop and SS hand files should be used to further negotiate the apical path. Correction/increase of the coronal taper

may often be beneficial in such cases. Coronal preflaring with hand files was reported to allow for a significantly increased number of rotary file uses before the occurrence of fracture (Berutti et al. 2004).

- Instrument should be advanced down the canal by a "pecking" or "watch-winding" motion (for hand instruments). These movements regularly disengage the instrument and allow it to return to its normal state before continuing the preparation.
- Instruments in the root canal should always be used in a wet environment.
- Pre-curved instruments should be used in curved root canal. The level of pre-curvature depends on the radiographic appearance of the degree of curvature of the root. Pre-curvature also prevents ledging, perforations, creation of false canal(s), and transportation of the foramen. A marked rubber stop should be oriented to match the file curvature.
- Instruments should always be used in sequence of sizes without skipping sizes.
- Instrumentation should be performed with instruments of the same manufacturing company and of the same design. Despite the existence of instrument standardization guidelines and the evolutions in manufacturing, significant variations in the diameters of instruments of nominally the same size are reported to exist within or between different manufacturers for both SS and NiTi instruments (Kerekes 1979; Serene and Loadholt 1984; Cormier et al. 1988; Johnson and Beatty 1988; Keate and Wong 1990; Stenman and Spangberg 1993; Zinelis et al. 2002; Lask et al. 2006; Hatch et al. 2008; Kim et al. 2014). Taper and size differences were mostly within the tolerance limit of ±0.02%, set by ISO 3630-1, 1992 specification (Zinelis et al. 2002). However, under such tolerance limits, there is a high possibility of either size overlapping or of great differences between two sequential sizes. Therefore, switching from the instruments of one company to the instruments of another in the course of the preparation of a root canal is risky and unreasonably complicates clinical manipulations. ISO standardization does not include the design and size of the handle of endodontic instruments. Differences in the design of the handle, combined with the effects of gloves on tactile discrimination (Masserann 1971; Girdler et al. 1987; Chandler and Bloxham 1990), can influence tactile sensitivity. A comparative study of the influence of the handle design on tactile sensitivity showed differences, although not statistically significant, and revealed a preference on the part of the practitioner for some types of handle design (Treble et al. 1993), an observation in favor of the view advocating the consistent use of instruments of the same manufacturing company. Instrument handle plastic sleeves that slip over handles to augment their size have been developed and advertised as increasing the operator's tactile sense. Despite the favorable comments by students participating in a trial evaluation of the two available sleeves, the octagonal Endoease (Precision Dental International, Chatsworth, CA, USA) and the hexagonal Endogrip (Svenska Dental AB, Solna, Sweden), the devices failed to deliver enhanced tactile discrimination (Warren and Chandler 1998). An electromyographic recording device was used to determine the influence of the handle diameter of endodontic instruments on forearm and hand muscles (Ozawa et al. 2001). Recordings

indicated that handle diameter has an effect on reaming time as well as on muscle activity, thus influencing operators' performance (Ozawa et al. 2001).

- Each instrument "should be rendered" loose in the root canal prior to the use of the next one.
- Care should be exercised to avoid instruments "cutting" with their entire length. The increased friction as a result of long engagement with canal walls results in an increased possibility of instrument fracture. Minimization of file engagement with root canal walls can be achieved by changing file tapers. Maximization of file engagement occurs if instrumentation with one file is followed by another of the same taper.
- During the use of an instrument, debris that has accumulated between its blades should be periodically removed. Thus the cutting flutes should be either (Parashos et al. 2004b):
  - Wiped with a sterilized gauge soaked in saline or an antiseptic solution (i.e., alcohol, sodium hypochlorite, 0.2% chlorhexidine) to remove debris and at the same time disinfect the instrument
  - Preferably wiped with a few vigorous strokes in a scouring or dense sponge soaked in a 0.2% chlorhexidine solution

The use of a sponge ensures that all sides of the instrument come into contact with the sponge simultaneously. Scouring sponges are the preferred sponges for the cleaning of rotary NiTi instruments because their coarse top layer consists of very fine, relatively stiff fibers that enter the instrument flutes, enabling effective removal of gross debris (Parashos et al. 2004b). Dense sponges and scouring sponges are preferable to porous sponges as they retain the chlorhexidine solution better (Parashos et al. 2004b). Natural sponges are unsuitable as a storage medium for endodontic instruments due to their large pore size. Moist sponges soaked with antimicrobial solution have been shown to be more effective in the mechanical cleaning of instruments when compared with dry sponges (Hubbard et al. 1975; Segall et al. 1977; Parashos et al. 2004b). The use of the sponge is also safer as wiping with gauze might result in a needlestick injury (Miller 2002; Zarra and Lambrianidis 2013). Endodontic sponges serving as a chairside storage and mechanical cleaning aid should be autoclaved before clinical use. Steam sterilization procedures are effective for sponges (Chan et al. 2016), and in an experimental study, they have actually provided the best results compared to chemical vapor sterilizers (chemiclaves) and dry heat sterilizers (Kuritani et al. 1993).

- Instruments should not be overused. This is mostly recommended for small-sized SS and NiTi instruments. These are extremely delicate and particularly susceptible to deformation-fracture. They should not be used therefore more than once or twice: they should be discarded very often even during their use in the same root canal (Ingle et al. 1985; Gabel et al. 1999; Bortnick et al. 2001). It may be prudent to view these instruments as disposables. There is still no consensus regarding a recommended number of uses for rotary instruments. Any decision to discard an instrument should take into account the fact that all uses of a file are not equal. A calcified canal stresses instruments more than a non-calcified one. The same applies to a curved canal as compared to a straight one. This is

Table 9.1 Cleaning protocol for endodontic instruments (Parashos et al. 2004b)

Steps	Procedure
First	Ten vigorous strokes in a scouring sponge soaked in 0.2% chlorhexidine solution
Second	30-min presoak in an enzymatic cleaning solution
Third	15-min ultrasonication in the same solution
Fourth	20-s rinse in running tap water

especially true when a NiTi rotary instrument is used in severe curvature conditions (Pruett et al. 1997). It is prudent to use new files in these cases. The policy of single-use endodontic instruments due to the difficulties encountered in their cleaning and sterilization is controversial. Those in favor of single-use instruments argue that reused instruments may act as a vehicle for disease transmission. They are particularly concerned about the prion protein, a pathogenic isoform of a common host cell receptor, which causes acquired iatrogenic Creutzfeldt-Jakob disease, a fatal neurodegenerative disease termed transmissible spongiform encephalopathy. The British and German dental associations, along with the Centers for Disease Control and Prevention and World Health Organization, regard such a policy as justifiable considering the risks posed by file reuse. The Joint AAE/CAE Special Committee on Single Use Endodontic Instruments in its final report in 2011 concluded "….. based upon best current scientific evidence and the very low risk of prion transmission to patients during endodontic treatment in the USA and Canada, the Special Committee on SUI feels that it is not currently warranted for clinicians to change the way in which they select endodontic files and reamers for re-use and sterilization (Hartwell et al. 2011). The Special Committee does recommend that practitioners prepare and sterilize instruments for re-use in accordance with 'best evidence' currently available" (McGibney 2016). A proposed (Parashos et al. 2004b) cleaning protocol for rotary nickel-titanium endodontic instruments that can be applied to all endodontic files (Table 9.1) and involves both mechanical and chemical cleaning procedures rendered, under experimental conditions, rotary NiTi files 100% free of stained debris. Therefore, these results do not support the recommendation for the single use of endodontic files based on an inability to clean files between uses.
- Sudden changes in rotary direction should be avoided.
- NiTi instruments should be inserted and withdrawn from a canal while rotating at a constant rotation speed.
- An instrument should never be burned in order to be sterilized.

9.2 Concluding Remarks

Prevention involves attention to detail and adherence to evidence-based approaches during endodontic procedures. Preventive measures reduce the frequency of instrument fracture and minimize the necessity for challenging management decisions.

Most contributory factors to endodontic instrument fracture are related to operator's clinical capacity and skills and can be minimized by proper training and extensive ex vivo practice prior to clinical application.

References

Alapati SB, Brantley WA, Svec TA, Powers JM, Nusstein JM, Daehn GS. SEM observations of nickel-titanium rotary endodontic instruments that fractured during clinical Use. J Endod. 2005;31(1):40–3.

Barbakow F, Lutz F. The 'Lightspeed' preparation technique evaluated by Swiss clinicians after attending continuing education courses. Int Endod J. 1997;30(1):46–50.

Berutti E, Negro AR, Lendini M, Pasqualini D. Influence of manual preflaring and torque on the failure rate of ProTaper rotary instruments. J Endod. 2004;30(4):228–30.

Booth JR, Scheetz JP, Lemons JE, Eleazer PD. A comparison of torque required to fracture three different nickel-titanium rotary instruments around curves of the same angle but of different radius when bound at the tip. J Endod. 2003;29(1):55–7.

Bortnick KL, Steiman HR, Ruskin A. Comparison of nickel-titanium file distortion using electric and air-driven handpieces. J Endod. 2001;27(1):57–9.

Chan HW, Tan KH, Dashper SG, Reynolds EC, Parashos P. Sterilization of rotary NiTi instruments within endodontic sponges. Int Endod J. 2016;49(9):850–7.

Chandler NP, Bloxham GP. Effect of gloves on tactile discrimination using an endodontic model. Int Endod J. 1990;23(2):97–9.

Cormier C, Von Fraunhofer J, Chamberlain J. A comparison of endodontic file quality and file dimensions. J Endod. 1988;14(3):138–42.

Gabel WP, Hoen M, Steiman HR, Pink FE, Dietz R. Effect of rotational speed on nickel-titanium file distortion. J Endod. 1999;25(11):752–4.

Girdler NM, Matthews RW, Scully C. Use and acceptability of rubber gloves for outpatient dental treatment. J Dent. 1987;15(5):209–12.

Hartwell G, Bowles W, Peters O, Peikoff M, Torneck C. Single use instruments. Chicago: Americal Association of Endodontists; 2011.

Hatch GW, Roberts S, Joyce AP, Runner R, McPherson JC III. Comparative study of the variability of 0.06 tapered rotary endodontic files to current taper standards. J Endod. 2008;34(4):463–5.

Hubbard TM Jr, Smyth RN, Pelleu GB Jr, Tenca JI. Chairside decontamination of endodontic files. Oral Surg Oral Med Oral Pathol. 1975;40(1):148–52.

Ingle J, Beveridge E, Glick D, Weichman J, Abou-Rass M. Modern endodontic therapy. In: Ingle JI, Taintor FJ, editors. Endodontics. 3rd ed. Philadelphia: Lea & Febiger; 1985. p. 1–53.

Johnson WB, Beatty RG. Clinical technique for the removal of root canal obstructions. J Am Dent Assoc. 1988;117(3):473–6.

Keate KC, Wong M. Comparison of endodontic file tip quality. J Endod. 1990;16(10):486–91.

Kerekes K. Evaluation of standardized root canal instruments and obturating points. J Endod. 1979;5(5):145–50.

Kim KW, Cho KM, Park SH, Choi KY, Karabucak B, Kim JW. A comparison of dimensional standard of several nickel-titanium rotary files. Restor Dent Endod. 2014;39(1):7–11.

Kosti E, Zinelis S, Molyvdas I, Lambrianidis T. Effect of root canal curvature on the failure incidence of ProFile rotary Ni-Ti endodontic instruments. Int Endod J. 2011;44(10):917–25.

Kuritani RH, McDonald NJ, Sydiskis RJ. Effect of sterilization on contaminated sponges. J Endod. 1993;19(2):68–70.

Lask JT, Walker MP, Kulild JC, Cunningham KP, Shull PA. Variability of the diameter and taper of size #30, 0.04 nickel-titanium rotary files. J Endod. 2006;32(12):1171–3.

Machtou P, Martin D. Utilisation raisonnee des Profile. Clinic. 1997;18:253–9.

Mandel E, Adib-Yazdi M, Benhamou LM, Lachkar T, Mesgouez C, Sobel M. Rotary Ni-Ti profile systems for preparing curved canals in resin blocks: influence of operator on instrument breakage. Int Endod J. 1999;32(6):436–43.

Masserann J. "Entfernen metallischer Fragmente aus Wurzelkanalen" (Removal of metal fragments from the root canal). J Br Endod Soc. 1971;5(3):55–9.
McGibney D. Ireland should follow U.K. practice by insisting on the single use of endodontic files. Ireland: University College Cork; 2016.
McGuigan MB, Louca C, Duncan HF. Endodontic instrument fracture: causes and prevention. Br Dent J. 2013;214(7):341–8.
McSpadden DDS. Mastering endodontic instrumentation. Chattanooga: Cloudland Institute; 2007. p. 1–197.
Miller CH. Tips on preparing instruments for sterilization. Am J Dent. 2002;15(1):66.
Ozawa T, Nakano M, Sugimura H, Kurayama H, Tahata K, Nakamura J, et al. Effects of endodontic instrument handle diameter on electromyographic activity of forearm and hand muscles. Int Endod J. 2001;34(2):100–6.
Parashos P, Gordon I, Messer HH. Factors influencing defects of rotary nickel-titanium endodontic instruments after clinical use. J Endod. 2004a;30(10):722–5.
Parashos P, Linsuwanont P, Messer HH. A cleaning protocol for rotary nickel-titanium endodontic instruments. Aust Dent J. 2004b;49(1):20–7.
Pruett JP, Clement DJ, Carnes DL Jr. Cyclic fatigue testing of nickel-titanium endodontic instruments. J Endod. 1997;23(2):77–85.
Sattapan B, Nervo GJ, Palamara JE, Messer HH. Defects in rotary nickel-titanium files after clinical use. J Endod. 2000;26(3):161–5.
Segall RO, del Rio CE, Brady JM, Ayer WA. Evaluation of debridement techniques for endodontic instruments. Oral Surg Oral Med Oral Pathol. 1977;44(5):786–91.
Serene TP, Loadholt C. Variations in same-size endodontic files. Oral Surg Oral Med Oral Pathol. 1984;57(2):200–2.
Stenman E, Spangberg LS. Root canal instruments are poorly standardized. J Endod. 1993;19(7):327–34.
Treble SJ, Chandler NP, Shaw JR. Tactile sensitivity of three endodontic instrument handles. Endod Dent Traumatol. 1993;9(2):77–8.
Warren CJ, Chandler NP. Influence of file handle attachments on tactile discrimination: an evaluation by dental students. Int Endod J. 1998;31(2):100–2.
Yared GM, Dagher FE, Machtou P, Kulkarni GK. Influence of rotational speed, torque and operator proficiency on failure of Greater Taper files. Int Endod J. 2002;35(1):7–12.
Yared G, Bou Dagher F, Kulkarni K. Influence of torque control motors and the operator's proficiency on ProTaper failures. Oral Surg Oral Med Oral Pathol Oral Radiol Endod. 2003;96(2):229–33.
Zarra T, Lambrianidis T. Percutaneous injuries amongst Greek endodontists: a national questionnaire survey. Int Endod J. 2013;46(3):264–74.
Zinelis S, Margelos J. In vivo aging of dental instruments and materials. In: Eliades G, Eliades T, Brantley W, Watts D, editors. Dental materials in vivo: aging and related phenomena. 1st ed. Chicago: Quintessence; 2003. p. 179–92.
Zinelis S, Magnissalis EA, Margelos J, Lambrianidis T. Clinical relevance of standardization of endodontic files dimensions according to the ISO 3630-1 specification. J Endod. 2002;28(5):367–70.

Index

T. Lambrianidis (ed.), *Management of Fractured Endodontic Instruments*,
DOI 10.1007/978-3-319-60651-4

FSC
www.fsc.org
MIX
Papier aus verantwortungsvollen Quellen
Paper from responsible sources
FSC® C105338

If you have any concerns about our products,
you can contact us on
ProductSafety@springernature.com

In case Publisher is established outside the EU,
the EU authorized representative is:
Springer Nature Customer Service Center GmbH
Europaplatz 3, 69115 Heidelberg, Germany

Printed by Libri Plureos GmbH
in Hamburg, Germany